Contact Lenses in
Ophthalmic Practice

Springer
New York
Berlin
Heidelberg
Hong Kong
London
Milan
Paris
Tokyo

Contact Lenses in Ophthalmic Practice

Mark J. Mannis, MD, FACS

Professor and Chair, Department of Ophthalmology, University of California, Davis, Sacramento, CA

Karla Zadnik, OD, PhD

Glenn A. Fry Professor of Optometry and Physiological Optics, Ohio State University, College of Optometry, Columbus, OH

Cleusa Coral-Ghanem, MD, PhD

Doctor of Ophthalmology, University of São Paulo (USP); Fellow in Cornea and Contact Lenses, University of São Paulo (USP); Hospital de Olhos Sadalla Amin Ghanem, Joinville, Santa Catarina, Brazil

Newton Kara-José, MD, PhD

Head, Department of Ophthalmology, University of São Paulo (USP); Head, Department of Ophthalmology, University of Campinas (UNICAMP), São Paulo, São Paulo, Brazil

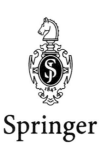

Springer

Mark J. Mannis, MD, FACS
Professor and Chair
Department of Ophthalmology
University of California, Davis
Sacramento, CA

Karla Zadnik, OD, PhD
Glenn A. Fry Professor of Optometry and
  Physiological Optics
Ohio State University
College of Optometry
Columbus, OH

Cleusa Coral-Ghanem, MD, PhD
Doctor of Ophthalmology
University of São Paulo (USP)
Fellow in Cornea and Contact Lenses
University of São Paulo (USP)
Hospital de Olhos Sadalla Amin Ghanem
Joinville, Santa Catarina, Brazil

Newton Kara-José, MD, PhD
Head, Department of Ophthalmology
University of São Paulo (USP)
Head, Department of Ophthalmology
University of Campinas (UNICAMP)
São Paulo, São Paulo, Brazil

Library of Congress Cataloging-in-Publication Data

Mannis, Mark J.
   Contact lenses in ophthalmic practice / Mark J. Mannis, Karla Zadnik.
     p. ; cm.
   Includes bibliographical references and index.
   ISBN 0-387-40400-7 (h/c : alk. paper)
   1. Contact lenses.   I. Zadnik, Karla.   II. Title.
   [DNLM: 1. Contact Lenses. WW 355 M284c   2003]
   RE977.C6M254   2003
   617.7'523—dc21
                                                                                          2003053883

ISBN 0-387-40400-7   Printed on acid-free paper

Printed in the United States of America.

9 8 7 6 5 4 3 2 1   SPIN 10938362

www.springer-ny.com

Springer-Verlag   New York Berlin Heidelberg
A member of BertelsmannSpringer Science + Business Media GmbH

To Judith and Kurt,
Lídia and Emir,
our anchors

Preface

Seven years ago, in Cancun, Mexico, at the meeting of the Pan-American Association of Ophthalmology, one of the editors came across a little book in Portuguese on contact lenses. Edited and written by two of Brazil's leaders in the specialty of contact lenses—Cleusa Coral-Ghanem, MD and Newton Kara-Jose, MD—this slim volume had already made a significant impact in Brazil. In a country where contact lens practice is already quite sophisticated, the book was designed as a learning tool for the new practitioner. Given its utility as a manual for the beginning contact lens practitioner, the notion that this book might be made available in English immediately came to mind. In the Foreword to the second edition in Portuguese, Rubens Belfort, a recognized leader in both Brazilian and international ophthalmology, wrote that "if this book were written in English, it would be recognized the world over" as a useful and practical tool for the contact lens practitioner. His comments were perhaps prescient. And so, the project to bring a new contact lens manual to English-speaking eye care practitioners was launched.

This book is a contact lens "primer." Originally signifying a small book for teaching children to read, the term *primer* now signifies any small book that is basic and introductory to a subject. There is already, of course, a spate of basic contact lens manuals on the market. Nonetheless, the present text is unique in at least two ways. First, it combines the somewhat quaint notion of a primer with the contemporary approach of FAQs—frequently asked questions. Guiding the novice stepwise into an acquaintance with the terminology and practice of contact lenses, it approaches questions as they arise in the "hands on" setting. Second, this new volume is the joint product of an ophthalmologist and an optometrist. Unfortunately, differences in clinical interests and political currents have swept the two disciplines apart, and often what is written by one is not read by the other. This project brings together a long collaboration between ophthalmology and optometry that capitalizes on the expertise of both disciplines. As such, it is designed to be of use to ophthalmology residents, optometry students, practitioners in both fields beginning or returning to contact lens practice, and to technicians and assistants working in contact lens practices.

We have attempted to adapt the excellent base established by our colleagues in Brazil for both ophthalmology and optometry and have expanded and updated the contents for the English-speaking professional readership. Primary credit for this book must go to Drs. Coral-Ghanem and Kara-José and to the contributors in Brazil and the United States who have updated and rendered the chapters clear and utilitarian. The original text was translated from Portuguese into English by Dr. Mannis and was further edited in English by Drs. Mannis and Zadnik. We hope that this text will answer the readers' questions—those you wanted to but perhaps were afraid to ask because they seemed so basic.

MARK MANNIS, MD
Sacramento, California

KARLA ZADNIK, OD, PhD
Columbus, Ohio

Foreword

The second edition of this book, still in the original Portuguese, was distinguished by an introduction by Mark Mannis. In his foreword to that edition, Dr. Mannis wrote "It is an extraordinary honor for me to be associated with the editors and authors of this essential text for Portuguese-speaking ophthalmologists. My only regret is that the book is not yet available to English-speaking contact lens practitioners." Now with this newly translated and substantially edited English edition that is enriched by the experience of two accomplished practitioners, Mark Mannis and Karla Zadnik, core information in contact lens practice that has always been the primary goal of this book is brought to English-speaking eye care professionals. As authors of the original text, we are honored to be associated with this new and updated English language version and its accomplished editors and contributors from both Brazil and the United States. The English edition encompasses a much broader collaboration of colleagues who have generously volunteered their hard work to make this book a valuable clinical tool.

The format of the book was conceived several years ago, when we were discussing the contact lens training of our residents and of new ophthalmic practitioners in Brazil. We noticed that their questions about contact lenses had common and recurrent threads. We were repeatedly faced with the same basic queries. Nonetheless, we were also well aware of the significant costs involved in the production of a conventional textbook in ophthalmology with lengthy text, numerous illustrations, and expensive paper that would make it prohibitive to a significant percentage of our target audience. The format, therefore, logically presented itself: straightforward questions and answers about the subjects of greatest concern to the new contact lens practitioner presented in a slim, compact, direct, and no-nonsense book. To our surprise, the book is now in its third edition in Portuguese. We are further delighted to witness its translation and updating in English—a language that will make it accessible to a much larger readership

Communicate comes from the Latin *communicare*, which means "to make common, to share." A nonfiction book communicates knowledge, makes it common, shares it. As physicians, we have two basic missions: to heal and to teach. We hope that this modest book effectively shares our own experience in contact lens practice with those who are new to the field. The original authors of *Lentes de Contato na Clínica Oftalmológica* are immensely thankful to Drs. Mannis and Zadnik for the opportunity of communicating and sharing with our English-speaking colleagues the world over.

CLEUSA CORAL-GHANEM, MD
Joinville, Brazil

NEWTON KARA-JOSÉ, MD
São Paulo, Brazil

Acknowledgments

We would like to thank Gary Campanile at the University of California, Davis, who kept this project superbly organized, managing all the manuscripts between Columbus and Sacramento. In addition, we appreciate the foresight and determination of Laurel Craven who perceived the value in bringing this edition to the English-speaking profession. The meticulous editing of Merry Post kept the project on track, and we thank her for her steadfastness in this task. Of course, the book could never have been completed without the contributing authors in Brazil and the United States to whom we are deeply grateful. And finally, we thank our families for their patience with this project—one of many that chip away at our time with them.

M.M.

K.Z.

Contents

Contributors

Milton Ruiz Alves, M.D, PhD
Doctor of Ophthalmology
University of São Paulo
Associate Professor, Director of
  Cornea and Contact Lens
  Service
University of São Paulo
São Paulo, SP, Brazil

Lisa Badowski, OD, MS
Assistant Professor of Clinical
  Optometry
The Ohio State University
College of Optometry
Columbus, OH

Melissa D. Bailey, OD MS
Postdoctoral Fellow
The Ohio State University
College of Optometry
Columbus, OH

Breno Barth, MD, PhD
Doctor of Ophthalmology
University of São Paulo
São Paulo, Brazil

Peter D. Bergenske, OD
Assistant Clinical Professor
Pacific University
College of Optometry
Forest Grove, OR

David A. Berntsen, OD
Fellow in Cornea and Contact
  Lenses
The Ohio State University
College of Optometry
Columbus, OH

Timothy B. Edrington, OD MS
Professor
Southern California College of
  Optometry
Fullerton, CA

Renato Giovedi Filho, MD, PhD
Doctor of Ophthalmology
University of São Paulo
Assistant Professor of Cornea
  and External Diseases
Santa Casa of São Paulo
São Paulo, SP, Brazil

Marizilda Andrade Giovedi,
    MD, PhD
Assistant Doctor of
    Ophthalmology
Santa Casa of São Paulo
Doctor of Ophthalmology
University of São Paulo (USP)
São Paulo, SP, Brazil

Cynthia H. Green, OD
Assistant Professor of Clinical
    Optometry
The Ohio State University
College of Optometry
Columbus, OH

Nilo Holzchuh, MD, PhD
Doctor of Ophthalmology
Director, Cornea and Contact
    Lens Department
University of Campinas
Director, Cornea Department
Santa Casa of São Paulo
São Paulo, SP, Brazil

LeVelle B. Jenkins, OD
Assistant Professor of Clinical
    Optometry
The Ohio State University
College of Optometry
Columbus, OH

Charlotte E. Joslin, OD
Assistant Professor
University of Illinois at Chicago
Department of Ophthalmology
    and Visual Sciences
Chicago, IL

Newton Kara-José, Jr., MD, PhD
Doctor of Ophthalmology
University of São Paulo
Director of Cataract Service
University of São Paulo
São Paulo, SP, Brazil

Claudia Assis Lima, MD
Assistant Doctor of
    Ophthalmology
State University of Campinas
    (UNICAMP)
Campinas, Brazil

Saly M. Bugmann Moreira, MD
Assistant Clinical Professor
Faculdade Evangélica do
    Paraná and Hospital
    Universitário Evangélico de
    Curitiba
Curitiba, Paraná, Brazil

Adamo Lui Netto, MD, PhD
Associate Clinical Professor
Medical Faculty of Santa Casa
Doctor of Ophthalmology
School of Medicine of Ribeirão
    Preto
São Paulo, SP, Brazil

Jason J. Nichols, OD, MS, MPH
Senior Research Associate
The Ohio State University
College of Optometry
Columbus, OH

Kelly K. Nichols, OD, MPH,
    PhD
Assistant Professor of Clinical
    Optometry
The Ohio State University
College of Optometry
Columbus, OH

Paulo Ricardo de Oliveira,
    M.D., PhD
Doctor of Ophthalmology,
    University of São Paulo
    (FMUSP)
Vice-President, International
    Contact Lens Society of
    Ophthalmology
Instituto Panamericano da
    Visão
Goiânia, Goiás, Brasil

Regina Carvalho de Salles
  Oliveira, B.A.
Ophthalmic Allied Personnel
  Program
University of São Paulo
São Paulo, SP, Brazil

Kaaryn Pedersen, OD
Co-Director, Contact Lens
  Service
University of California, Davis
Department of Ophthalmology
Sacramento, CA

Ari de Souza Pena, MD, PhD
Director, Cornea and Contact
  Lens Department
Fluminense University of Rio
  de Janeiro
Doctor of Ophthalmology
Federal University of Rio de
  Janeiro
Niterói, Rio de Janeiro, Brazil

Marjorie J. Rah, OD, PhD
Assistant Professor of
  Optometry
New England College of
  Optometry
Boston, MA

Dede Reyes, FCLSA
Contact Lens Fitter
University of California, Davis
Department of Ophthalmology
Sacramento, CA

Eric R. Ritchey, OD, MS
Fellow in Cornea and Contact
  Lenses
The Ohio State University
College of Optometry
Columbus, OH

Jeffery M. Schafer, OD, MS
Fellow in Cornea and Contact
  Lenses
The Ohio State University
College of Optometry
Columbus, OH

Muriel Schornack, OD
Mayo Clinic
Department of Ophthalmology
Rochester, MN

Loretta B. Szczotka-Flynn, OD,
  MS
Associate Professor
Case Western Reserve
  University
Department of Ophthalmology
Cleveland, OH

Michael D. Twa, OD, MS
Postdoctoral Fellow
The Ohio State University
College of Optometry
Columbus, OH

Ricardo Uras, MD
Adjunct Professor
Department of Ophthalmology
Federal University of São Paulo
São Paulo, SP, Brazil

Jeffrey J. Walline, OD, PhD
Research Scientist
The Ohio State University
College of Optometry
Columbus, OH

1

Design and Nomenclature of Contact Lenses

Renato Giovedi Filho, Marizilda Andrade Giovedi, and Jason J. Nichols

1. What types of contact lenses exist?

Contact lenses can be classified by the nature of the material from which they are made, by their wearing schedule, by their purpose, or by their design.

Nature of the Material

1. Hard
2. Rigid gas permeable
2. Hydrogel
3. Hybrid

Wear and Replacement Schedule

1. Daily wear (removed daily and not utilized during sleep).
2. Continuous or extended wear (utilized both during waking and sleep hours for a specified number of days continuously). These lenses are generally made from high water content or high DK material.
3. Flexible wear (utilized during the day and occasionally overnight).
4. Traditional/conventional: replaced annually.
5. Disposable or planned replacement (discarded after a specified wearing period defined by manufacturer's guidelines). Can be disposed of daily, weekly, biweekly, monthly, bimonthly, or quarterly.
6. Occasional (indicated for occasional use, e.g., athletic or social activities).

Purpose

1. Therapeutic (for protection or healing of the cornea).
2. Cosmetic (for modification of the color of the eye or to improve the appearance of a disfigured eye).
3. Optical (for correction of refractive errors and/or regularization of the corneal surface).

Design

1. Spherical (having anterior and posterior spherical surfaces).
2. Aspheric (different radii of curvature in the center and periphery, simulating the structure of the cornea).
3. Toric (two principal meridians have different radii of curvature; this may be the anterior or posterior surfaces of the lens or both). Used to correct astigmatism.
   - Front surface toric lenses
   - Back surface toric lenses
   - Bitoric lenses (when both the anterior and posterior surfaces are toric)
4. Bifocal
5. Progressive
6. Multicurve (two or more posterior curves). See Figure 1.1.
7. Reverse curve (a central posterior curve, which is flatter, utilized primarily for fitting after refractive surgery for myopia or orthokeratology). See Figure 1.2.

2. What is a rigid gas permeable lens?

A rigid gas permeable lens is made of a material with a molecular structure that permits the passage of oxygen and carbon dioxide gas

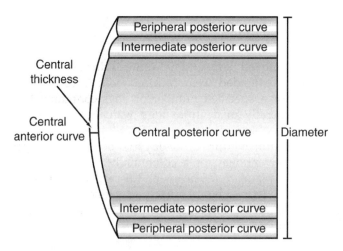

Figure 1.1. Configuration of a single cut contact lens.

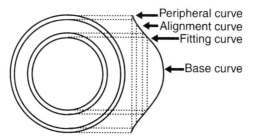

Figure 1.2. Reverse geometry lens design.

but contains no water. The general categories of gas permeable materials are:

1. Cellulose acetate butyrate
2. Pure silicone
3. Silicone acrylate (siloxymethacrylate copolymer)
4. Fluorocarbonate (fluoromethacrylate siloxy copolymer)

3. What is the design of a single-cut lens?

The anterior surface of a single-cut contact lens is a continual curvature, the front optic zone radius, associated with the anterior optic zone.

The posterior surface of a tricurve lens is formed of three or more curves:

1. The central posterior curve, or base curve, is designed to fit the curvature of the cornea.
2. The secondary posterior curve provides a transition between the base curve and the peripheral posterior curve. Multicurve contact lenses may have more than one intermediate posterior curve in order to create a gradual transition.
3. A peripheral (tertiary) curve is designed to create a smooth transition between the base curve and the edge of the lens, facilitating the exchange of tear film under the lens with each blink.

4. What is a "blend," and what is its importance?

To smooth the junction between adjacent curves on the back surface of a lens, blending is performed. A blend does not induce a new curve on the posterior surface of a lens. Blending is a smoothing of these different curves at their junctions, removing the rigidly demarcated zones of transition to permit better exchange of tear film under the lens.

5. What are the types of edge design and what are their purposes?

The shape of the outermost portion ($\approx$0.2 mm in from the edge) of the lens is referred to as the edge contour. It is difficult to quantify, so descriptors such as rounded, blunt, sharp, knife edge, square, or tapered are used. The edge contour can be modified in order to diminish or augment attachment of the lens to the lid in the contact lens fitting process. An additional reason for modifying edge contour is to improve patient comfort (Figure 1.3).

6. What is a base curve?

A base curve is the radius of curvature of the central region of the posterior surface of the contact lens, selected based on the curvature of the corneal apex.

7. What is sagittal depth?

Sagittal depth is the distance between a superficial plane over which the contact lens is placed and the center of the optical zone diameter (Figure 1.4). To increase sagittal depth, one must increase the optic zone diameter or diminish the radius of curvature of the lens.

8. What is the relationship between contact lens center thickness and dioptric power?

Contact lens center thickness varies with lens power (minus lenses are thinner), diameter (smaller diameter lenses are thinner), and refractive index (higher refractive index lenses are thinner). Central contact lens thickness is important in contact lens fitting, because it may influence stability, flexibility, edge thickness, and oxygen transmission.

9. What is the wetting angle?

The wetting angle is the angle formed at the surface of the contact lens material when a drop of liquid is placed on the surface (Figure 1.5).

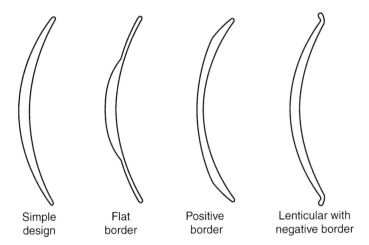

| Simple design | Flat border | Positive border | Lenticular with negative border |

Figure 1.3. Types of rigid contact lenses.

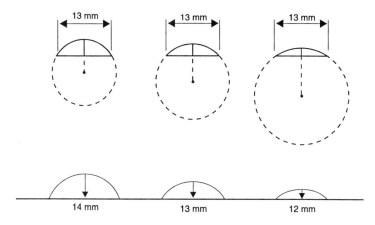

Figure 1.4. The relationship between sagittal depth and diameter.

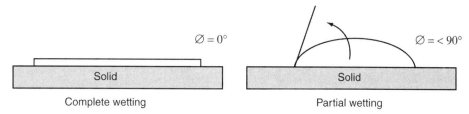

Figure 1.5. Wetting angle.

The extent of the angle is related to the cohesive and adhesive properties of a lens material. When the wetting angle is greater, the material is more hydrophobic. For example, polymethylmethacrylate (PMMA) is a relatively hydrophobic material with a wetting angle of approximately 60 degrees.

10. What are prism ballast, truncation, and dynamic stabilization?

Contact lenses may have rotational movement with blinking. In general, the inferior edge of the lens moves laterally and/or up with a blink. In the fitting of a toric contact lens, this is not desirable, because the axis of the cylinder needs to remain in the same position. There are various methods of stabilization (Figure 1.6 A–C).

1. Prism ballast: The inferiorly thickened portion of the lens at the 6 o'clock position acts as a weight.
2. Truncation: The inferior portion of the contact lens is cut off horizontally, forming a thicker edge that is supported by the inferior lid margin.
3. Dynamic stabilization: The superior and inferior borders of the contact lens are beveled so that the thinnest portion of the lens is positioned under the lid margin, preventing rotation of the lens.

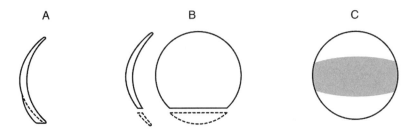

Figure 1.6. A: Contact lens with prism ballast. B: Truncated contact lens. C: Contact lens with beveled superior and inferior borders.

11. What is the water content (degree of hydration) of a hydrophilic contact lens?

The water content represents the percent water contained in the polymer matrix and ranges from 35% to 80% in hydrogel contact lenses. Hydrophilic contact lenses can be classified in two categories based on water content:

1. Low water content (less than 50% water)
2. High water content (greater than 50% water)

The oxygen transmissibility of a hydrophilic contact lens is directly related to its water content and inversely related to its thickness.

12. What is the significance of the ionic content of hydrogel contact lenses?

Contact lenses may also be classified by their ionic nature. Ionic materials are negatively charged and therefore more reactive, whereas nonionic materials are electrically neutral. The ionic lenses are more prone to protein deposition on the surface of the lens.

Selected Readings

Mandell RB. *Contact Lens Practice*, 4th ed. Springfield, IL: Charles C. Thomas, 1988.

Phillips AJ, Speedwell L. *Contact Lenses*. Oxford: Butterworth Heinemann, 1997.

Stein HA, Slatt BJ, Stein RM, Freeman MI. *Fitting Guide for Rigid and Soft Contact Lenses*, 4th ed. St. Louis: Mosby, 2002.

2

Indications, Contraindications, and Selection of Contact Lenses

Claudia Assis Lima, Newton Kara-José, and Jason J. Nichols

1. What are the principal indications for contact lens use?

A thorough examination of each patient's history, medical conditions, expectations and responsibility, refractive needs, and response to trial fitting determines whether contact lenses are appropriate. The principal indications for contact lens fitting are as follows.

Optical Indications

Most contact lens wearers fall into this group. The great majority are myopic with or without astigmatism.

Medical Indications

Keratoconus

Keratoconus is a bilateral, but asymmetric, progressive thinning of the cornea. Such cases are generally fitted with rigid gas permeable contact lenses to correct myopia and irregular astigmatism resulting from the corneal irregularity and ectasia.[1-3] The contact lens does not inhibit the progression of the disease and is used only when the visual acuity obtained with glasses becomes unsatisfactory.[3]

Irregular Astigmatism and/or Corneal Opacification

Rigid contact lenses provide an excellent means of correcting irregular astigmatism associated with corneal opacification by eliminating the aberrations and glare, leading to better visual acuity.[4] The fitting of a contact lens in these cases is almost always undertaken prior to considering corneal transplantation. For the most part, rigid gas permeable lenses provide better results, although hydrophilic lenses may have utility in selected cases.

Anisometropia

Anisometropia exists when there is a difference in the refraction of generally more than two diopters between the two eyes. Uncorrected anisometropia in the infant may lead to amblyopia, especially when one eye is hypermetropic. In the adult, differences of greater than three diopters generally are not tolerated with spectacle correction. In such cases, a contact lens may be indicated in order to reduce the development of amblyopia and anisometropic aniseikonia.

Unilateral Aphakia

Unilateral aphakia induces significant disparity in image size (aniseikonia). Anisometropic correction with glasses produces intolerable aniseikonia, with a difference in image size of approximately 30%. The contact lens diminishes the aniseikonic image difference to approximately 7%—a difference generally not perceptible to the visual cortex. This reduces the magnifying effect of the positive lens, permitting binocular vision.

Nystagmus

When it is necessary to correct ametropia in patients with nystagmus, contact lenses offer advantages over glasses, because contact lenses follow the movement of the eye and, in many cases, permit better visual acuity.

After Refractive Surgery

Patients with significant residual ametropia after surgery may have their ametropia corrected with a contact lens.[5-7] Contact lens fitting may be initiated 3 to 6 months after surgery. In most cases, rigid gas permeable lenses are appropriate, and a reverse-curve design is most commonly used.[8] Special care must be taken to consider the degree of corneal topography, vascularization (e.g., at keratotomy incisions), and the possibility of epithelial erosions.

After Penetrating Keratoplasty

A contact lens is indicated in cases with large refractive errors, anisometropia, or irregular astigmatism after corneal transplantation.[8-13] Fitting is usually initiated no sooner than 3 months and often 6 to 12 months after surgery, and contact lenses are primarily used when there is persistent regular or irregular astigmatism after removal of the sutures.

Cosmesis

Prosthetic, tinted lenses are often used in patients with a disfiguring corneal scar or an iris coloboma to improve the aesthetics of a nonseeing eye or to occlude an iris coloboma. Cosmetic lenses may also simply be used to alter the color of the eye.

Therapeutic Lenses

Although every contact lens may be considered "therapeutic," therapeutic lenses are those that are applied specifically for treatment of a corneal disease.[10,14–17]

2. What is the routine examination prior to contact lens use?

Many factors determine whether a patient is a good candidate for the use of contact lenses. First, a detailed history and ocular examination are necessary prior to fitting a contact lens. The history collects information about the patient's general medical health, ocular health, family history of eye disease, and previous use of contact lenses.

Motivation is one of the most important factors for the success of fitting. Patients with moderate to high refractive errors may be better candidates for contact lens wear than those with low degrees of refractive error. A good way to make this judgment is to evaluate the number of hours per day that the patient wears glasses. Patients who are minimally dependent on glasses in general have a low degree of success with contact lens fitting. Poorly motivated patients frequently may not care for their contact lenses adequately and may not adapt to the lenses, particularly rigid gas permeable lenses.

General Health

Allergies

The patient should be questioned about allergies to medications, foods, and other substances. The allergic patient is more susceptible to adverse reactions to contact lenses and their maintenance products.[18,19]

Diabetes

In moderate or severe cases of diabetes, there is occasionally corneal hypesthesia, leading to a greater propensity for corneal erosion and infection. Diabetic patients are not candidates for extended-wear contact lens use.[20]

Pregnancy and Menopause

Pregnant women with water retention may be intolerant of a contact lens. In general, contact lens fitting should be avoided during pregnancy. Some patients in menopause may present significant changes in the quality and quantity of the lacrimal tear film that may cause contact lens intolerance.

Chronic Respiratory Disease

Patients with chronic respiratory disease such as asthma, sinusitis, and other similar conditions may have difficulty in fitting a contact lens. During respiratory crises they may have conjunctival hyperemia, tearing, light sensitivity, and generalized discomfort that is aggravated by the use of contact lenses.

Psychological Conditions

It is essential that the contact lens wearer be sufficiently responsible to follow medical instructions, including information about the duration of wear, contact lens maintenance, understanding of the signs and symptoms of contact lens–related problems, the risks of contact lens wear, and an understanding of when prompt assistance must be obtained.

Medication Use

The contact lens wearer must be informed also of the medications, either topical or systemic (such as nasal decongestants, diuretics, benzodiazepines, immunosuppressants, etc.), that may alter the tear film and that may contraindicate or make difficult contact lens use.[21]

Ocular Health

One must ask about the following issues:

1. Any previous ocular injury
2. Lid infection
3. Conjunctivitis
4. Cataract
5. Glaucoma (including family history)
6. Dry eye
7. Any surgery to the eye or ocular adnexa
8. Previous contact lens use
9. Medication intolerance

Contact Lens History

The following contact lens information should be obtained:

1. Types of contact lens previously worn
2. Success and complications with previous lenses

3. Reasons for the use of contact lens (cosmetic, spectacle intolerance, aphakia, keratoconus, improvement of visual acuity)
4. Patient occupation (to determine if the patient is exposed to chemical products or works in a dirty or dusty environment)
5. Previous refractive correction
6. Sports and recreational activities

Ophthalmic Examination

Manifest Refraction

Corneal Curvature
The procedure most commonly employed is manual or automated keratometry, which measures the central corneal curvature. One may also use photokeratoscopy or computed topography.

Biomicroscopy
The biomicroscope is used to evaluate the lid, conjunctiva, tear film, cornea, iris, pupil, and anterior chamber.

Tear Film Evaluation (See Chapter 5.)

Measurement of Palpebral Aperture Height
The opening of the normal palpebral fissure ranges from 7 to 13 mm (average is approximately 10 mm). The size of the palpebral fissure may contribute to or detract substantially from stabilization of the lens, especially rigid gas permeable contact lenses. Measurement of the palpebral aperture height is done at the slit lamp, with the patient looking at the examiner's ear. It may be accomplished in the following ways:

- Noting in millimeters, with the help of a ruler, the distance between lids.
- Noting the position of the lid in relationship to the limbus, the lid at the limbus is annotated as zero; covering the corner, it is notated in millimeters of area covered (for example, $+1$, $+2$ mm), and if sclera is left exposed, it is noted as -1, -2 mm, etc.[7]

Lid Tone
Lids that are extremely tense or tight may alter the movement of the contact lens. There is no precise clinical method to measure lid tension. One can estimate lid tension by grasping the lid between the index finger and thumb and pulling it away from the globe. It can then be classified as loose or tight. Studies have found a relation among lid tension, palpebral aperture height, and contact lens fitting characteristics.[22]

Blinking
The examiner should evaluate the frequency and thoroughness of the blink. An incomplete blink may change the movement of the lens on the eye and the distribution of the tear film, with consequent desiccation of the cornea and/or conjunctiva and lens intolerance.[23-27] Normal frequency of blinking is 12 to 15 times per minute, which is increased

with head movement and is diminished during states of attention, such as reading, watching television, driving, and computer use.[28,29]

Corneal Diameter

The average horizontal diameter is approximately 11.7 mm (varying generally between 11 and 12.5 mm).[30,31] The vertical diameter is approximately 1 mm less.[31] This is an important measurement in the determination of lens diameter.

Corneal Sensation

Corneal sensation may be diminished in systemic diseases such as diabetes, intrinsic eye disease (herpes simplex keratitis, for example), pregnancy, the menstrual cycle, the use of topical or systemic medications, or as a result of corneal surgery.[32–40] Contact lens wear may also induce decreased corneal sensation.[41–43] Contact lens wearers with decreased corneal sensation may be more prone to corneal erosion and/or infection. Corneal sensation can be grossly evaluated using a wisp of cotton or, more precisely, with the esthesiometer of Cochet-Bonnet.[44]

3. What are the criteria for selecting candidate patients for the use of an extended wear hydrophilic lens?

The choice of the appropriate patient for hydrogel extended wear is based on careful evaluation. Patients must be generally free of both systemic and ocular disease. Patients with a history of ocular infections or inflammation are not good candidates for the overnight wear of contact lenses. Although the overnight wear of contact lenses is convenient, it is necessary that patients are aware of the risk and responsibilities associated with this modality including:

1. Increased probability of complications, including infection such as corneal ulceration.[45,46]
2. The importance of good ocular and general health and strict adherence to regimens of contact lens care.
3. Attending a scheduled follow-up examination every 6 months.
4. Recognition of and immediate attention to the first symptoms of complications.
5. Removal of the lenses at the first sign of ocular irritation.

4. When should rigid gas permeable contact lenses be used?

Rigid contact lenses are indicated in the following cases:

1. Regular astigmatism greater than one diopter
2. Irregular astigmatism
3. Patients with difficulty manipulating a hydrophilic contact lens
4. Postsurgical fits (e.g., post–refractive surgery, post–penetrating keratoplasty)
5. Corneal opacification
6. Myopia control

5. When should spherical hydrophilic contact lenses be used?

Hydrophilic contact lenses may be primarily indicated in the following situations:

1. Ametropia with minimum astigmatism
2. Rigid contact lens intolerance
3. Athletes
4. Infants with ocular pathologies such as aphakia
5. Patients with nystagmus
6. Excessively wide interpalpebral fissure
7. Patients with large iridectomies

6. What are the primary ocular contraindications to the use of contact lenses?

Before initiating any contact lens fitting for the purposes of optical correction, it is important to evaluate the patient's motivation, ocular needs, and ocular and medical history. Unmotivated patients tend not to adhere to the prescribed methods and care regimens for the contact lens, putting them at greater risk of complications.

Contraindications

1. Any acute or subacute inflammation of the anterior segment of the eye
2. Acute and chronic ocular infections
3. Any eye disease affecting the cornea, conjunctiva, and lids (e.g., epithelial fragility, endothelial failure, dry eye, allergy, pinguecula, pterygium)
4. Corneal hypesthesia
5. Uncontrolled glaucoma
6. Vitreocorneal touch in aphakia
7. Psychological intolerance to the placement of a foreign body in the eye

All of these contraindications are relative. If any contraindication is eliminated, the patient can be reevaluated, remembering that a successful fitting is almost always based on a strong indication.

7. What are the general contraindications to the use of a contact lens for optical purposes?

1. Any systemic or allergic illness that affects the eye and may be exacerbated by the contact lens

2. Inability to follow the instructions for cleaning, storage, and asepsis of the contact lens
3. Poor personal hygiene (particularly hands and nails)
4. Inability to understand the risks associated with contact lens use
5. Low refractive error in a patient reluctant to use glasses
6. Immunosuppressed patients
7. The use of systemic medications that may cause changes in the quality of the tear film
8. Pregnancy, nursing, and menopause—circumstances that may be associated with contact lens intolerance and refractive instability. It may be better to wait until the end of pregnancy and lactation in order to fit a contact lens
9. Very old or very young patients who cannot manage insertion, removal, or contact lens care without assistance

8. What are the relative contraindications to the use of hydrophilic contact lenses?

1. Poor vision secondary to uncorrected astigmatism
2. Problems with handling the contact lens (elderly patients or patients with Parkinson's disease, hemiplegia, or rheumatoid arthritis with hand malformations)
3. Exposure to unfavorable environments (extremely dry atmosphere, exposure to volatile chemicals, etc.)
4. Difficulty adhering to the prescribed regimen of contact lens care

9. What are the relative contraindications for the use of rigid contact lenses?

1. Sports activities—rigid contact lenses may easily dislocate with abrupt movements
2. Discomfort of the rigid contact lenses
3. Sporadic use

10. What are the primary professional contraindications to the use of contact lenses for optical purposes?

Such contraindications include:

1. Workers in polluted environments (e.g., mechanics, farm workers, bricklayers)
2. Environments with chemical products (e.g., insecticides, chemical fertilizers)
3. Exceedingly dry atmosphere
4. Handling of volatile materials

References

1. Rabinowitz YS. Keratoconus. *Surv Ophthalmol.* 1998;42:297–319.
2. Mannis MJ, Zadnik K, Miller MR, Marquez M. Preoperative risk factors for surface disease after penetrating keratoplasty. *Cornea.* 1997;16:7–11.
3. Smiddy WE, Hamburg TR, Kracher GP, Stark WJ. Keratoconus. Contact lens or keratoplasty? *Ophthalmology.* 1988;95:487–492.
4. McMahon TT, Devulapally J, Rosheim KM, Putz JL, Moore M, White S. Contact lens use after corneal trauma. *J Am Optom Assoc.* 1997;68(4):215–224.
5. Yeung KK, Olson MD, Weissman BA. Complexity of contact lens fitting after refractive surgery (1). *Am J Ophthalmol.* 2002;133:607–612.
6. Bufidis T, Konstas AG, Pallikaris IG, Siganos DS, Georgiadis N. Contact lens fitting difficulties following refractive surgery for high myopia. *CLAO J.* 2000;26:106–110.
7. Zadnik K. Contact lens management of patients who have had unsuccessful refractive surgery. *Curr Opin Ophthalmol.* 1999;10:260–263.
8. Lim L, Siow KL, Sakamoto R, Chong JS, Tan DT. Reverse geometry contact lens wear after photorefractive keratectomy, radial keratotomy, or penetrating keratoplasty. *Cornea.* 2000;19:320–324.
9. Arora R, Gupta S, Taneja M, Raina UK, Mehta DK. Disposable contact lenses in penetrating keratoplasty. *CLAO J.* 2000;26:127–129.
10. Lim L, Tan DT, Chan WK. Therapeutic use of Bausch & Lomb Pure Vision contact lenses. *CLAO J.* 2001;27:179–185.
11. Eggink FA, Nuijts RM. A new technique for rigid gas permeable contact lens fitting following penetrating keratoplasty. *Acta Ophthalmol Scand.* 2001; 79:245–250.
12. Beekhuis WH, van Rij G, Eggink FA, Vreugdenhil W, Schoevaart CE. Contact lenses following keratoplasty. *CLAO J.* 1991;17:27–29.
13. Genvert GI, Cohen EJ, Arentsen JJ, Laibson PR. Fitting gas-permeable contact lenses after penetrating keratoplasty. *Am J Ophthalmol.* 1985;99:511–514.
14. Baum J, Dabezies OH Jr. Pathogenesis and treatment of "sterile" midperipheral corneal infiltrates associated with soft contact lens use. *Cornea.* 2000;19:777–781.
15. Hayworth NA, Asbell PA. Therapeutic contact lenses. *CLAO J.* 1990;16: 137–142.
16. McDermott ML, Chandler JW. Therapeutic uses of contact lenses. *Surv Ophthalmol.* 1989;33:381–394.
17. Mackie IA. Contact lenses in dry eyes. *Trans Ophthalmol Soc UK.* 1985;104 (pt 4):477–483.
18. Kari O, Teir H, Huuskonen R, Bostrom C, Lemola R. Tolerance to different kinds of contact lenses in young atopic and non-atopic wearers. *CLAO J.* 2001;27:151–154.
19. Lea SJ, Neugebauer MA, Smith RG, Vernon SA. The incidence of ophthalmic problems in the contact lens wearing population. *Eye.* 1990;4(pt 5): 706–711.
20. O'Donnell C, Efron N, Boulton AJ. A prospective study of contact lens wear in diabetes mellitus. *Ophthalmic Physiol Opt.* 2001;21:127–138.
21. Lemp MA. Report of the National Eye Institute/Industry workshop on Clinical Trials in Dry Eyes. *CLAO J.* 1995;21:221–232.
22. Carney LG, Mainstone JC, Carkeet A, Quinn TG, Hill RM. Rigid lens dynamics: lid effects. *CLAO J.* 1997;23:69–77.
23. Abelson MB, Holly FJ. A tentative mechanism for inferior punctate keratopathy. *Am J Ophthalmol.* 1977;83:866–869.

24. Collins M, Heron H, Larsen R, Lindner R. Blinking patterns in soft contact lens wearers can be altered with training. *Am J Optom Physiol Opt.* 1987; 64:100–103.
25. Doane MG. An instrument for in vivo tear film interferometry. *Optom Vis Sci.* 1989;66:383–388.
26. Korb DR. Tear film-contact lens interactions. *Adv Exp Med Biol.* 1994;350: 403–410.
27. Lam BL, Steinemann TL. Blink-associated eye movements with contact-lens wear. *Am J Ophthalmol.* 1993;116:240–241.
28. Doughty MJ. Consideration of three types of spontaneous eyeblink activity in normal humans: during reading and video display terminal use, in primary gaze, and while in conversation. *Optom Vis Sci.* 2001;78:712–725.
29. Doughty MJ. Further assessment of gender- and blink pattern-related differences in the spontaneous eyeblink activity in primary gaze in young adult humans. *Optom Vis Sci.* 2002;79:439–447.
30. Matsuda LM, Woldorff CL, Kame RT, Hayashida JK. Clinical comparison of corneal diameter and curvature in Asian eyes with those of Caucasian eyes. *Optom Vis Sci.* 1992;69:51–54.
31. Kwok LS. Measurement of corneal diameter. *Br J Ophthalmol.* 1990;74:63–64.
32. Benitez-del-Castillo JM, del Rio T, Iradier T, Hernandez JL, Castillo A, Garcia-Sanchez J. Decrease in tear secretion and corneal sensitivity after laser in situ keratomileusis. *Cornea.* 2001;20:30–32.
33. Brennan NA, Bruce AS. Esthesiometry as an indicator of corneal health. *Optom Vis Sci.* 1991;68:699–702.
34. Campos M, Hertzog L, Garbus JJ, McDonnell PJ. Corneal sensitivity after photorefractive keratectomy. *Am J Ophthalmol.* 1992;114:51–54.
35. Inoue K, Kato S, Ohara C, Numaga J, Amano S, Oshika T. Ocular and systemic factors relevant to diabetic keratoepitheliopathy. *Cornea.* 2001; 20:798–801.
36. Lawrenson JG. Corneal sensitivity in health and disease. *Ophthalmic Physiol Opt.* 1997;17 (suppl 1):S17–22.
37. Norn MS. Dendritic (herpetic) keratitis. IV. Follow-up examination of corneal sensitivity. *Acta Ophthalmol (Copenh).* 1970;48:383–395.
38. Patel S, Perez-Santonja JJ, Alio JL, Murphy PJ. Corneal sensitivity and some properties of the tear film after laser in situ keratomileusis. *J Refract Surg.* 2001;17:17–24.
39. Riss B, Riss P. Corneal sensitivity in pregnancy. *Ophthalmologica.* 1981;183: 57–62.
40. Riss B, Binder S, Riss P, Kemeter P. Corneal sensitivity during the menstrual cycle. *Br J Ophthalmol.* 1982;66:123–126.
41. Millodot M. Effect of soft lenses on corneal sensitivity. *Acta Ophthalmol.* 1974;52:603–608.
42. Millodot M. Effect of hard contact lenses on corneal sensitivity and thickness. *Acta Ophthalmol (Copenh).* 1975;53:576–584.
43. Millodot M. Effect of the length of wear of contact lenses on corneal sensitivity. *Acta Ophthalmol (Copenh).* 1976;54:721–730.
44. Millodot M. Corneal sensitivity. *Int Ophthalmol Clin.* 1981;21:47–54.
45. Schein OD, Glynn RJ, Poggio EC, Seddon JM, Kenyon KR. The relative risk of ulcerative keratitis among users of daily-wear and extended-wear soft contact lenses. A case-control study. Microbial Keratitis Study Group. *N Engl J Med.* 1989;321:773–778.
46. Schein OD, Poggio EC. Ulcerative keratitis in contact lens wearers. Incidence and risk factors. *Cornea.* 1990;9(suppl 1):S55–58; discussion S62–53.

3

The Routine Contact Lens Examination

Newton Kara-José, Jr., Cleusa Coral-Ghanem, and Jeffery Schafer

1. What are the chief components of the ocular examination geared specifically to the contact lens patient?

The routine eye examination for the potential contact lens wearer includes taking a careful history, performing a complete examination, and evaluating the patient as a candidate for contact lens wear.

History

Present illness

1. Chief complaint
2. Systemic and topical medications used
3. Allergies (seasonal or chronic)

Previous Medical History and General Health

Previous Ocular History

1. History of spectacle use
   - Reason for using glasses
   - Activities for which glasses are used
   - Date of spectacle prescription and the last examination
2. History of contact lens use
   - Contact lens type
     - Polymethylmethacrylate (PMMA)
     - Rigid gas permeable (RGP)
       —Spherical/toric
       —Single vision/monovision/multifocal

- ■ Hydrophilic (soft contact lens)
  - —Spherical/toric
  - —Single vision/monovision/multifocal
  - —Cosmetic
  - —Therapeutic
- ● Wearing Schedule
  - ■ Daily wear
  - ■ Flexible wear
  - ■ Extended wear
  - ■ Occasional wear
- ● Additional contact lens history
  - ■ Satisfaction with vision and comfort
  - ■ Average wearing time (hours/day)
  - ■ Lens replacement schedule (if disposable or planned replacement)
  - ■ Disinfection regimen
  - ■ Reasons for changing the type of contact lens or discontinuation of use in the past
  - ■ Previous contact lens- or solution-related complications

Family History (Systemic and Ocular)

Evaluation of the Candidate for Contact Lenses

1. Reasons for interest in contact lens wear
   - ● Cosmesis
   - ● Sports and hobbies
   - ● High refractive error, irregular corneas, and/or poor refractive surgery outcomes
   - ● Improved vision
2. Personal hygiene
3. Psychological and physical condition
4. Work environment
5. Manual dexterity
6. Financial cost
7. Patient expectations
8. Recognition by the user of:
   - ● Risks and cautionary measures
   - ● Importance of lens care
   - ● Importance of follow-up

2. What are the important aspects of the ophthalmic examination in the contact lens patient?

The ophthalmic examination of the contact lens patient should assess visual acuity, binocular vision, refraction, and visual field and should include examination of the ocular adnexa, the anterior segment, and the dilated fundus. The fit of the contact lenses should be evaluated. Patient education on proper lens care and handling should be addressed and follow-up visits scheduled.

Visual Acuity

1. Right, left, and both eyes
2. With and without correction
3. Distance and near vision

Binocular Vision Assessment

1. Extraocular muscle function
2. Cover test
3. Test of accommodation
4. Ocular dominance

Refractive Assessment

1. Manifest refraction with binocular balance
2. Baseline keratometry/corneal topography
   - Quality of mires

Examination of the Anterior Segment and Ocular Adnexa

External Examination

1. Entropion/ectropion
2. Horizontal visible iris diameter
3. Rate and quality of blinks
4. Palpebral aperture position and size (measured in mm)
5. Lacrimal puncta (position and reflux)
6. Pupil size and function

Biomicroscopy

1. Tear film
   - Tear breakup time
   - Schirmer test
   - Lacrimal lake assessment
2. Bulbar conjunctiva
3. Tarsal conjunctiva
4. Cornea
   - Fluorescein staining
   - Limbal vasculature
   - Endothelium
5. Intraocular pressure

Visual Field Evaluation

Dilated Fundus Examination

Contact Lens Fit Evaluation

1. Measure current contact lens parameters.
   - Base curve
   - Power
   - Diameter
   - Thickness
2. Observe at the slit-lamp biomicroscope.
   - Centration
   - Movement
   - Central fluorescein pattern
   - Edge lift
   - Lid and lens interactions
3. Evaluate fit and wearing capacity.
   - Comfort
   - Patient satisfaction
   - Ocular reactions to the contact lens
     - Tearing
   - Photophobia
   - Measurement of visual acuity at distance and near

Patient Education

1. Always wash hands before handling lenses.
2. Perform training in the correct care and handling of the contact lens, including insertion and removal.
3. Explain the importance of cleaning and maintenance.
4. Provide the patient with written instructions and educational materials.
5. Explain importance of follow-up care.
6. Remove lens immediately for pain or red eye.
7. Recommend return visit at any sign or symptom of ocular irritation.
8. Reinforce proper care at every visit.

Follow-Up Visits

1. Measure visual acuity.
2. Evaluate lens performance.
   - Lens fit
   - Surface inspection
   - Over-refraction
3. Evaluate ocular health with slit-lamp biomicroscope.

4. Confirm care and handling instructions.
5. Confirm the parameters of the contact lens.

Selected Readings

Bennett ES, Henry VA. *Clinical Manual of Contact Lenses,* 2nd ed. Philadelphia: Lippincott Williams & Wilkins, 2000.

Hom MM. *Manual of Contact Lens Prescribing and Fitting,* 2nd ed. Boston: Butterworth Heinemann, 2000.

Phillips AJ, Speedwell L. *Contact Lenses,* 4th ed. Boston: Butterworth Heinemann, 1997.

4

The Role of the Ophthalmic Assistant in Contact Lens Practice

Dede Reyes, Newton Kara-José, and Regina Carvalho de Salles Oliveira

1. What is the role of the ophthalmic assistant in the fitting of contact lenses?

The ophthalmic assistant plays a vital role in ensuring patient satisfaction and successful adaptation to contact lenses. He or she gathers information as well as educates the patient. The information gleaned by the assistant helps the fitter select appropriate patients and make appropriate lens choices. The assistant also educates the patient on recommended lens use, compliance, appropriate follow-up, and good communication with the lens fitter. Normally, the assistant has more time available to listen to patient complaints, concerns, and anxieties. His or her role can increase productivity and contribute to the quality of the care rendered. This, in turn, increases patient satisfaction and good doctor–patient relations.

2. How should the assistant present himself or herself to the patient?

The assistant needs to be knowledgeable and should present himself or herself to the patient confidently. He or she should be well versed in contact lenses and lens care products and should have a working knowledge of wearing schedules, contact lens designs, and replacement schedules.

Grooming is also important. The assistant should perform hand washing in front of each patient prior to contact and should have short, clean fingernails. The assistant should avoid the use of hand creams or lotions, because these can damage the contact lenses and/or cause allergic reactions in the patient. Perfumes should likewise be avoided.

3. What is the function of the ophthalmic assistant in relationship to the new contact lens user?

The relationship begins during the history-taking process. The assistant obtains information that is vital in making contact lens–related decisions. During the history-taking process, the assistant has the opportunity to observe patient characteristics that may be important in contact lens use: personal hygiene, profession, age, maturity, and the necessity of a contact lens. Patient expectations, motivation for lens wear, previous contact lens experience, fears and insecurities, all play a role in lens design selection. In addition, information collected about the patient's ocular health is also vital. Items such as previous ocular surgeries, ocular disease, eye medications, dry eye, previous infection, systemic medications, and other ocular dysfunction also affect contact lens–related decisions.

   The assistant may also gather technical information such as keratometry readings, corneal diameter, and palpebral fissure measurements.

   During the trial lens fitting process, after an ideal lens has been selected by the fitter, the assistant may place the lens in the eye, instruct the patient on the lens design chosen, and teach the patient about care and handling of the contact lens. The assistant may then make note of the position and mobility of the lenses and measure the patient's visual acuity. Notes regarding the patient's initial reaction to the lens may also be made.

4. What is the function of the ophthalmic assistant relative to the experienced contact lens user?

The assistant may begin with the history, much as with the new wearer, including visual acuity with lenses. Information such as wearing time, both the regular routine as well as wearing time on the day of the examination, time spent not wearing lenses, routine cleaning habits, lens solutions, use of eye drops, status of vision after lens removal with or without glasses, lens comfort, current source of lenses, verification of lens condition and parameters, and any history of contact lens complications or difficulties must be gathered. If the patient is wearing a disposable or planned replacement lens regimen, replacement schedule and lens type are also important.

   The assistant may then answer any questions the patient may have regarding the contact lenses, care regimen, or wearing schedule.

5. Can the assistant prescribe contact lenses?

The assistant cannot prescribe contact lenses, just as he or she cannot prescribe eye drops, ophthalmic ointments, and other prescription medications. The contact lens must be fitted by a physician, optometrist, or certified contact lens fitter. All of the data collected by the assistant must be communicated to the eye care practitioner, who then supervises the remainder of the fitting and follow-up care.

6. What is the function of the assistant in relation to the contact lens laboratory?

The assistant must be prepared to maintain a good relationship with the contact lens laboratory. The laboratory provides many services for the eye care practitioner including materials, fitting sets, solutions, samples, inventory and consulting services, when needed. Ordering contact lenses, checking delivery status and availability, stock lens and solution ordering and maintenance, and keeping track of new lenses and care products available on the market are important functions of the assistant.

7. What are the concerns of the assistant for the contact lens fitting areas?

The assistant should keep a well-organized, well-stocked, and clean fitting area. This will ensure good organization and hygiene.

Basic Materials

A contact lens fitting room should include a hand washing facility including liquid soap, lint-free towels, a drain cover, a large magnifying mirror, and good lighting. It is the assistant's responsibility to maintain a clean, organized work area. Educational materials such as brochures, literature, and videos should also be readily available.

Contact lenses used for fitting purposes should be disinfected after each use unless they are disposable. All reusable lenses should be inspected routinely for damage, contamination, or expiration.

8. What is the assistant's role in follow-up examination of contact lens patients?

In general, return visits are largely handled by the assistant. On these occasions, the assistant has the opportunity to obtain information on the condition and management of the patient's contact lenses. Assistance with problem solving; contact lens handling, including storage, asepsis, and adaptation; cautions concerning the use of homemade saline and tap water; signs of complications; and recognition of danger signals may also be reinforced. Any concerns or the detection of abnormal findings are then reported immediately to the eye care practitioner.

9. What role does the assistant play in patient compliance?

By educating the patient in how to avoid contact lens complications and reinforcing this with literature, the assistant has the opportunity to increase patient compliance. Reaffirming with the patient the appropriate use of solutions, wearing schedule, and signs of contact lens–related complications also increases compliance.

The assistant needs to be available to answer questions, should they arise. In cases of complications, where medications are prescribed, the assistant may review the prescription with the patient and explain, step by step, how to use the prescribed medication or instill drops or ophthalmic ointments.

10. Can the assistant help in problem solving for the patient over the phone?

The patient should be instructed to telephone the office if questions or complications arise. The assistant can answer questions, clarify misunderstandings, and triage complication calls for the eye care practitioner.

Symptoms of complications include, but are not limited to, pain, redness, inflammation, halos, vision loss (with or without lenses), excessive secretions, and post–contact lens blur. Depending on the type of complaint, the assistant should not hesitate to communicate concerns to the ophthalmologist or optometrist. Should the patient develop symptoms of pain, hyperemia, halos, vision decrease, excessive secretions, or post–contact lens blur, all of which may indicate more urgent danger signals, the technician should communicate with the ophthalmologist or optometrist immediately.

11. How does the ophthalmic assistant maintain competence?

Continuing education is the key to maintaining competence. The assistant may participate in continuing education courses, use Web sites, attend meetings, or read books or trade magazines. National, state, or local contact lens education organizations may provide local continuing education courses.

Selected Readings

Castro RS, Kara-Jose N. Anamnese dirigida. In: Belford R Jr, Kara-Jose N, eds. *Cornea Clinica-cirurgica.* Sao Paulo: Roca, 1997:99.

Holyk PR, Atwood JD. Starting a contact lens practice. In: Kastl PR, ed. *Contact Lenses The CLAO Guide to Basic Science and Clinical Practice.* Iowa: Kendall Hunt, 1995:263–275.

Norman CW. Practice management. In: *Advanced Contact Lens Manual, A Comprehensive Study and Reference Guide,* vol II. Contact Lens Society of America, 1998:222–255.

Oliveira RCS, Kara-Jose N. *Auxiliar de Oftalmologia.* Sao Paulo: Roca, 2000 (Serie Oftalmologia USP):297–305.

Stein AS, Slatt BJ, Stein RM. Management of a contact lens practice. In: ——. *Fitting Guide for Rigid and Soft Lenses,* 3rd ed. St. Louis: C.V. Mosby, 1990: 489–498.

5

The Importance of Tear Film Evaluation in the Candidate for Contact Lens Wear

Milton Ruiz Alves,
Newton Kara-José,
and Kelly K. Nichols

1. What is the importance of tear film in the patient being considered for contact lens wear?

In contact lens wear, the tear film provides a smooth optical surface anterior to the contact lens. In addition to optical qualities, the tear film lubricates the ocular surface, provides antimicrobial function, helps to remove bacteria and devitalized epithelial cells, and acts as a vehicle for the diffusion of oxygen, nutrients, and local growth factors to the ocular surface. Individuals with symptoms of dry eye should not be excluded categorically from the use of contact lenses. However, their symptoms may be exacerbated by contact lens use, ambient conditions, or specific activities. Careful evaluation of the tear film, both prior to and during contact lens wear, is beneficial in promoting success with contact lens wear.

2. When is tear film evaluation indicated in a candidate for contact lens use?

A complete evaluation of the tear film is indicated at each new fitting, and a modified evaluation is recommended at follow-up visits. Ancillary testing is warranted with symptomatic complaints. The diagnostic workup for dry eye precedes the fitting of the contact lens and can avoid problems or indicate measures to be taken or specific contact lenses in such patients. Evaluation of the tear film in contact lens patients with complaints of ocular irritation can help define the problem and can help determine appropriate management and treatment if needed.

3. What are the examinations to evaluate the tear film in symptomatic patients or those with diseases commonly associated with keratoconjunctivitis sicca?

Tests of the tear film can be divided into routine clinical tests and accessory or specialty tests.

Routine Clinical Tests

Symptom Assessment

All contact lens patients should be asked if they experience symptoms of irritation, either with or without contact lens wear. Dryness and discomfort with contact lenses worsen with increasing hours of wear time; therefore, examining patients in the afternoon or asking about dry eye symptoms after several hours of lens wear can help identify mild dry eye patients. Contact lens wearers with reduced contact lens wearing time can have mild dry disease.

Slit-Lamp Biomicroscopy

At the slit lamp, one can observe debris in the tear film; mucous fragments; corneal and conjunctival epithelial changes; conjunctival vasodilation; tear meniscus height; and lid, lash, and blink irregularities. These evaluations are best performed with white, diffuse light.

Tear Meniscus Height

The inferior tear lake (or prism) accumulates at the junction of the bulbar conjunctiva in the inferior lid margin and is approximately 0.3 to 0.4 mm in height in normal individuals. Significant diminution or absence of the tear meniscus, frequently with accumulation of debris, is suggestive of lacrimal deficiency. Increased tear debris may also be associated with an unstable tear film. A measurement scale in the reticule or an adjustable slit beam height can be used to measure tear meniscus height.

Tear Breakup Time

The fluorescein tear breakup time test evaluates the stability of the precorneal tear film. Following the instillation of sodium fluorescein (either one drop of liquid 2% sodium fluorescein or fluorescein from a saline wetted fluorescein strip), the cobalt filter on the slit lamp is used to examine the tear film. The examiner asks the patient to hold the eye open after blinking several times. A 3- to 4-mm wide beam is used to scan the tear film for the first breakup, or black spot. Tear breakup time is considered borderline if it is less than 10 seconds and frankly abnormal if it is less than 5 seconds. A noninvasive test can also be performed to determine tear breakup time. Several instruments can be used, such as the TearScope, the Xeroscope, or the keratometer. The time in seconds until distortion in the ring image or keratometric mires is observed. Noninvasive tear breakup measurements are generally longer than fluorescein-based tear breakup time.

Fluorescein Staining

Fluorescein dye is used to detect epithelial defects on the anterior surface of the eye. It is generally accepted that fluorescein penetrates only the corneal epithelium at sites of interrupted continuity of the epithelial surface.[1] In a normal sample, the inferior cornea is the most common location for fluorescein staining, followed by the nasal cornea.[2] The evaluation of corneal staining with sequential instillations of fluorescein[3] also revealed that nasal and inferior regions of staining were the most common and occurred more frequently in the morning and late afternoon. While some degree of corneal staining is frequent in contact lens wearers,[4] moderate to severe staining may warrant contact lens modification or therapeutic management. Fluorescein staining is enhanced with the use of a No. 12 Wratten barrier filter that blocks extraneous light and highlights staining patterns.[5]

Rose Bengal or Lissamine Green Staining

Devitalized cells on the cornea and conjunctiva and mucus in the tear film are detected using 1% rose bengal or 1% lissamine green (liquid or wetted strip). The areas of compromise are highlighted by red punctate staining (rose bengal) or blue-green punctuate stain (lissamine green) in the exposed areas of the cornea and conjunctiva. Rose bengal stings slightly on instillation, which does not occur with lissamine green dye. Lissamine green is suitable for staining degenerate cells, mucus, and dead cells with identical staining patterns to rose bengal.[6] Rose bengal staining patterns are classically graded on a 0 to 3 graded scale proposed by van Bijesterveld, where three regions of the interpalpebral ocular surface are assessed (the triangular wedge of the nasal interpalpebral conjunctiva, the corneal surface, and the wedge of the temporal conjunctiva). The grade of each region is summed, and a score greater than 3.5 is considered indicative of dry eye.[7]

The Schirmer Test

The Schirmer test measures tear secretion from the lacrimal gland and measures both the basal and reflex tear production. The result is normal when, after 5 minutes, 10 mm or more of the filter paper strip is saturated with tears. Schirmer results with anesthesia are lower than results without anesthesia; therefore, the use of anesthetic with the Schirmer test is generally not recommended.[8] The Schirmer I test is generally considered to be a measurement of total (reflex and basic) tear secretion, while the Schirmer II test is regarded as a test of induced reflex secretion.[9] Historically, the Schirmer I test is performed with an open eye. The Schirmer II test requires irritation of the nostril on the same side with a cotton swab fiber.[8] Schirmer values of less than 5 mm/5 minutes have been considered to indicate low tear production; however, many authors report different cutoff values ranging from ≤3[10] to ≤10 mm/5 minutes.[11] Many attempts have been made to improve the accuracy of the Schirmer test, and controversy exists over its usefulness. Despite this disagreement, the Schirmer test remains the primary method of assessing tear production.

Phenol Red Thread Test

The phenol red thread test, first described in 1977, is an alternative to the Schirmer test.[12] The thread test was developed in response to two main problems inherent in the Schirmer test: the length of time necessary to perform the Schirmer test (5 minutes) and the potential influence of reflex tears secondary to irritation of the palpebral conjunctiva. Hamano and coworkers[13] developed a test using a No. 40/2 thread impregnated with phenol red dye. The thread is 70 mm in length, and the test is 15 seconds in duration, with the eye open. Recently, the Zone Quick phenol red thread test has become commercially available from Menicon, Inc. and is fast and easy to perform. The abnormal values for the phenol red thread test are ≤10 mm wetting per 15 seconds in the open eye condition.

Accessory Dry Eye Tests

Lacrimal Clearance Test

This test constitutes a variation on the Schirmer II test. In this test, one instills a drop of topical anesthetic, and, after removing the excess, a drop of sodium fluorescein 0.25% is placed in the inferior cul-de-sac while the patient blinks normally. One then proceeds with a Schirmer test for 1 minute every 10 minutes. Clearance is normal when the color clears after the second paper strip. After 30 minutes, one should perform nasal stimulation and a new Schirmer test. Basal secretion is considered normal if the first two strips of paper are wet to at least 3 mm. Reflex secretion is considered normal if, at the last test, the paper is wetter than the two previous tests.

Osmolarity

Increased osmolarity of the tear film may lead to interpalpebral surface damage and, therefore, dry eye. The concentration of the tear film due to increased evaporation of the tear film results in increased osmolarity of the tear film over the ocular surface and has been associated with keratoconjuctivitis sicca.[14] The rise in tear film osmolarity is proposed to cause the movement of fluid out of the epithelial calls and lead to cellular damage.[15] The cutoff point proposed by Gilbard for dry eye diagnosis is 312 mOsm/L, with higher values reflecting dry eye. Newer nanoliter osmometers are more portable, require smaller tear samples, and have automated calibration, all of which indicate potential clinical promise in dry eye diagnosis.

Lysozyme Agar Diffusion Test

This test employs disks of No. 41 Whatman filter paper that have been soaked in tears and are placed on agar previously inoculated with a suspension of *Micrococcus lysodeikticus*. A zone of lysis surrounding the disk of paper in 24 hours indicates the antibacterial activity of tear lysozyme. The production of lysozyme parallels lacrimal secretion and is a test that provides information on the function of the lacrimal glands. Lysozyme disappears prematurely in Sjögren syndrome. The test is well correlated with the concentration of tear lactoferrin.

Lactoferrin Level Measurement with Lactoplate™ or the Touch Tear MicroAssay System™

Lactoferrin is one of the principal proteins secreted by the lacrimal gland. Its concentration can be determined by measuring concentric circular precipitate after 72 hours of incubation at room temperature. There is a correlation between the concentration of lactoferrin and the quantity of tears secreted. It is both sensitive and specific in the evaluation of cases of keratoconjunctivitis sicca. In using lactoferrin analysis, a measurement of ≤ 0.9 mg/μL is indicative of dry eye and has been highly associated with moderate to severe dry eye patients.[16] The Touch Tear MicroAssay System™ is also a solid-phase enzyme immunoassay that requires a tear sample of 1 to 2μL. Once collected, tear samples can be stored up to 14 days. The instrument requires 15 minutes for the process.

Conjunctival Impression Cytology

Millipore filter paper of cellulose acetate (with 0.02-μm pores) can be employed to assess conjunctival goblet cell density. The filter paper is cut into strips approximately $5 \times 5 \times 10$ mm in size. After instillation into the inferior cul-de-sac of one drop of proparacaine or a similar anesthetic, with the aid of a forceps, the pieces of filter paper are pressed against the nasal, temporal, inferior, and superior bulbar conjunctiva. Pressure is applied to the paper for 2 to 3 seconds. The filter paper containing the conjunctival specimen is then fixed for 10 minutes in a mixture of 70% ethyl alcohol, 37% formaldehyde, and glacial acetic acid in a proportion of 20:1:1. Subsequently, each paper containing the material to be studied is stained, using periodic acid–Schiff (PAS), hematoxylin and eosin, and Papanicolaou. Under the light microscope ($200\times$), the epithelial cells are evaluated for morphology and density. Nelson (1988) classified impression cytology of the conjunctiva in grades: Grade 0 denotes small, round endothelial cells with eosinophilic cytoplasm with a nuclear cytoplasmic ratio of 1:2 and abundant goblet cells. Grade 3 is large, polygonal endothelial cells with basophilic cytoplasm and a nuclear cytoplasmic ratio of less than 1:6 and the number of goblet cells reduced or absent. Grades 1 and 2 are considered normal.

Serologic Testing

Approximately 80% of individuals with severe dry eye have antinuclear antibodies (ANAs) and antibodies A and B in Sjögren syndrome (SS-A and SS-B). Approximately 50% of patients with keratoconjunctivitis sicca without evidence of connective tissue disease are ANA and rheumatoid factor positive, and SS-A and SS-B antibodies are found in one third of these individuals. Serologic studies for infection with Epstein-Barr virus in patients with Sjögren syndrome suggested recurrent infections in some of these patients.

Salivary Gland Biopsy

This is the most specific test for confirmation of Sjögren syndrome. Histologically, the finding of lymphocytic foci in the accessory salivary glands is virtually diagnostic of the disease. There is a correlation between the number of lymphocytic foci and the severity of the disease.

4. When do the results of tear film evaluation contraindicate the use of contact lenses?

In mild dry eye patients, contraindication to the use of contact lenses is relative. The user may have mild-to-moderate discomfort while wearing lenses and limitations with regard to wearing time. In addition, rigorous daily lens hygiene may be needed. If tear function is clearly inadequate, hydrophilic contact lenses tend to dry the eye further, form deposits on their surface, and irritate the corneal surface. Artificial tears can be instilled to maintain adequate lens hydration and corneal lubrication. In such cases, the fitting of a low-water-content lens may encourage complete and frequent blinking and so avoid the use of drugs that interfere with lacrimal secretion. Proclear Compatibles™ (Cooper Vision) and Extreme H^2O (Hydrogel Vision Corp.) are two hydrogel lenses marketed toward the mild-to-moderate dry eye patient. Silicone hydrogel lenses are also being used as a dry eye alternative. Certain situations can be improved by changing systemic medication, teaching the patient to blink more frequently and completely, or even surgically correcting an excessively large interpalpebral space. The presence of severe dry eye constitutes an absolute contraindication to the use of contact lenses (with the exception of therapeutic contact lenses in selected cases).

5. What short-term changes in the tear film are induced by the use of a contact lens?

The insertion of a contact lens into the tear film causes short-term fluctuations in the stability of the tear film, with a possible decrease in osmolarity due to the contact lens storage solutions and reflex tearing due to lens insertion. There are also mild short-term fluctuations in the tear film pH. It is thought that the pre–contact lens tear film differs from the post-lens tear film once the tear film has stabilized. The pre-lens tear film is postulated to be lipid and slightly aqueous, while the post-lens layer is composed of mucin and aqueous.

6. What is the effect of the "lacrimal pump" on corneal oxygenation?

A supply of oxygen to the cornea is a prerequisite for the maintenance of aerobic metabolism, which supplies energy for the maintenance of the cornea's normal state of deturgescence. The oxygen arrives at the cornea from the atmosphere as well as through the bloodstream. Oxygenation is associated with blinking and is a factor of minor importance in the case of a hydrophilic contact lens when less than 5% of the tears is exchanged with each blink. This is different from what occurs in the rigid contact lens, in which case 20% of the tear volume is exchanged with each blink. Nevertheless, the lacrimal pump has importance even in hydrophilic contact lens wear because it permits removal of the debris and other products of the metabolism of the surface.

7. What contact lens materials are most likely to develop surface deposits?

Deposits can occur in all types of contact lenses, although deposits are more likely to form on the surface of hydrogel contact lenses. There are two classification systems for hydrogel lens materials worldwide: the U.S. Food and Drug Administration (FDA) and the European International Standards Organization (ISO) system. In using the FDA system, FDA group IV (high water, ionic) hydrogel lenses are likely to develop protein deposits, while FDA group II (high water, nonionic) hydrogel lenses deposit predominately lipid. The polymethylmethacrylate (PMMA) contact lens is not subject to deposits except in cases of corneal surface irregularity. Deposits easily adhere to the rigid gas permeable lens due to problems with wetting of the surface.

8. From what parts of the tear film do contact lens deposits originate?

The substances responsible for the formation of deposits may originate in any of the layers of the tear film. The aqueous layer of the tear film is composed of 98% water; 2% is mineral content, including electrolytes such as potassium, chloride, and calcium, as well as organic compounds. Included in these organic compounds are proteins, and of these proteins, lysozyme has a special attraction to the materials from which hydrophilic contact lenses are made. Lipids produced by the meibomian glands also deposit on contact lenses, as do products of the mucin layer.

9. What types of deposits are encountered on contact lenses?

Organic Deposits

1. Proteins (lysozyme, lactoferrin, albumin, immunoglobulin A [IgA], IgG)
2. Lipids
3. Mucin
4. Carbohydrates
5. Mixed-composition substances (calculi = lipid, calcium, protein)
6. Microorganisms
7. Pigments (e.g., melanin)

Inorganic Deposits

1. Calcium salts
2. Salts of iron oxides
3. Mercury
4. Color changes (e.g., pigmentation due to dyes, makeup, tobacco smoke)

10. What organic deposits are most commonly encountered in contact lenses?

Proteins

The most common deposit is lysozyme, which is attracted by the ionic content of the material of hydrophilic lenses. Protein deposition appears as a white, partially opaque deposit that is very thin and superficial. It can also be transparent and recognizable only when it starts to separate from the lens surface or as the lens dries. Protein deposits are primarily on the lens surface but can penetrate the lens matrix of high water content lenses. The adherence of protein is stimulated by dry zones on the lens surface, which can be caused by poor lubrication or incomplete blinking. The presence of these deposits can lead to giant papillary conjunctivitis.

Lipids

When deposited on contact lenses (the tears contain abundant quantities of lipid), lipid facilitates the formation of other types of deposits and decreases the wetting of the contact lens, causing poor distribution of the tears on the anterior surface. Lipid deposition can be prevented with the daily use of surfactant cleaning solution and lid hygiene.

Mucopolysaccharides

Of mixed composition (carbohydrates, mucin, proteins, and inorganic substances), mucopolysaccharide deposits range in color from white to amber and can produce significant discomfort.

Pigments

In hydrophilic contact lenses, most pigment deposits vary in coloration from yellow to brown. They generally begin at the borders and move gradually, covering the entire contact lens. It is thought that these pigments originate from melanin. Their removal with oxidizing agents may alter the structure of the contact lens.

Microorganisms

The bacteria most commonly associated with the use of contact lenses are *Pseudomonas aeruginosa, Staphylococcus aureus,* and *Staphylococcus epidermidis.* Fungi can deposit on the surface, followed by filamentary growth that can penetrate the contact lens and destroy it. Fungi can often be seen with a loupe or with the slit lamp. Deposits on the contact lens provide nutrients for colonization by microorganisms. In recent years, infections with *Acanthamoeba* associated with soft contact lens wear have gained importance because of their gravity.

References

1. Norn MS. Micropunctate fluorescein vital staining of the cornea. *Acta Ophthalmol.* 1970;48:108–118.
2. Schwallie JD, McKenney CD, Long WD, McNeil A. Corneal staining patterns in normal non-contact lens wearers. *Optom Vis Sci.* 1997;74:92–98.
3. Josephson JE, Caffery BE. Corneal staining characteristics after sequential instillations of fluorescein. *Optom Vis Sci.* 1992;69:570–573.
4. Nichols KK, Mitchell GL, Simon KM, Chivers DA, Edrington TB. Corneal staining in hydrogel lens wearers. *Optom Vis Sci.* 2002;79:20–30.
5. Eliason JA, Maurice DM. Staining of the conjunctiva and conjunctival tear film. *Br J Ophthalmol.* 1990;74:519–522.
6. Norn MS. Lissamine green. Vital staining of the cornea and conjunctiva. *Acta Ophthalmol.* 1973;51:483–491.
7. Van Bijsterveld OP. Diagnostic tests in the sicca syndrome. *Arch Ophthalmol.* 1969;82:10–14.
8. Norn M. Diagnosis of dry eye. In: Lemp M, ed. *The Dry Eye.* New York: Springer-Verlag, 1992:134–182.
9. Doughman DJ. Clinical tests. *Int Ophthalmol Clin.* 1973;13(1):199–217.
10. Lamberts DW, Foster CS, Perry HD. Schirmer test after topical anesthesia and the tear meniscus height in normal eyes. *Arch Ophthalmol.* 1979;97: 1082–1085.

11. Mathers WD Lane JA. Meibomian gland lipids, evaporation, and tear film stability. *Adv Exp Med Biol.* 1998;438:349–360.
12. Kurihashi K. Diagnostic tests of lacrimal function using cotton thread. In: Holly FJ, ed. *The Preocular Tear Film in Health, Disease, and Contact Lens Wear.* Lubbock, TX: Dry Eye Institute, Inc., 1986:89–114.
13. Hamano H, Hori M, Hamano T, et al. A new method for measuring tears. *CLAO J.* 1983;9:281–289.
14. Refojo MF, Rolando M, Belldegrün R, Kenyon KR. Tear evaporimeter for diagnosis and research: In: Holly FJ, ed. *The Preocular Tear Film in Health, Disease, and Contact Lens Wear.* Lubbock, TX: Dry Eye Institute, Inc., 1986:117–123.
15. Gilbard JP. Tear film osmolarity and keratoconjunctivitis sicca. In: Holly FJ, ed. *The Preocular Tear Film in Health, Disease, and Contact Lens Wear.* Lubbock, TX: Dry Eye Institute, Inc., 1986:127–139.
16. McCollum CJ, Foulks GN, Bodner B, et al. Rapid assay of lactoferrin in keratoconjunctivitis sicca. *Cornea.* 1994;13:505–508.

6

Corneal Topography and Contact Lenses

Michael Twa, Cleusa Coral-Ghanem, and Breno Barth

1. What is the shape of the normal cornea?

The shape of the normal cornea is not spherical but aspheric (Color Plate 1). The central 6-mm portion of the cornea, called the central corneal cap, is approximately spherical. However, the corneal curvature flattens progressively toward the periphery. The resulting shape is a prolate aspheric surface, (Figure 6.1). The average shape of the anterior corneal surface is a prolate asphere with a central radius of 7.7 mm that is slightly steeper (7.95 mm) in the vertical meridian.[1,2] The prolate shape effectively reduces spherical aberration of the eye. Although this aspheric shape has optical benefits, it complicates contact lens design.

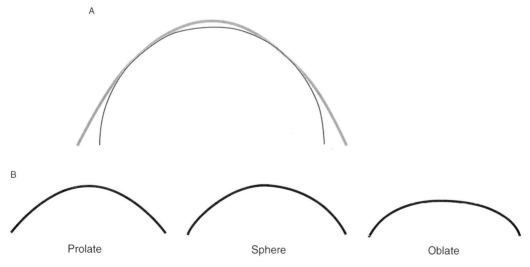

Figure 1. Diagram demonstrating the shape relationship of the aspheric prolate cornea to a sphere. B: Diagram illustrating the relationships among the shapes.

Consequently, contact lenses consist of a central optical portion and a peripheral portion designed to provide proper alignment, position, and adequate movement of the lens on the eye. There is great variation in corneal shape within the normal population due to corneal size, astigmatism, influence of eyelids, and other factors. Videokeratography is a useful tool for describing the form of this important optical structure of the eye.

2. What are the methods for evaluating the anterior profile of the cornea?

The most common methods of measuring corneal shape are keratometry, videokeratography, and anterior segment analysis.

Keratometry

Keratometry measures central corneal curvature at two points within the central 2 to 4 mm (3 mm on average) of the cornea and does not measure the mid-peripheral or peripheral cornea. Keratometry is a rapid and accurate method of determining curvature of the central corneal cap that is useful for estimating the overall optical power of the cornea. Keratometry measurements are less repeatable with abnormal corneal shapes distorted by injury or diseases that distort corneal shape such as keratoconus. While keratometry normally provides no information about the peripheral corneal shape, the normal clinical procedure can be modified to measure peripheral corneal curvature.[3]

The principle of keratometry relies on the reflective optical properties of the cornea. The reflective surface of the cornea produces a virtual image the size of which is a function of the corneal radius of curvature. The keratometer employs the doubling principle. The reflected image is split into two images using a semisilvered mirror and a series of prisms. The relative displacement of the two images is then adjusted until the top of one image is coincident with the bottom of the second, as described below.

The figure demonstrates the mires as viewed from the practitioner's side of a conventional keratometer. The task is to align the mires at the 9 o'clock position of the lower right hand circle to measure the horizontal meridian and at the 12 o'clock position of the lower right hand circle to measure the vertical meridian.

The specific procedure is as follows:

1. Ask the patient to place his or her chin in the chin rest and forehead against the headrest.
2. Have the patient fixate on the reflected image of his or her eye or the target in the instrument.
3. With the keratometer in the straight-ahead position, sight down the instrument vertically until the leveling sight is aligned with the patient's temporal canthus.
4. Occlude the eye not being tested. Release the knob for locking the instrument and rotate the instrument until it points directly at the

eye to be tested. Instruct the patient to look into the instrument where he or she sees a reflection of his or her own eye.

5. Adjust the focus of the instrument until the image of the mires is clear.
6. Make fine vertical and horizontal adjustments necessary to place the reticule cross near the center of the lower right mire image.
7. Lock the instrument in place.
8. Rotate the instrument (to locate the horizontal or near horizontal principal meridian) until the horizontal bars of the two crosses to the left of the focusing mire are aligned. Maintain clarity of the image during this step by continual refinement of the focus.
9. Turn the horizontal measuring knob (on the left of the instrument) until these two crosses are superimposed.
10. Direct attention to the two horizontal lines above the focusing mire and turn the vertical measuring knob (on the right of the instrument) until these lines are superimposed.
11. Record the median readings as, for example:
   - 43.00/44.75 @ 090, mires regular or distorted, or
   - 43.00 @180, 44.75 @ 090, mires regular or distorted

The keratometer measures an area of the central cornea with a diameter of approximately 3.50 to 3.75 mm. Curvatures approaching 50.00 D should raise the suspicion of keratoconus, and inferior steepening and/or excess superior flattering may indicate a keratoconus suspect. If the corneal curvature is too steep, a plus lens can be placed over the opening on the mire face of the standard keratometer and secured with tape or special lens holder. A minus lens can be placed for curvature flatter than the standard range. Conversion tables are available for extending the range of the keratometer using these lens additions. A hand-held keratometer (Alcon Laboratories, Ft. Worth, TX) is also available for general patient use in bedridden, obese, aged, or young patients who may be difficult to position behind a standard table mounted device.

Videokeratography

Also commonly referred to as corneal topography, computer-assisted videokeratography instruments measure approximately 95% of the corneal surface. These measurements produce elevation and curvature maps of the anterior corneal surface. A circular pattern of concentric rings known as a Placido disk is the basis of most clinical instruments (Figure 6.2). Corneal shape is derived from distortion of the reflected circular rings. (Figure 6.3). Other instruments such as the Orbscan II (Bausch & Lomb, Rochester, NY) or CTS (Medtec, Columbus, OH) measure the shape of the corneal surface directly by triangulating individual points on the cornea. The CTS projects a grid onto the corneal surface and corneal shape is calculated from deflection of the grid by triangulation of grid intersections (Figure 6.4). The Orbscan records diffuse reflection of slit-illumination scans of the cornea. Corneal shape is reconstructed from triangulation of points along these edges. Re-

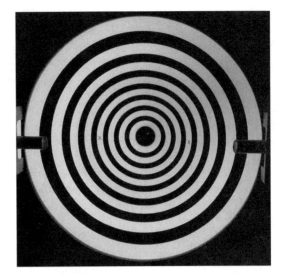

Figure 2. Placido disk.

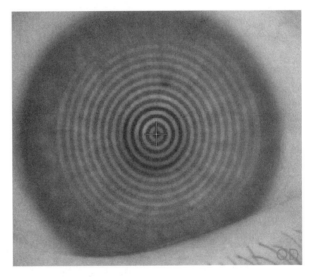

Figure 3. Placido disk rings reflected off the cornea.

gardless of method, it is possible to generate both elevation and curvature maps from any of these clinical instruments.

Anterior Segment Analysis

Clinical instruments are now available that can measure anterior curvature, posterior curvature, total corneal thickness, and anterior chamber depth. The Orbscan II (Figure 6.5) was the first instrument to provide this additional information. The Astramax (Figure 6.6) is another instrument designed to measure the anterior and posterior corneal shape, corneal thickness, pupil size, and anterior chamber depth.

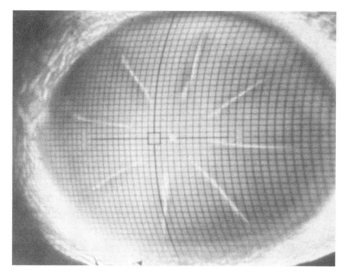

Figure 4. CTS image.

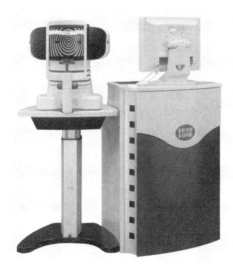

Figure 5. Orbscan.

3. What are the indications for computed topography of the cornea?

1. Refractive instability
2. Reduced best spectacle corrected visual acuity
3. Contact lens wear, especially rigid lenses
4. Design and simulation of rigid contact lens fitting
5. Diagnosis of contact lens–induced corneal distortion
6. Management of therapeutic and refractive corneal surgeries
7. Diagnosis and management of corneal disease such as keratoconus

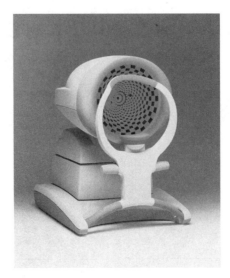

Figure 6. Astramax.

8. Determination of corneal power for correct intraocular lens (IOL) power calculation in cataract surgery
9. Evaluation of corneal surface abnormalities and determination of their affect on the optical quality of the eye

4. What is a good way to interpret videokeratography maps?

Orient yourself to videokeratography maps before attempting interpretation.

- First, determine the type of map. The three most common maps are axial curvature, tangential curvature, and elevation maps. Each map provides different information about corneal shape and will have a different appearance even for the same eye. Color Plate 2 shows an example demonstrating the variety of possible maps for the same eye.
- Second, determine the numerical range and size of the steps represented by the color scale associated with the corneal map. The color scale is like the map legend; without it, one has no idea what value the colors represent. The color scale is crucial to correct interpretation. The units of a color scale for elevation maps is usually microns; curvature maps are normally represented in either diopters or millimeters.
- Third, consider possible artifacts that may explain unusual maps when clinical findings from videokeratography are inconsistent with expectations and other clinical test results. Several common artifacts can influence the appearance of videokeratography maps including eyelids and eyelashes, tear debris, contact lens wear, instrument alignment, and focus. Clinicians should always consider these factors during map interpretation. It is easier to identify these artifacts when

the raw video image of the eye is included in the printout. For example, in Color Plate 5A and 5B, the same eye is presented with the instrument in correct focus and in poor focus with the Placido mires too far away from the eye. Artifacts can be caused by tear debris and eyelashes.

5. What is the difference between the different types of corneal topography maps?

Axial radius of curvature for any point on the corneal surface is defined by the radius of a sphere fit to that point and centered on the instrument axis (Figure 6.7A). Tangential curvature maps do not force the center of curvature of the best fitting sphere to lie along the instrument axis

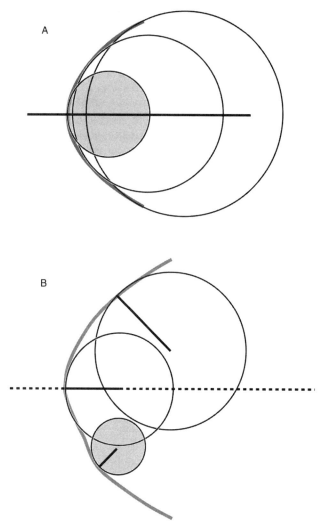

Figure 7. Axial radius of curvature. B: Tangential radius of curvature.

(Figure 6.7B). Elevation maps commonly represent deviation of the corneal surface from a reference spherical surface (Figure 6.1A).

Axial Curvature Maps

Areas of greater curvature are represented by red and orange (warm) colors and regions of flatter curvature are represented by green and blue (cool) colors. In standard keratometry, the size of a reference object reflected from the corneal surface is proportional to the curvature of the outer eye. Axial curvature maps approximate corneal curvature by applying these same principles and assume that all corneal surface features have a center of curvature lying on the measurement axis of the instrument. This assumption results in curvature maps that change more gradually from center to periphery. Axial curvature maps describe the mean shape of the cornea well but do not detect localized surface features very well. The axial curvature map of a normal corneal surface with a prolate aspheric shape is shown in Color Plate 1.

   With axial curvature maps, corneal astigmatism produces a symmetric pattern called a "bow tie" (Color Plate 3). The orientation of the steep meridian of this axial bow tie indicates the axis of the correcting lens in plus cylinder notation. Corneal toricity that is steeper in the vertical meridian represents with-the-rule astigmatism. Against-the-rule astigmatism occurs when the steep meridian is oriented horizontally. Regularity and symmetry of this pattern is an indication of normal corneal shape. Abnormal corneal shape altered by disease, trauma, or even contact lens wear is typically more irregular and has asymmetric patterns that are more easily seen with other maps.

Tangential Curvature Maps

Tangential curvature maps describe localized changes of corneal curvature more accurately than the axial maps. A red color on a tangential curvature map represents areas of greater curvature, while blue represents less curvature. Also known as local curvature, tangential curvature maps are useful to demonstrate the location and dimensions of corneal surface features. Tangential maps are useful for locating the apex of corneal steepening in keratoconus, boundaries of a treatment zone after corneal refractive surgery, pterygia, and corneal scarring. One disadvantage is that tangential curvature maps are susceptible to artifacts and overinterpretation. Even minor surface anomalies caused by mucus, tear breakup, or other tear debris can influence corneal shape in tangential curvature maps.

Elevation Maps

Elevation maps are interpreted differently from axial or tangential curvature maps. An average cornea may have as much as 0.25 mm or 250 µm of sagittal depth from apex to periphery. To appreciate this relatively small variation in elevation occurring over a 9-mm corneal diameter, the anterior corneal surface is usually compared to the best fit of a sphere (Figure 6.1A). The resulting elevation map values represent the difference between the front surface of the cornea and the spherical reference surface.

It is important to remember that colors do not represent curvature in elevation maps. In elevation maps, the red color signifies elevation above an established reference surface but can correspond with either steep or flat curvature. In fact, for an astigmatic corneal surface, the meridian of steeper curvature often corresponds to elevation below a spherical reference surface, and regions of flatter corneal curvature correspond to elevation above a best fit reference sphere. The "bow-tie" pattern of an axial curvature map of an eye with astigmatism becomes a "biscuit" shape on the elevation map. Elevation maps are useful when interpreting fluorescein patterns beneath a rigid contact lens and also for making a differential diagnosis of corneal ectasia.

6. What are the most commonly used maps for contact lens fitting?

Axial (sagittal), tangential (local) curvature, and elevation maps are all commonly used for contact lens fitting. Each of these methods has advantages and specific applications for contact lens fitting.

Axial curvature maps provide good information about the average shape of the cornea. Thus, axial curvature maps can be very useful for selecting contact lens parameters especially posterior curvature during a rigid contact lens fitting. Corneal astigmatism significant enough to influence contact lens design (>1.00 D) is easily seen in axial curvature maps.

Tangential curvature maps are helpful for locating the size, shape, and position of specific features on the corneal surface. Tangential maps can guide contact lens design by providing a better estimate of the location and severity of surface features that might require special attention. Some of the features that can be easily identified are pterygia, keratoconus, and corneal scars. The better resolution of tangential curvature maps can also give clinicians a basis for judging the impact of local surface features on vision.

Elevation maps provide an excellent way to simulate contact lens alignment to the corneal surface. Most videokeratography instrument manufacturers include contact lens fitting modules that simulate fluorescein pooling patterns behind rigid contact lenses. These software modules estimate the elevation difference (in microns) between the back surface of the contact lens and the corneal surface elevation map.

Example

A 34-year-old man with normal ocular health presented for cosmetic rigid gas permeable contact lens fitting. Both tangential and axial curvature maps were generated from a videokeratography examination.

There were no irregular surface features detectable by tangential curvature maps. The mean shape of the cornea was prolate, with a 6-mm diameter spherical central corneal cap and a central curvature of 43 D. Posterior central curvature of the first trial lens was selected from the axial curvature value measured 2.5 mm from center (5-mm diameter). A 9-mm diameter lens with a 6.2-mm optical zone was designed with flatter intermediate and peripheral curves. The fit to the corneal surface was simulated using an elevation map. Simulated fluorescein patterns suggested the lens design would provide good alignment centrally with pooling in the periphery. Simulated fluorescein patterns for lenses steeper and flatter than alignment are seen in Color Plates 4 and 5.

7. What are the specific programs for fitting contact lenses?

Refractive surgery and contact lens design were the two primary applications that drove the development of videokeratography technology.[4,5] The availability of affordable powerful personal computers and video cameras accelerated the development of this imaging technology in the late 1980s.[6] Software programs for the fitting of contact lenses are included by every equipment manufacturer; each has its own specific options and advantages.

There are several ways to use these programs. For inexperienced contact lens fitters, the software routines can offer a flexible, inexpensive, and friendly environment for simulating the effects of contact lens modifications on lens alignment. Experienced contact lens fitters may find these programs inefficient for routine fitting. However, despite their limitations, even experienced users may find fit simulations provide valuable insight for challenging cases with irregular corneal surfaces.

Use of these programs is helpful and may reduce the number of lens design changes required during trial fitting. Most contact lens design programs suggest optimal design parameters based on measured corneal shape, provide the details of these design parameters, allow modification of lens design using custom parameters, and even provide simulations of the expected fluorescein pattern. Most automated fitting routines suggest a central posterior curve for the contact lens, the diameter of the optical zone, lens power, and the type of material. Another benefit of contact lens design through videokeratography software is the option to submit orders directly to manufacturing laboratories. One of the most significant limitations of fitting contact lenses by this approach is an inability to account for lens mass, translation, and lid interactions.

Each program has a variety of options and additional features, and all have continued to evolve over time. Following is a description of some of the more common programs used for contact lens fitting.

Keratron Scout (Optikon 2000, Rome, Italy)

The Keratron is currently produced as a tabletop instrument and as a portable hand-held instrument. The software used to analyze video-keratography images and calculate contact lens parameters is the same for both instrument platforms.

The contact lens design module is flexible, allowing clinicians to create their own library of fitting lenses from 32 different materials, choose lenses from standardized fitting sets, or design contact lenses using custom lens parameters. Default lens parameters are recommended by the software based on curvature or elevation criteria selected by the user. Toric lens design parameters are suggested by the software above a user-defined threshold of corneal astigmatism.

The Keratron contact lens software allows the user to simulate lens decentration and recalculates the predicted fluorescein pattern for the new lens location. In addition, lid effects or other mechanical influences on lens alignment can be estimated using tilt buttons located at the edge of the lens to simulate pressure at four peripheral locations. Other contact lens design programs are available to work in conjunction with the Keratron instrument. Using the same corneal shape data, software designers have created plug-in software design modules that create advanced contact lenses for orthokeratology, bifocals, bitorics, and other designs.

TMS-1 (Topographical Mapping System 1, Computed Anatomy, Inc.)

The TMS program makes it possible for the contact lens designer to choose one of three types of contact lens: Boston™, Paragon™, or Menicon™. Depending on the type of contact lens chosen, the software, based on proprietary algorithms, supplies the diameter, base curve, peripheral zone, and refractive power of the contact lens. These data can be found on the fluorescein map that appears on the monitor. In another quadrant of the map, one may observe fluorescein clearance represented graphically and demonstrating the relationship between the anterior cornea and the posterior surface of the contact lens in all of the meridians. The parameters provided in this diagram include the diameter of the contact lens, the diameter of the posterior optical zone in millimeters, central posterior curvature in diopters, and the keratometry. With the data provided by this software, one can choose a trial lens for the patient and examine the lens at the slit lamp. The fluorescein pattern expected should be similar to that seen on the monitor. One study that evaluated the role of corneal topographers in contact lens fitting concluded the TMS-1 program is useful in choosing the contact lens type but emphasized that the clinical evaluation is absolutely necessary for successful fitting.[7]

Fitscan

This is the contact lens fitting software of the Orbscan II(™) (Bausch & Lomb Surgical, Rochester, NY). This program is a rigid contact lens fitting software module. By setting the software to individual preferences, the user can constrain the initial lens selection to match the corneal surface features as closely as possible. The two methods of defining lens fit characteristics are:

1. Selecting minimum and maximum posterior lens clearance from the corneal surface.
2. Assigning default lens parameters such as optical zone radius, secondary and peripheral zone width, and curvature values.

The software calculates and displays a simulated fluorescein pattern of the resulting lens. These values are a good starting point for most patients. However, the user may modify these lens parameters and recalculate the simulated fluorescein pattern to improve the fit.

The Fitscan software also allows simultaneous display of the simulated fluorescein pattern as well as the videokeratography map that is useful for comparing elevation or curvature maps with the simulated contact lens design. When the simulated contact lens fitting is complete, a summary screen containing the final contact lens design specifications can be printed or e-mailed directly to the contact lens manufacturing lab.

EyeSys System 2000 Pro-Fit Software (v. 4.0)

The EyeSys Pro-Fit program performs a sagittal analysis that considers the contact lens sagittal depth and touch in all meridians for the specific patient. The system calculates a central posterior curve, an optical zone, and a fluorescein pattern. These data are obtained by way of formulas developed for the anterior surface of the cornea and the posterior surface of the contact lens. The contact lens parameters are based on measurements of both the central and peripheral corneal shape.

Humphrey Atlas MasterVue Contact Lens Module (v. A6)

This program employs algorithms to calculate data on corneal elevation and the thickness profile of the tear film. It uses adjusted keratometry based on simulated keratometry (Sim K). Contact lens design is based on the corneal "shape factor," which describes how aspheric the curvature is relative to a normal cornea. This is especially useful for eyes that have had refractive surgery for the correction of myopia (oblate corneas) or hyperopia (increased prolate shape).

One study comparing the efficiency and accuracy of two rigid gas permeable contact lens fitting programs—Humphrey and EyeSys—demonstrated equal success with the two systems: 82% in the Humphrey system and 82.9% in the EyeSys.[8] The lens specifications most often modified from the suggested software design were contact lens power in both systems and optical zone in the Humphrey Atlas.

Dicon CT-200

The contact lens module of this instrument makes contact lens design and ordering very simple. There are two screens for this process. The first screen is the fitting guide. The second screen is the order form. In the fitting guide, the user enters the patient's prescription and chooses the lens type. In addition to selecting lens type, the user also chooses a fitting strategy such as flat, steep, or alignment to the cornea.

After the lens type is chosen and a fitting strategy is selected, the order form is displayed, which shows the recommended lens parameters. These recommendations are a good starting point. However, experienced users may choose to customize the lens design further. Choosing to customize a rigid gas permeable contact lens will display simulated fluorescein patterns and allow the user to see the effects of changing lens design on lens alignment to the corneal surface. After the final lens is chosen, the order form may be faxed or printed for ordering, and saved for future reordering.

8. What is the relationship between corneal topography and fluorescein patterns?

Fluorescein patterns are most directly related to elevation topography maps. The patterns visible on elevation maps are created by deviation of the shape of the cornea from a spherical reference surface. This corresponds with the thickness of the tear layer between the surface of the cornea and the posterior curvature of the contact lens. Fluorescein patterns beneath the contact lens are more directly related to elevation maps than curvature maps. Some examples follow.

Fluorescein Patterns in Astigmatism

In corneal astigmatism greater than 1.00 D, one observes a fluorescein pattern in the shape of a dumbbell. The thickness of the tear layer gradually increases near the edge in the steepest meridian. Fluorescein pooling is less along the flatter meridian, tear thickness diminishes near the periphery, and the contact lens is in contact with the cornea at the optical zone. A difference in the thickness of the tear layer along the two primary meridians can give some indication of the amount of corneal astigmatism. A dumbbell pattern of fluorescein becomes exaggerated as corneal toricity increases.

With-the-Rule Astigmatism

The curvature map (Color Plate 6) demonstrates a bow-tie shape with a symmetric pattern, and the elevation map (Color Plate 7) has a biscuit shape. Color Plate 8 demonstrates fluorescein pooling in the vertical meridian (the green areas) with alignment, or touch, in the horizontal meridian (dark areas).

Against-the-Rule Astigmatism

The curvature map in against-the-rule astigmatism (Color Plate 9) shows a horizantal bow-tie pattern. The contact lens fit would demonstrate pooled fluorescein in the horizontal meridian with alignment, or touch, in the vertical meridian.

Oblique Astigmatism

Oblique astigmatism may be represented by a dumbbell pattern at the 45° or 130° meridian with accumulation of fluorescein under the lens over the steeper meridian when the contact lens is fitted on the flattest K. Figure 6.3 A demonstrates an oblique dumbbell with alignment in the 130° and 310° meridian and an accumulation of fluorescein in the 30° and 210° meridian.

Topographic Analysis After Refractive Surgery

Topographic analysis is very helpful for contact lens fitting after refractive surgery. The central corneal curvature is often dramatically changed by treatment. This change in central corneal curvature can be measured by manual keratometry. However, most of contact lens bearing on the corneal surface occurs in the mid-periphery where relatively little change occurs. For this reason, central corneal curvature measurements do not provide the most useful measurements for contact lens fitting after corneal refractive surgery. Corneal topography provides important information about the shape of the peripheral cornea for successful contact lens fitting.

There are two common concerns when fitting contact lenses after corneal refractive surgery. First, the primary profile of the cornea has changed. After most forms of myopic corneal refractive surgery, the shape of the cornea is no longer prolate. Instead, the curvature of the cornea is flatter centrally and steeper peripherally. This shape is known as oblate asphericity (Fig. 1). Hyperopic corneal refractive surgery can exaggerate the natural prolate asphericity of the cornea. A second consideration is the outer boundary of the treatment zone after corneal refractive surgery. This boundary is often visible on videokeratography as a red ring. This junction between treated and untreated tissue is sometimes referred to as the "surgical knee" of the cornea. This boundary is often defined by an abrupt increase in curvature that can influence the fit and position of a contact lens.

Soft and rigid contact lenses are equally common after corneal refractive surgery. However, corneal surface irregularities caused by surgical complications are most often managed with rigid gas permeable (RGP) contact lenses. Curvature maps are most useful after corneal refractive surgery. Tangential curvature maps can provide important diagnostic information about surface irregularities including their location, exact dimensions, and severity. It is often possible to infer the impact that a corneal irregularity may have on vision from tangential curvature maps. Axial curvature maps are useful for describing the general shape of the cornea even after cornea refractive surgery. The central posterior curvature of a rigid contact lens is best selected from the axial curvature map. Initial lens curvature selected from the 5 mm diameter zone was a successful starting point for fitting RGP contact lenses after myopic excimer laser treatments.[8]

Post–Radial Keratotomy

Both the curvature maps (Color Plate 10) and the elevation map demonstrate an oblate cornea. Color Plate 11 shows the fluorescein pattern of an aspheric contact lens fit:

1. Apical pooling
2. Compression zone in the mid-periphery in four quadrants
3. Edge clearance adequate for this case

Post-LASIK

The curvature maps (Color Plate 12) demonstrate an oblate cornea, and Color Plate 13 demonstrates the fluorescein pattern of an aspheric contact lens fit:

1. Apical pooling
2. Compression in the mid-peripheral zone and discrete temporal decentralization, causing edge lift

In the Post-transplant Cornea

Topographic changes after corneal transplant are profound. There are several sources of distortion to corneal shape after penetrating keratoplasty:

1. Oversized graft
2. Uneven suture tension
3. Uneven donor bed
4. Differences in curvature between the donor and recipient tissues.

Apposition of a donor corneal button frequently alters the natural asphericity of the cornea, causing a "step" at the junction. This sloped surface can complicate the fitting of rigid contact lenses, depending on its location and severity. If the steepest area is inferior, it is best to fit the RGP lens with a flatter, superior cornea, permitting more vertical movement of the contact lens. As an alternative, one can try to avoid the inferior irregularity by decreasing overall lens diameter. If this is not successful, large-diameter RGP contact lenses can be used to bridge this irregular region. However, one must be careful not to let the lens bear too heavily on any one spot or to create inflammation with lens adherence. Steepening of the graft that is nasal or temporal can often cause lens dislocation accompanied by significant edge lift. Contact lens fitters should be cautious about excessive lens bearing that could lead to peripheral corneal neovascularization.

9. What is the importance of videokeratography in keratoconus?

Computed topography provides an excellent way to confirm the diagnosis of keratoconus, even when the disease does not present with the characteristic biomicroscopic signs.[9–13] Localization of the apex of the cone and progression of the disease can be visualized easily when the color maps are analyzed sequentially. The most useful videokeratography map for detection of keratoconus is the tangential curvature map. While there is no accepted standard for diagnosis of keratoconus by videokeratography alone, the following are the most common patterns associated with keratoconus:

1. Prominent central steepening greater than 50 D that is centrally symmetric
2. Asymmetric steepening that is greater inferiorly
3. Irregular bow-tie pattern of astigmatism that is often oblique

10. How is keratoconus diagnosed from videokeratography?

Indices for the Diagnosis of Keratoconus

In 1989 Dingeldein et al.[4] described the first quantitative index for corneal topography analysis. Prior to that time and even as recent as 1999, others suggested diagnostic classifications of corneal topography based on the recognition of color patterns or shapes from curvature maps.[14] In 1989, Rabinowitz and McDonnell[15] suggested several topographic criteria for the diagnosis of keratoconus:

1. Central curvature reading greater than 47 D
2. A difference of 3 D or more between two points situated 3 mm superior to and 3 mm inferior to the corneal center (I-S value)
3. An asymmetry between central keratometry of the two eyes greater than 1 D

These criteria were subsequently modified and designated as the Rabinowitz indices.[12,13] These indices suggest keratoconus if:

1. The Central K is greater than 47.2 D.
2. The I-S value is greater than 1.4 D.

These indices are diagnostic for keratoconus when:

1. The Central K reading is greater than 48.2 D.
2. The I-S value is greater than 1.6 D.

Simulated keratometry is an index that quantifies the central curvature; the I-S value quantifies the dioptric difference between the superior and inferior paracentral cornea that occurs in keratoconus.

Derivation of the KISA% Index

The KISA% index quantifies the topographic characteristics seen in patients with clinical keratoconus.[13] It is derived from the product of four indices: keratometry; I-S value; the AST index, which quantifies the degree of regular corneal astigmatism (simulated flat and steep keratometry values, Sim K1 and Sim K2); and SRAX, which is an expression of irregular astigmatism.

The KISA% index has demonstrated high sensitivity and specificity for the diagnosis of keratoconus. Between 60% and 100% of patients with a high KISA% index qualify as keratoconus suspects. This index is currently the most useful in classifying patients with keratoconus topographically among candidates being considered for refractive surgery.[13] These indices and the methods by which they are derived were described by Rabinowitz in 1995.[12]

Indices of Maeda and Klyce

The keratoconus-prediction index (KPI) is derived from eight other quantitative videokeratographic indices. The authors suggest that a value greater than 0.23 is indicative of keratoconus.[9]

Classification Scheme by Schwiegerling and Greivenkamp

Schwiegerling and Greivenkamp[16] described a keratoconus classification scheme based on Zernike polynomial coefficients that could be used with any topography instrument and compared this method with several of the methods described above. Their results showed good classification accuracy based on features that represented inferior steepening and asymmetry. This method has not been adopted by instrument manufacturers; however, we mention this novel approach because we are likely to see other similar methods in the future.

The Dicon CT-200

The Dicon CT-200 has a peak detection algorithm that locates areas of corneal steepening relative to peripheral curvature readings. This feature provides the location, maximum detected power, size of the steeper region, as well as an index related to a proprietary severity scale.

11. What is the topographic pattern most commonly encountered in patients with contact lens–induced corneal distortion?

The most frequent topographic pattern demonstrates flattening adjacent to the point at which the decentralized contact lens rests against the cornea: flattening the superior meridian and increasing inferior curvature, which can be confused with some types of keratoconus. In brief, it is possible to distinguish this from early keratoconus by considering corneal thickness, posterior corneal curvature (obtained by Orbscan™), stability of corneal curvature after removal of contact lenses, and normalization of shape over time.[17,18] Studies of the topographic characteristics of contact lens–induced corneal deformity in an eye with a superiorly displaced rigid contact lens demonstrated four patterns:[18–20]

1. Irregular central pattern.
2. Increase of the peripheral curve on the side opposite the decentralized contact lens.
3. Arcuate flattening at the margin of the contact lens.
4. Flattening in the superior region adjacent to the corneal lens touch with increased inferior curvature, which is the most commonly encountered.

12. How can one differentiate between contact lens–induced abnormalities of corneal curvature and true ectasia?

Suspected cases can be evaluated and clarified by the use of elevation maps. Consistent with the study of Lebow and Grohe,[17] corneal distortion can be differentiated from ectasia by analyzing three geometric corneal indices:

1. Shape factor (SF)—related to the aspheric shape of the cornea
2. Irregularity (CIM)—measurement of corneal irregularity
3. Apical toricity (TKM)—measure of central corneal astigmatism

In this study, eyes with true keratoconus in relationship to those with contact lens–induced distortion presented as follows:

1. The shape factor was greater and more variable.
2. CIM was greater and more variable.
3. Apical toricity: The flatter Keratometric reading was steeper with major variations in axial curvature and maximal variations in the tangential areas.
4. Major corneal toricity and greater variability.
5. Steeper reference spheres.
6. Maximal elevation greater and steeper than the reference spheres.

   In the elevation maps, which demonstrate the posterior corneal curve, it is easier to make this differential diagnosis because keratoconus also induces changes in the posterior corneal surface, while contact lens–induced deformation in the cornea begins with the anterior surface and rarely alters the posterior surface.

   In the changes induced by contact lenses, the axial map may demonstrate an asymmetric pattern, but the pachymetry should be regular and symmetrical with a normal corneal thickness. In keratoconus, the pattern is both asymmetrical and eccentric, demonstrating steep curves greater than 48 D. In the pachometry map, the thinnest point is generally eccentric and localized inferotemporally. The pachometry demonstrates a thickness of less than 540 μm. Besides this, in the biomicroscopic examination, one may not see corneal distortion and the typical signs of keratoconus such as corneal thinning, a Fleischer ring, Vogt's striae, and apical scarring. The pachometry map is an important tool for the evaluation of cases with possible corneal ectasia or considering refractive surgery. Risk factors include a thinnest point less than 500 μm that is eccentrically located and not coincident with the corneal apex.[19–23]

References

1. Carney, Mainstone, Henderson. Corneal topography and myopia. A cross-sectional study. *Invest Ophthalmol Vis Sci.* 1997;38:311–320.
2. Kiely, Smith, Carney. The mean shape of the human cornea *Opt Acta.* 1982; 28:1027–1040.
3. Mandell. *Contact Lens Practice.* Springfield, IL: Charles C. Thomas, 1988.
4. Dingeldein, Klyce, Wilson. Quantitative descriptors of corneal shape derived from computer-assisted analysis of photokeratographs. *Refract Corneal Surg.* 1989;5:372–378.
5. Reynolds. Corneal topography as found by photo-electric keratoscopy. *Contacto.* 1959;3:229–233.
6. Buratto. *Corneal Topography: The Clinical Atlas.* NJ: Slack, 1996.
7. Bufidis, Konstas, Mamtziou. The role of computerized corneal topography in rigid gas permeable contact lens fitting. *CLAO J.* 1998;24:206–209.
8. Jani, Szczotka. Efficiency and accuracy of two computerized topography software systems for fitting rigid gas permeable contact lenses. *CLAO J.* 2000;26:91–96.
9. Maeda, Klyce, Smolek, Thompson. Automated keratoconus screening with corneal topography analysis. *Invest Ophthalmol Vis Sci.* 1994;35:2749–2757.
10. Maguire, Bourne. Corneal topography of early keratoconus. *Am J Ophthalmol.* 1989;108:107–112.
11. McMahon, Robin, Scarpulla, Putz. The spectrum of topography found in keratoconus. *CLAO J.* 1991;17:198–204.
12. Rabinowitz. Videokeratographic indices to aid in screening for keratoconus. *J Refract Surg.* 1995;11:371–379.
13. Rabinowitz, Rasheed. KISA% index: a quantitative videokeratography algorithm embodying minimal topographic criteria for diagnosing keratoconus *J Cataract Refract Surg.* 1999;25:1327–1335.
14. Karabatsas, Cook, Sparrow. Proposed classification for topographic patterns seen after penetrating keratoplasty *Br J Ophthalmol.* 1999;83:403–409.
15. Rabinowitz, McDonnell. Computer-assisted corneal topography in keratoconus. *Refract Corneal Surg.* 1989;5:400–408.
16. Schwiegerling, Greivenkamp. Keratoconus detection based on videokeratoscopic height data. *Optom Vis Sci.* 1996;73:721–728.
17. Lebow, Grohe. Differentiating contact lens induced warpage from true keratoconus using corneal topography. *CLAO J.* 1999;25:114–122.
18. Novo, Pavlopoulos, Feldman. Corneal topographic changes after refitting polymethylmethacrylate contact lens wearers into rigid gas permeable materials. *CLAO J.* 1995;21:47–51.
19. Maeda, Klyce, Hamano. Alteration of corneal asphericity in rigid gas permeable contact lens induced warpage. *CLAO J.* 1994;20:27–31.

20. Wilson, Lin, Klyce, Reidy, Insler. Topographic changes in contact lens–induced corneal warpage. *Ophthalmology.* 1990;97:734–744.
21. Amoils, Deist, Gous, Amoils. Iatrogenic keratectasia after laser in situ keratomileusis for less than −4.0 to −7.0 diopters of myopia. *J Cataract Refract Surg.* 2000;26:967–977.
22. Pallikaris, Kymionis, Astyrakakis. Corneal ectasia induced by laser in situ keratomileusis. *J Cataract Refract Surg.* 2001;27:1796–1802.
23. Vinciguerra, Camesasca. Prevention of corneal ectasia in laser in situ keratomileusis. *J Refract Surg.* 2001;17(2 suppl):S187–189.

7

How to Fit Rigid Spherical Contact Lenses

Peter Bergenske and Saly Moreira

1. What are the principal characteristics of the polymers used in rigid contact lenses?

Polymethylmethacrylate (PMMA) is the material from which rigid corneal contact lenses were made for the first several decades of modern contact lens practice. It is a relatively stable polymer that is easily molded and machined. The contact lens made of PMMA generally had excellent optics, was durable, easy to maintain, and relatively inexpensive. Its primary disadvantage was a lack of gas permeability. Modern rigid lenses are made of gas permeable polymers. Their permeability to gases is primarily a function of the quantity of silicone and fluorine contained in the molecules.

2. How does one express the terms "permeability to gases" and "oxygen transmissibility"?

Gas permeability (P) is a property of certain polymers expressed as the product of the coefficient of diffusion (D) and the coefficient of solubility (k).

$$P = Dk$$

Oxygen transmissibility (t) is the quantity of oxygen that passes across a specific contact lens and depends on the Dk value of the polymer and is inversely proportional to the thickness (L) of the lens:

$$t = \frac{Dk}{L}$$

3. What parameters should be specified in prescribing a spherical rigid contact lens?

1. Contact lens type (material, design)
2. Base curve (BC) = the central posterior curve

3. Power
4. Total diameter

Other parameters such as optic zone diameter, peripheral curve(s), and center thickness may be specified by the fitter; however, they are generally determined by standards used by the laboratories that make the contact lenses.

4. What is the general fitting philosophy for rigid contact lenses?

Using the keratometry of the flatter meridian of the cornea (K) as a reference point, fitting can be chosen to be either equal to K, flatter than K, or steeper than K. Depending on the lens–cornea relationship, the fitting can result in:

1. Apical alignment
2. Apical touch
3. Apical clearance

Generally, the goal is to achieve a lens–cornea relationship that causes the lens to bear lightly in the mid-periphery (3 to 4 mm from center) of the horizontal meridian of the cornea and allows the lens to move in the vertical meridian.

5. What anatomic factors are taken into consideration in choosing the most appropriate method for contact lens fitting?

The position of the lids and the axis, the amount of corneal astigmatism, and the corneal diameter are of considerable importance in choosing a fitting method. When the superior lid covers the superior portion of the cornea (a narrow palpebral fissure), one should aim to fit the lens so that it parallels the central cornea and remains in a slightly superior, "lid attachment" position. When the superior lid covers only the superior corneal limbus or remains above it, a more centered, "interpalpebral" fit may be necessary (employing a contact lens with a curvature somewhat steeper than K and with a smaller diameter). In the presence of mild or moderate with-the-rule astigmatism, lenses fitted slightly steeper than flat K normally provide a desirable fitting relationship. (See section on base curve selection that follows.) When the corneal astigmatism is against-the-rule, fitting on alignment with the horizontal meridian is often not satisfactory. In such cases, one may try an interpalpebral fit, a lens with an aspheric posterior surface, or, alternatively, a toric base curve lens.

6. How does one select a trial rigid contact lens?

It is often helpful to place a trial contact lens on the eye to aid in determination of an optimal fit. The trial contact lens should be, if possible, of the same material as the lens to be prescribed, although this is not absolutely necessary.

Parameters

Diameter (D)

The first parameter that needs to be determined is the diameter of the contact lens. Selection of the diameter of the contact lens is based on the diameters of the visible iris and the pupil as well as the corneal curvature. The choice of the diameter should be made after measurement of the horizontal visble iris diameter (HVID), which can be classified as small, medium, or large (Table 7.1). As a general rule, lens diameter is chosen to be approximately 2.5 mm smaller than HVID.

In general, rigid gas permeable contact lenses are fitted with diameters between 8.8 and 9.8 mm with an optical zone of 7.4 to 8.4 mm. Larger diameters may be chosen to provide a larger optical zone for large pupil diameter. The optical zone is typically 1.0 to 1.4 mm smaller than the overall diameter.

Base curve (BC)

The base curve is the radius of curvature of the central area of the posterior surface of the contact lens. The first trial lens's base curve is generally on K or slightly steeper than K, depending on the degree of astigmatism present and the diameter of the lens. Some professionals prefer to choose a base curve for the first trial lens, using the average K; that is, half the difference between the measurements of the two principal meridians of the cornea added to the flat K. (A nomogram for choosing base curve using diameter and astigmatism as variables follows; see question 10.)

A criterion commonly used in the course of trial fitting contact lenses is evaluation of the contact lens movement on the cornea. At the slit lamp, one should examine the position of the contact lens on the cornea as well as its movement. The evaluation criteria depend on one's experience with fitting and observation of the lenses. A contact lens of appropriate diameter should not cross the limbus, nor should it reach the inferior pupillary margin with blinking.

Power

The dioptric power of the primary trial contact lens is ideally close to the spherical component of the minus cylinder form of the manifest refraction.

Table 7.1. Examples of determination of diameter of a rigid gas permeable contact lens

	Small	Medium	Large
Horizontal visible iris	11.00	11.50	12.00
Contact lens diameter (mm)	8.5	9.0	9.5
D = HVID − 2.5			

7. What is the relationship between base curve and diameter of the contact lens?

Changes in contact lens diameter may alter the choice of radius of the base curve. Increasing the diameter without altering the base curve increases the sagittal depth, effectively steepening the fit. Reducing the diameter of the contact lens without changing the radius of curvature alters the sagittal depth so that the contact lens fit is flatter. To maintain the same sagittal depth, the radius of curvature must be increased (made flatter) as the diameter is increased. For every modification of 0.2 mm in diameter, the radius of the base curve is altered by 0.125 D or 0.023 mm.

8. How does one calculate the power of rigid contact lenses?

The prescription of rigid contact lens power can be made after refraction and keratometry alone, although the ideal method is to make this calculation after overrefraction of a known and well-fitting trial lens. In prescribing the power, one needs to take into consideration the "tear lens" formed between the cornea and the posterior surface of the rigid contact lens. The power of the "tear," or lacrimal, lens is the difference between the base curve of the contact lens (in diopters "K") and the keratometric reading of the flatter meridian of the cornea. When the refraction is greater than ±4 D, the vertex distance must also be taken into consideration.

Power Determination

It is possible to predict the expected power of the final lens based on the refraction in minus cylinder form and on the keratometric readings. The cylindrical component of the manifest refraction is optically eliminated by the lacrimal lens. The spherical component represents the dioptric power of the flatter meridian of the cornea. When the lens is fit with the base curve "on K," the lacrimal lens power is plano and the power of the lens should be the same as the vertex-corrected spherical component of the refraction in minus cylinder form. When the contact lens is fitted with a base curve steeper than K, a lacrimal lens with a positive dioptric power is formed. To compensate for this added plus power, an equal amount of minus should be added to the spherical power of the spectacle refraction when converting to a contact lens power.

Example

Base curve steeper than the flatter K with a minus refraction.

Manifest refraction	= $-3.00 - 1.00 \times 180°$
Keratometry	= 43.00×44.00 diopters

Base curve	=	43.50 (0.50 diopters steeper than K − the tear lens has a positive power, so −0.50 is added to the sphere of the spectacle power)
Final power of the contact lens	=	−3.00 −0.50 = −3.50 diopters

Example

Base curve steeper than the flatter keratometric meridian in a plus refraction.

Manifest refraction	=	+3.00 −1.00 × 180°
Keratometry	=	43.00 × 44.00 diopters
Base curve	=	43.50 (0.50 diopters steeper than K − the tear lens has a plus power, so again, −0.50 is added to the sphere of the refraction)
Final power of the contact lens	=	+3.00 diopters −0.50 diopters = +2.50 diopters

When the contact lens is fitted flatter than K, a tear lens of minus power is formed, and therefore plus power is added to the spherical component of the spectacle refraction.

Example

Base curve flatter than K in a minus refraction.

Manifest refraction	=	−3.00 −0.75 × 180°
Keratometry	=	43.00 × 43.75 diopters
Base curve	=	42.50 (0.50 D flatter than K)
Final contact lens power	=	−3.00 + 0.50 = 2.50 diopters

Example

Base curve flatter than K in a plus refraction.

Spectacle refraction	=	+3.00 −0.75 × 180°
Keratometry	=	43.00 × 43.75 D
Base curve	=	42.50 (0.50 D flatter than K)
Final contact lens power	=	+3.00 +0.50 = +3.50 diopters

Power Determination by Overrefracting a Trial Lens

When a trial lens is evaluated on the eye, one should perform an over-refraction to aid in prescribing the final lens power. If the base curve of the prescribed lens is the same as that of the trial lens, the final power is the sum of the trial lens power and the overrefraction. If the base curve ordered is steeper or flatter than that of the trial lens, the lacrimal lens effect should be accounted for as in the preceding examples. An advantage of this method is that it is independent of the accuracy of the manifest refraction and keratometry reading. It is of particular value when refraction and keratometry readings are difficult or suspect, as with an irregular cornea.

Example:

Trial lens parameters: D 9.2/B.C. 43.00/power	− 3.00
Overrefraction:	+ 1.50
Power prescribed (BC 43.00):	− 1.50

9. What is the vertex distance?

This is the distance between the corneal apex and the center of the correcting spectacle lens, typically 12 mm. It is necessary to compensate for vertex distance when the refraction is greater than ±4.00 D. For powers less than 4.00 D the effect is minimal and can be ignored. In practice, one uses tables to compensate for vertex distance in the power determination. Vertex correction means that contact lens powers are greater than spectacle powers for plus refractions and less than spectacle powers for minus refractions.

Example

Compensating for vertex distance in a high plus contact lens fitted on K:

Spectacle prescription	=	$+13.00 - 2.00 \times 090°$
Keratometry	=	41.75×44.00
Base curve	=	41.75 (on K, so no lacrimal lens effect)
Adjustment for vertex distance		+ 13.00 at 12 mm is equivalent to + 15.50 at the corneal plane
Final contact lens power	=	15.50 diopters with a diameter of 9.7 mm

10. What is the nomogram for choice of a base curve for rigid gas permeable contact lenses?

The nomogram is shown in Table 7.2.

Table 7.2. Nomogram for determination of base curve for rigid gas permeable contact lenses

Corneal cylinder	8.5-mm diameter	9.0-mm diameter	9.5-mm diameter
0.00 to 0.50 D	0.25 D STK	On K	0.25D FTK
0.75 to 1.25 D	0.50 D STK	0.25 D STK	On K
1.50 to 2.00 D	0.75 D STK	0.50 D STK	0.25 D STK
2.25 to 2.75 D	1.00 D STK	0.75 D STK	0.50 STK
3.00 to 3.50 D (note sphere not likely, may need toric base curve)	1.25 STK	1.00 STK	0.75 STK

STK = steeper than K.
FTK = flatter than K.

11. How does one proceed with evaluation of the trial lens?

A trial contact lens is selected based on the parameters closest to the theoretical calculations of diameter, base curve, and power as described in the preceding sections. Once the patient has adapted to the presence of the lens and there is no further tearing, the fitting can proceed. For patients new to rigid lenses, it may be helpful to first instill a drop of topical anesthetic. The lens should be reasonably comfortable and have appropriate movement to determine the dioptric power adequately. A spherical overrefraction is performed. Fluorescein dye is placed on the eye. At the slit lamp, one should observe:

1. The contact lens position, its mobility during blinking, its location in relationship to the corneal apex, and the fluorescein pattern, both static and dynamic.
2. With rigid contact lenses on K or slightly steeper, the tear film should be uniform with light central pooling and mid-peripheral touch along the horizontal meridian.
3. When there is with-the-rule astigmatism, the tear film should demonstrate fluorescein in the central optical zone with a decrease in the intermediate zone and an increase in the periphery along the horizontal meridian, and greater pooling of fluorescein along the steeper, vertical meridian.
4. In a tight or very steep contact lens, there is concentration of fluorescein in the tear film in the central zone (apical clearance) and absence or minimal fluorescein accumulation in the periphery. A lens that is too steep will not move properly along the vertical meridian.
5. In a loose or flat contact lens, there is an absence of fluorescein pooling at the apex (apical touch) and excessive pooling of fluorescein in the intermediate and peripheral zones.

12. How does one accomplish the final fitting of a trial rigid contact lens?

After placement of the rigid gas permeable contact lens and the cessation of tearing, one evaluates with fluorescein the position of the lens and the lens–cornea relationship.

Position

The position of the contact lens is considered ideal when the border of the contact lens is at or near the superior limbus and is secured by the upper lid throughout the blinking cycle. The most desirable rigid gas permeable contact lens fit is slightly superior or central without excessive movement induced by the lid.

Movement

The contact lens should have unrestricted veritcal movement with the blink. When movement is minimal, the contact lens interferes with the lacrimal exchange. When the movement is excessive, it may produce discomfort and interfere with vision.

Visual Quality

The vision should be sharp and stable. With overrefraction, one can arrive at the final refraction. The power of the overrefraction is added to the power of the diagnostic lens. One needs to compensate for the vertex distance only if the overrefraction is greater than ±4.00 D.

Evaluation of the Fluorescein Pattern

For rigid contact lenses, the ideal fluorescein pattern should demonstrate a uniform lacrimal film or at least slight central clearance with touch in the mid-periphery of the horizontal meridian. Because many polymers contain an ultraviolet filter it is helpful use a yellow (Wratten or Tiffen) filter designed to enhance viewing of fluorescein patterns.

13. What is the suggested trial set for rigid gas permeable lenses?

It is useful to have a variety of trial contact lenses for the correction of myopia, hyperopia, aphakia, and keratoconus. To achieve the greatest success in fitting, it is helpful to have available contact lens trial sets of different diameters, for example, diameters of 9.2, 9.6, and 9.8 mm. There are many commercially available trial lens sets. It is of greatest value to have trial lenses manufactured by the same laboratory that will be providing the prescribed lenses. Tables 7.3, 7.4, 7.5, and 7.6 are examples of trial sets. Significant confusion and error can occur if trial sets are not carefully maintained. The fitter should routinely verify that trial lenses used in prescribing are correctly labeled.

14. Is trial fitting necessary?

Trial fitting can improve chances of "first fit" success; however, it is time-consuming and dependent on the availability of trial lenses close to correct parameters. In cases of warped or irregular corneas, where keratometry and refraction data are spurious, trial lens fitting may be the only means of determining a lens prescription. For eyes with regular astigmatism and stable refractions, empirical ordering of lenses can be successful, particularly if topography is employed to determine overall corneal shape. An advantage of empirical fitting is that the first lens the patient experiences is one that should fit well and have proper

Table 7.3. Trial set of 50 lenses

Number	Diopters	Radius	Power	Diameter	Number	Diopter	Radius	Power	Diameter
01	40.00	8.44	−2.00	8.9	26	46.25	7.30	−3.00	8.6
02	40.25	8.36	−2.00	8.9	27	46.50	7.26	−3.00	8.6
03	40.50	8.33	−2.00	8.9	28	46.75	7.22	−3.00	8.6
04	40.75	8.28	−2.00	8.9	29	47.00	7.18	−3.00	8.6
05	41.00	8.23	−2.00	8.9	30	47.50	7.10	−3.00	8.5
06	41.25	8.18	−2.00	8.9	31	48.00	7.03	−5.00	8.5
07	41.50	8.13	−2.00	8.8	32	48.50	6.96	−5.00	8.5
08	41.75	8.08	−2.00	8.8	33	49.00	6.89	−5.00	8.5
09	42.00	8.03	−2.00	8.8	34	50.00	6.75	−5.00	8.5
10	42.25	7.99	−2.00	8.8	35	51.00	6.62	−5.00	8.5
11	42.50	7.94	−2.00	8.8	36	52.00	6.49	−5.00	8.5
12	42.75	7.89	−2.00	8.6	37	53.00	6.37	−5.00	8.4
13	43.00	7.85	−2.00	8.6	38	54.00	6.25	−5.00	8.4
14	43.25	7.80	−2.00	8.6	39	55.00	6.13	−5.00	8.4
15	43.50	7.76	−2.00	8.6	40	56.00	6.03	−5.00	8.4
16	43.75	7.71	−2.00	8.6	41	41.00	8.23	−12.0	9.0
17	44.00	7.67	−2.00	8.6	42	42.00	8.04	−12.0	9.0
18	44.25	7.63	−2.00	8.6	43	43.00	7.85	−12.0	9.0
19	44.50	7.58	−2.00	8.6	44	44.00	7.67	−12.0	9.0
20	44.75	7.54	−2.00	8.6	45	45.00	7.50	−12.0	9.0
21	45.00	7.50	−2.00	8.6	46	41.00	8.23	+12.0	9.0
22	45.25	7.46	−2.00	8.6	47	42.00	8.04	+12.0	9.0
23	45.50	7.42	−2.00	8.6	48	43.00	7.85	+12.0	9.0
24	45.75	7.38	−2.00	8.6	49	44.00	7.67	+12.0	9.0
25	46.00	7.33	−2.00	8.6	50	45.00	7.50	+12.0	9.0

Table 7.4. Trial set for spherical rigid gas permeable contact lenses for myopia with a diameter of 9.2 mm

Number	Diopters	Radius of curvature	Power	Diameter
01	40.00	8.44	−3.00	9.2
02	40.50	8.33	−3.00	9.2
03	41.00	8.23	−3.00	9.2
04	41.50	8.13	−3.00	9.2
05	42.00	8.04	−3.00	9.2
06	42.50	7.94	−3.00	9.2
07	43.00	7.86	−3.00	9.2
08	43.50	7.76	−3.00	9.2
09	44.00	7.67	−3.00	9.2
10	44.50	7.58	−3.00	9.2
11	45.00	7.50	−3.00	9.2
12	45.50	7.42	−3.00	9.2
13	46.00	7.43	−3.00	9.2
14	46.50	7.26	−3.00	9.2
15	47.00	7.18	−3.00	9.2

Table 7.5. Trial contact lens set for spherical rigid gas permeable contact lenses for myopia with a diameter of 9.6 mm

Number	Diopters	Radius of curvature	Power	Diameter
01	40.00	8.44	−2.00	9.6
02	40.50	8.33	−2.00	9.6
03	41.00	8.23	−2.00	9.6
04	41.50	8.13	−2.00	9.6
05	41.75	8.08	−2.00	9.6
06	42.00	8.04	−2.00	9.6
07	42.25	7.99	−2.00	9.6
08	42.50	7.94	−2.00	9.6
09	42.75	7.90	−2.00	9.6
10	43.00	7.85	−2.00	9.6
11	43.25	7.85	−2.00	9.6
12	43.50	7.76	−2.00	9.6
13	43.75	7.71	−2.00	9.6
14	44.00	7.67	−2.00	9.6
15	44.25	7.63	−2.00	9.6
16	44.25	7.58	−2.00	9.6
17	44.75	7.54	−2.00	9.6
18	45.00	7.50	−2.00	9.6

Table 7.6. Trial contact lens set for spherical rigid gas permeable contact lenses for hyperopia

Number	Diopters	Radius of curvature	Power	Diameter
01	40.00	8.44	+3.00	9.2
02	40.50	8.33	+3.00	9.2
03	41.00	8.23	+3.00	9.2
04	41.50	8.13	+3.00	9.2
05	42.00	8.04	+3.00	9.2
06	42.50	7.94	+3.00	9.2
07	43.00	7.85	+3.00	9.2
08	43.50	7.76	+3.00	9.2
09	44.00	7.67	+3.00	9.2
10	44.50	7.58	+3.00	9.2
11	45.00	7.50	+3.00	9.2
12	45.50	7.42	+3.00	9.2
13	46.00	7.34	+3.00	9.2

optical power. Potential confusion caused by mislabeled trial lenses is avoided. In addition, significant chair time can be saved using the empirical method.

Selected Readings

Campbell RC, Connelly S. Rigid gas-permeable contact lens fitting. In: Kast PR, ed. *The CLAO Guide to Basic Science and Clinical Practice.* IA: Kendall/Hunt, 1995:11–49.

Fletcher LJ, Lupelli L, Rossi AL. *Contact Lens Practice.* Oxford: Blackwell Scientific, 1994:1772.

Girard LJ, Soper JW, Sampson WG. Follow up visits. In: Girard LJ, ed. *Corneal Contact Lenses.* St. Louis: CV Mosby, 1970:229–268.

Gordon JM, Hanish SJ. Fitting techniques for gas-permeable rigid lenses. In: Aquavella JV, Rao GN, ed. *Contact Lenses.* Philadelphia: JB Lippincott, 1987: 39–46.

Hales RH. *Contact Lenses, a Clinical Approach to Fitting.* Baltimore: Williams & Wilkins, 1982:351.

Stein HA, Freeman MI, Stein RM. *The CLAO Residents' Contact Lens Curriculum Manual.* Kellner/McCaffery Associates, 15 Fifth Avenue, New York: 1996: 72–86.

Stein HA, Slatt BJ. *Fitting Guide for Rigid and Soft Contact Lenses,* 3 rd ed. St. Louis: CV Mosby, 1990.

8

Follow-Up After Fitting Rigid Gas Permeable Lenses

Cleusa Coral-Ghanem and Lisa Badowski

The most important factor for successful long-term contact lens use is careful attention to the patient after the initial contact lens fit. The eye care professional must clearly indicate to the patient what symptoms might dictate the need for return visits that may result in modification or changing of the lens. By the same token, follow-up is important to verify lens hygiene, to look for toxic or allergic reactions to chemical products in lens care solutions, and to examine the cornea for physiologic changes that may decrease a patient's comfort or wearing time.

1. How often should follow-up visits for rigid gas permeable lens patients be scheduled?

Follow-up of the contact lens patient actually begins with the contact lens dispensing visit. The dispensing visit is usually scheduled about 1 or 2 weeks after the initial examination/fitting to allow sufficient time for the finishing laboratory to fabricate the ordered contact lens. Following contact lens dispensing, a short-term visit at about 1 to 2 weeks should be scheduled. At this visit, the patient's adaptation to the new lenses and compliance with instructions are monitored. Changes to lens fit or power may also be made at this time, if indicated. If any changes are made to the contact lens fit or power, then another short-term dispensing/follow-up visit should be scheduled. A medium-term visit should then be scheduled 1 to 3 months later. At this point, the patient should be fairly well adapted to the lenses and should be monitored for any physiologic changes secondary to the contact lens wear. After the patient is deemed a successful contact lens wearer, the patient should then be seen for long-term follow-up visits at intervals of 6 to 12 months.

2. What clinical tests should be done at a follow-up visit?

There are three primary goals at dispensing/follow-up visits:

1. Evaluating contact lens performance
2. Evaluating ocular physiology
3. Educating the patient

First, one should establish that the newly dispensed lens performs in the same manner as predicted by the diagnostic lens at the fitting visit. In subsequent follow-up visits, the lens should continue to perform in the same manner and meet the patient's visual needs. Appropriate tasks to achieve this goal include (but are not limited to) taking a case history, testing visual acuity with the contact lens at the appropriate distances to establish the patient's functional performance, testing the overrefraction to confirm the contact lens power, doing a slit-lamp evaluation of the lens fit with fluorescein, and evaluating the contact lens surface. The case history should include questions about the patient's subjective evaluation of vision and comfort, average wearing time of the contact lenses, and lens care routine.

The ocular physiology evaluation includes a detailed anterior segment slit-lamp biomicroscopic examination that includes fluorescein staining of the cornea and evaluation of the tarsal conjunctiva with lid eversion. A yellow Kodak Wratten No. 12 or yellow No. 2 camera filter over the objective of the slit-lamp biomicroscope enhances the fluorescence of the fluorescein stain when evaluating rigid gas permeable lens fits or corneal staining. Corneal topography, keratometry, or refraction may be reevaluated if corneal distortion is suspected.

Patient education is an ongoing process. New patients need to understand the initial instructions that were provided. Misunderstandings can often be corrected at early follow-up visits. Established patients can become complacent and start to omit steps essential to proper lens care or otherwise misuse their lenses. The importance of maintaining the prescribed contact lens wearing schedule and following the prescribed lens care routine needs to be reinforced at every patient encounter to ensure patient compliance.

3. What are the common symptoms after rigid gas permeable contact lens fitting?

1. Sensation of "wet" eyes with increased tearing
2. Photophobia
3. Mild lid irritation
4. Incomplete blink (to decrease awareness from the edge of the lens against the lid)
5. Excessive blinking
6. Difficulty with upgaze
7. Intermittent visual blurring

4. What problems are most commonly encountered after initiating contact lens wear?

Visual Symptoms

Verify Contact Lens Parameters

Regardless of how careful the fitter is, mistakes can occur, both in the specifications of the lens as well as its ordering/manufacture. There can be an inadvertent use of an incorrect lens from the trial set or errors in power determination and/or other parameters.

Relatively simple instruments are used to verify rigid gas permeable lenses:[1]

1. The radiuscope is used to verify base curve.
2. Lensometry with a specially designed stage for a rigid gas permeable lens is used to measure the dioptric power of the contact lens and to detect any problems with the optical quality of the lens.
3. A millimeter rule or a 7× to 10× hand-held magnifier with a millimeter scale is used to verify the diameter and observe the blend between the base and peripheral curves.
4. A stereomicroscope, slit-lamp biomicroscope, radiuscope, or a hand-held magnifier is used to verify the optical quality of the surface and edge of the rigid gas permeable lens.
5. A lens thickness gauge is used to measure central thickness of the lens. Upon receipt of the lenses, their measurement should be verified and then labeled with the patient's name to avoid the inadvertent switching of contact lenses. Prior to dispensing the final contact lens, overrefraction and evaluation of the lens–cornea fitting relationship with the slit-lamp biomicroscope should be performed.

Diameter of the Optical Zone

A small optical zone, especially in dim illumination, may provoke glare and difficulty with vision. This complaint is most commonly encountered with night driving because of the light reflections from oncoming cars. This symptom is also commonly known as "flare."

Decentration of the Contact Lens

Lens decentration may induce symptoms similar to a small optical zone, as mentioned above. The same complaints are sometimes found in aphakic patients with a sector iridectomy who are fitted with a lenticular contact lens that has a small lenticular zone. One might also encounter other problems, including corneal drying,[2] corneal distortion,[3] a poor contact lens-cornea fitting relationship, and other visual symptoms.

Reversed Contact Lenses

Contact lenses inadvertently placed in the wrong eye can produce visual symptoms, corneal changes, and other symptoms associated with a poorly fitting contact lens. The inadvertent placement of lenses in the wrong eye can be minimized using different-colored lenses in each eye or by marking the right lens with a black dot.

Flexure

On-eye flexure of the contact lens can be the result of pressure from the upper lids during blinking or can occur on a toric cornea as a result of a steep contact lens fit, a contact lens with a very thin central thickness, a lens with a very large optical zone, or a contact lens material that is very flexible.[4-6] Flexure can be diagnosed by performing keratometry over the contact lens on the patient's eye, which measures toricity, even though the contact lens is spherical.

Hydrophobic Contact Lens

Poor surface wettability of a rigid gas permeable lens can be either acquired over time or present initially on a newly dispensed lens. Acquired problems may be the result of alterations in the tear film, contamination by cosmetics or lotions, the use of solutions that are not compatible with the material, or the development of surface scratches or deposits. Initial wettability issues may be the result of manufacturing debris/residue, skin oils from lens handling, or improper polishing during manufacture.[7] Regardless of cause, a poorly wetting lens may produce both discomfort and foggy or hazy vision.[6,7] Identifying the specific cause and then addressing it best solves acquired problems. A change in the care and handling routine may help prevent recurrences. To decrease initial wettability problems, a new contact lens should be cleaned with a laboratory cleaner after all verification is completed to remove debris or residue and skin oils. It should also be soaked in an appropriate rigid lens wetting/soaking solution for at least 24 hours prior to dispensing.[7]

Incomplete Blinking

Decreased or incomplete blinking, particularly during concentrated work such as computer use or prolonged near tasks may produce drying of the ocular surface and the cornea, causing blurred vision and symptoms of discomfort. Lubricating drops helps alleviate these symptoms. The patient should also be instructed to take frequent visual breaks and to be conscious of blinking regularly and completely.

Difficulty Reading

When a patient with moderate or high myopia converts from spectacles to contact lenses, he or she no longer has the base-down prism that is normally induced with down gaze through a spectacle lens. For this reason, more effort is required for accommodation and convergence. In young patients, this problem becomes insignificant after a few hours of wear. However, the presbyopic patient requires a reading prescription or bifocal contact lens design to improve reading comfort. The borderline presbyope may find that he or she has more difficulty with near tasks while wearing the contact lenses than with spectacles.

Complaints of Discomfort

Contact Lens Shape

The overall shape of the contact lens is determined by the relationship between the edge and center thicknesses and can greatly influence how the lens centers on the eye and interacts with the upper lid. All plus powered contact lenses have a plus shape so that the center thickness is greater than the edge thickness. Moderate and high minus lenses (approximately greater than -4.00 D) have a minus shape, so that the edge thickness is greater than the center thickness. Unlike spectacle lenses, contact lenses have peripheral curves cut on the posterior lens surface, which results in a reduced edge thickness.[8] This leads to a lens shape anomaly in that low minus contact lenses actually have an edge thickness that is less then the center thickness, resulting in a plus shape.

Plus shaped lenses are problematic and can ride low on the cornea. Their general shape creates a lens with an anteriorly displaced center of gravity and a thick center that leads to a high overall mass.[9] This shape lends itself to be squeezed out from under the lids due the "watermelon seed effect." The use of a lenticular carrier design in any plus shaped lens decreases the center thickness and overall mass, moves the center of gravity posteriorly, and decreases the "watermelon seed" shape, resulting in a lens with much improved vertical centration on the cornea.

Contact Lens Decentration

Lateral decentration generally results from against-the-rule astigmatism, a decentered corneal apex, or a flat base curve. Superior decentration may occur when there is flattening of the superior cornea, tight lids, a very flat base curve, excessive edge lift, or a thick edge. Inferior decentration most often results from a steep base curve, incomplete blinking, loose lids, increased mass due to high specific gravity materials,[10] corneal surface irregularities, or from nonlenticulated, plus shaped lenses.

Edges

The edge of the lens should be smooth, thin, and tapered from the front.[11] In a contact lens with moderate to high negative power, a front taper or lenticular curve (myodisk) may be necessary to decrease the edge thickness. This will improve lens comfort and reduce lid interaction with the thick edge.[12] To avoid chipping the lens edge, for example from dropping the lens on a rigid surface, it is advisable to moisten the tip of the finger with a drop of wetting solution. Another recommendation to avoid edge chipping is to assure that the lens is in the center of the case prior to closing the cap.

Lens Thickness

A thick contact lens tends to decenter inferiorly. When prescribing low minus and low plus lenses, a regular carrier or minus carrier lenticular should be used[8] to help decrease center thickness, aid centration, and to achieve adequate vertical movement. When one fits moderate to high astigmatism, it is often necessary to increase the center thickness to prevent contact lens flexure in minus shaped lenses. In these cases, a stiff material that is more flexure resistant is preferred to minimize lens thickness. A back surface/bitoric lens design should also be considered.

Sudden Movement

Sudden contact lens movements can be caused by a decentered corneal apex, a very large optical zone, or a poorly fited contact lens.

Excessive Movement

Excessive movement is generally caused by a loose contact lens that irritates the upper lid and limbus.

Alterations in the Tear Film

The sensation of dry eye or a dry contact lens can be caused by insufficient lubrication, excessive evaporation of fluid from the ocular surface, or poor blinking. An insufficient tear film may be the result of the use of systemic medications, including birth control pills,[13] antihistamines,[14] isotretinoin,[15] beta-blockers,[16–18] anticholinergic agents,[16] diuretics, as well as others less frequently used. Hormonal alterations (i.e., menopause or pregnancy[19]) and systemic illnesses, notably rheumatoid arthritis and thyroid disease, may also alter the tear film.

Sensitivity to Chemical Products

The preservatives in contact lens solutions may cause toxic or allergic reactions that result in ocular irritation, conjunctival hyperemia, and punctate keratitis.

Refitted Rigid Gas Permeable Contact Lenses

When a polymethylmethacrylate (PMMA) wearer is refitted with rigid gas permeable lenses, he or she may recover more normal corneal sensation and may be more sensitive to environmental pollutants and debris.

Complaints of Photophobia/Glare

Mild photophobia and glare may occur as a normal symptom in the first 2 weeks after contact lens fitting. Some contact lens wearers require sunglasses even on cloudy days, and others are more sensitive to fluorescent lights. If these symptoms persist, the contact lens design should be reviewed, including the width of the optical zone in relationship to the pupillary diameter and the lens–cornea relationship. The cornea should be carefully examined for the presence of corneal edema, and if necessary the lens material should be changed to one with a higher *Dk* (see Chapter 7). Nonprescription sunglasses should be recommended to the patient as well.

5. What are the most common long-term problems?

In addition to the problems outlined above, which can persist beyond the fitting period, one may encounter the following problems:

Changes in Power

A change in ametropia may be natural, may be produced as the result of corneal edema, or may result from topographic alterations of the cornea. At each consultation, the practitioner should do an overrefraction over a clean contact lens of known parameters. After removal of the lens, the refraction and keratometry or corneal topography should be reviewed to detect any change that may have occurred.

Changes in the Parameters of the Contact Lens

Other factors that can produce warpage of a rigid gas permeable lens include excessive digital pressure during the cleaning process,[20] exposing the lens to excessive heat, and continued use with a tense upper lid. Cleaning the contact lens in the palm of the hand rather than between two fingers will help decrease the incidence of lens warpage.

Corneal Warpage

Corneal warpage is primarily associated with rigid gas permeable lenses (both PMMA and rigid gas permeable) of low DK. Nonetheless, one can also see corneal warpage associated with hydrophilic lenses, especially toric lenses with prism ballast. The visual symptoms are most notable when the patient removes the contact lenses and puts on glasses. When corneal distortion is detected, a refit should be undertaken. A back surface toric/bitoric design should be considered for patients with high corneal cylinder who have shown sphericalization due to the use of a spherical base curve radius.

Deficient Blinking

Infrequent blinking or incomplete blinking may produce drying of the contact lens and the cornea, causing punctate keratitis, drying (3 to 9 o'clock staining), and corneal erosion. To alleviate the symptoms, a wetting agent should be used as well as blinking exercises and possibly a redesign of the contact lens.

Dry Contact Lens

To maximize comfort, the contact lens should be stored wet in an appropriate solution. This will help to preserve the stability of its parameters.

Contact Lens Deposits

The surface of the contact lens may become hazy due to deposits. Normal tear film constituents as well as inadequate cleaning and maintenance may cause deposits. Some patients use saliva or other products not designed specifically for contact lens use that will alter rigid gas permeable materials or simply do not properly clean the contact lens. Deposited lenses can cause blurred vision, changes in refractive power, and the sensation of dryness. The process of cleaning and disinfection should be reviewed at each visit with the patient to enhance compliance. The choice of lens care system should be tailored to best suit the patient needs. In general, firmly bound protein deposits tend to accumulate more on silicone acrylate (SA) materials than on fluorosilicone acrylate (FSA) materials. The FSA materials may be more prone to lipid deposits.[21] Heavy protein depositors benefit from abrasive daily cleaners and regular enzyme cleaning, while lipid depositors do better with surfactant and/or alcohol-based cleaners that are formulated for use with rigid gas permeable materials.[6,22,23]

Slit-Lamp Findings

Superficial Punctate Staining (SPK)

This finding presents as diffuse or patchy areas of punctate staining. It is most commonly caused by protein buildup on the posterior surface of the contact lens, solution toxicity, foreign bodies under the contact lens, hypoxia, or intense ultraviolet (UV) exposure. The patient's symptoms vary by cause and may range from none to noticeable irritation that results in decreased wearing time.

Corneal Arc Staining

When the posterior surface peripheral curve junctions are not properly blended, they may mechanically abrade the corneal surface and result in an arc-shaped area of staining. This is more likely to occur when there are large differences between the two curve radii. It is usually most noticeable in the mid-periphery of the cornea just about the pupil.

Peripheral Corneal Desiccation Staining (3 to 9 O'Clock Staining)

When the lid blinks over the contact lens, proper tear exchange should spread a new layer of tears across the corneal surface. If there is an area near the lens edge where a gap exists, preventing proper tear exchange, corneal desiccation will occur and staining will result. This may result from chronic low-riding lenses, interpalpebral fits with minimal movement, thick edges, either inadequate[24,25] or excessive edge lift, poor-quality tears, poorly wetting contact lenses, or inadequate/improper blinking patterns. This staining is seen most often just outside the lens edge in the 3 to 9 o'clock or 4 to 8 o'clock positions. Conjunctival injection adjacent to the corneal staining areas is often present. Long-term, heavy desiccation staining can result in scarring, neovascularization, or dellen formation.[26] Management requires refitting to a lens design that allows better tear exchange[27] and/or improving the tear quality and quantity. Larger diameter lenses with moderate edge lift may be beneficial.[25] This condition is generally chronic and progressive in nature.[28] In early stages, the patient is usually fairly asymptomatic. As the condition progresses, the patient often notices the conjunctival hyperemia and may report symptoms of burning, drying, and increased lens awareness, resulting in decreased wearing time.[29]

Vascularized Limbal Keratitis[6,29,30]

Vascularized limbal keratitis is also associated with desiccation staining as previously discussed. However it is a progressive inflammatory condition that appears also to have a mechanical etiology due to epithelial chafing. It is most often associated with contact lens fits that incorporate large overall diameters, low edge lift, and apical clearance worn for extended wear. Its clinical presentation also includes staining in the 3 to 9 o'clock positions of the cornea, but it may extend more peripherally and include both the limbus and adjacent conjunctival area. There is also corneal vascularization that leads to a raised peripheral corneal infiltrate. The patient reports symptoms of lens awareness and/or pain, conjunctival hyperemia, and photophobia, resulting in decreased wearing time. These symptoms generally intensify as the condition progresses. Treatment includes discontinuing contact lens wear until the inflammation is quelled, refitting the contact lens to a flatter base curve, modifying peripheral curves to increase edge lift, decreasing overall diameter, heavy blending of peripheral curve junctions, and using ocular lubricants and vasoconstrictors.

Dimple Veiling

A collection of trapped bubbles under the contact lens will result in small temporary depressions into the epithelium.[26] Fluorescein stain collects in these depressions, resulting in a staining pattern of circular or oval spots with sharp borders. These are not epithelial breaks and generally resolve with lens removal; however, chronic formation of the dimples in the same area can result in decreased vision and corneal damage.

6. How should one proceed with the dissatisfied contact lens patient who has been fitted by another professional?

Obtain a detailed case history, which includes:

1. Current and previous complaints
2. Onset of contact lens use
3. Reason for the contact lens fitting
4. Type of contact lens used
5. Reason for and/or time course of the lens changes
6. Methods of cleaning and disinfection that are used
7. Compliance with the lens care recommendations
8. The patient's expectations in relationship to contact lens use.

With the answers to these questions, it is possible to determine whether the basic problem is related to the contact lens, the fitter, or the wearer. After a complete ophthalmic examination, which includes a corneal examination with fluorescein staining, lid eversion to evaluate the tarsal conjunctiva, keratometry, and corneal topography, as well as other appropriate ophthalmic testing, one should do the following:

1. Check the contact lens parameters
2. Place the contact lens on the patient's eye
3. Evaluate the integrity of the contact lens surface
4. Evaluate the overall contact lens fit
5. Overrefract

When the problem is identified, one can refit the patient and dispense new contact lenses of the appropriate design and materials. The patient needs to be reeducated with regard to lens maintenance, because many of these patients may not have received suitable instruction in lens maintenance or did not comply with instructions. This patient requires special attention if contact lens wear is to be continued.

7. How often should gas permeable contact lenses be replaced?

A rigid gas permeable lens generally lasts approximately 1 to 2 years, but this is highly variable and depends on lens material and patient handling. Excessive scratches, heavy depositing, or power changes are indications for lens replacement. As mentioned earlier, patient handling may also induce contact lens base curve warpage and/or power changes. If this results in decreased vision or an altered contact lens fit, then the lens should be replaced and the patient should be educated in proper lens handling.[6] A stiffer, more durable lens material may also be considered for the replacement lens.

8. Can patients wear gas permeable contact lenses overnight?

Although the modality is not nearly as common as with soft contact lenses, rigid gas permeable contact lenses can be worn safely for overnight wear under very specific circumstances determined by the patient's corneal health, visual needs, and available lens materials.[27] Materials in the high to hyper-Dk range should be utilized for best oxygen transmission, and a more aggressive follow-up schedule must be carefully adhered to. The patient should be seen early in the morning after initial overnight wear. Patients should be successful with daily wear of contact lenses first before starting overnight wear.

References

1. Moreira SMB, Moreira H. *Controle de Qualidade das Lentes Rigidas,* 2nd ed. Lentes de Contato. Rio de Janeiro: Cultura Medica, 1998:94–99.
2. Henry VA, Bennett ES, Forrest JF. Clinical investigation of the Paraperm EW rigid gas-permeable contact lens. *Am J Optom Physiol Opt.* 1987;64: 313–320.

3. Wilson SE, et al. Rigid contact lens decentration: a risk factor for corneal warpage. *CLAO J.* 1990;16:177–82.

4. Bennett ES. Silicone acrylate lens design. *ICLC.* 1985;12:45–53.

5. Bennett ES, Egan DJ. Rigid gas-permeable lens problem solving. *J Am Optom Assoc.* 1986;57:504–511.

6. Grohe RM. Rigid gas-permeable problem solving. *Contact Lens Spectrum.* 1990;5:82–99.

7. Grohe RM, Caroline PJ. RGP non-wetting lens syndrome. *Contact Lens Spectrum.* 1989;4:32–44.

8. Lowther GE. Review of rigid contact lens design and effects of design on lens fit. *ICLC.* 1988;15:378–389.

9. Carney LG, Hill RM. Center of gravity of rigid lenses: some design considerations. *ICLC.* 1987;11:431–436.

10. Quinn TG, Carney LG. Controlling rigid lens centration through specific gravity. *ICLC.* 1992;19:84–88.

11. La Hood D. Edge shape and comfort of rigid lenses. *Am J Optom Physiol Opt.* 1988;65:613–618.

12. Moore CF, Mandell RB. The design of high-minus contact lenses. *Contact Lens Spectrum.* 1989;4:43–47.

13. Frankel SH, Ellis PP. Effect of oral contraceptives on tear production. *Ann Ophthalmol.* 1978;10:1585–1588.

14. Crandall DC, Leopold IH. The influence of systemic drugs on tear constituents. *Ophthalmology.* 1979;86:115–125.

15. Fraunfelder FT, LaBraico JM, Meyer SM. Adverse ocular reactions possibly associated with isotretinoin. *Am J Ophthalmol.* 1985;100:534–537.

16. Scott D. Another beta-blocker causing eye symptoms? *Br Med J.* 1977;2:1221.

17. Mackie IA, Seal DV, Pescod JM. Beta-adrenergic receptor blocking drugs: tear lysozyme and immunological screening for adverse reaction. *Br J Ophthalmol.* 1977;61:354–359.

18. Almog Y, et al. The effect of oral treatment with beta blockers on the tear secretion. *Metab Pediatr Syst Ophthalmol.* 1982;6:343–345.

19. Imafidon CO, Imafidon JE. Contact lens wear in pregnancy. *J BCLA.* 1991; 14:75–78.

20. Carrell BA, et al. The effect of rigid gas permeable lens cleaners on lens parameter stability. *J Am Optom Assoc.* 1992;63:193–8.

21. McLaughlin R. Fluoro-silicone-acrylate RGPs vs. silicone-acrylate RGPs. *Contact Lens Spectrum.* 1989;4:74–75.

22. Ames KS. The surface characteristics of RGP lenses. *Contact Lens Spectrum.* 1991;5:45–48.

23. Terry R, Schnider C, Holden BA. Rigid gas permeable lenses and patient management. *CLAO J.* 1989;15:305–309.

24. Andrasko GJ. The effect of varying edge lift on rigid gas permeable extended wear. *Optom Vis Sci.* 1989;66:197.

25. Schnider CM, Terry RL, Holden BA. Effect of lens design on peripheral corneal desiccation. *J Am Optom Assoc.* 1997;68:163–170.

26. McMahon TT. Dellen and dimple veiling. *Contact Lens Spectrum.* 2002;17:52.

27. Schnider CM. Rigid gas permeable extended wear: a viable alternative to hydrogel extended wear. *Contact Lens Spectrum.* 1990;101–105.

28. Andrasko GJ. Peripheral corneal staining: incidence and time course. *Contact Lens Spectrum.* 1990;5:59–62.

29. Davis LJ, Lebow KA. Noninfectious corneal staining. In: Silbert JA, ed. *Anterior Segment Complications of Contact Lens Wear.* Butterworth Heinemann, 2000:67–93.

30. Grohe RM, Lebow KA. Vascularized limbal keratitis. *ICLC.* 1989;16:197–208.

9

Fitting Spherical Hydrophilic Soft Contact Lenses for Daily and Extended Wear

Ricardo Uras and Marjorie J. Rah

1. What are the characteristics of hydrophilic soft contact lenses?

The majority of hydrophilic soft contact lenses (or hydrogel lenses) are made of hydroxyethyl methacrylate (HEMA) and maintain a water content that is more or less constant when they are immersed in saline solution or tears. The water content of hydrogel lenses ranges from approximately 38% to approximately 76%. For this reason, they should not be stored dry.

The pore size in the polymers used in these lenses is greater than many microorganisms, necessitating daily disinfection as prophylaxis against contamination. In addition, tear proteins adhere easily to the hydrophilic polymers. Regular cleaning of the contact lenses is necessary. Mechanical friction and enzymatic cleaners are used to maintain the surface quality of the lenses. The enzymatic cleaners break down protein molecules and reduce the adherence of tear proteins.

In 1999, silicone hydrogel lenses were introduced. These lenses represent a hybrid lens material that combines the oxygen permeability of silicone with the hydrophilic HEMA of traditional soft lenses. The water content of silicone hydrogel lenses is relatively low at approximately 20% to 40%, depending on the brand of the lenses. The oxygen transmissibility (Dk/t) of silicone lenses is much higher (greater than 100×10^{-9} cm mL O_2/s mL mm Hg) than traditional hydrogel soft lenses, making them the best choice for patients who prefer extended wearing schedules.

2. How are hydrophilic soft contact lenses classified?

Hydrophilic soft contact lenses are classified according to:

- Method of manufacture. They are spin-cast contact lenses that are lathed, molded, and mixed (one surface lathed and one surface spin-cast).

- Water content. Low, medium, and high water content lenses are, respectively, 38%, 55%, and 75% water.
- Permeability: medium and high permeability, Dk less than or greater than 50, respectively.
- Transmissibility: The transmissibility to oxygen will depend on the Dk of the primary material and the thickness of the lens, as in rigid gas permeable lenses.
- U.S. Food and Drug Administration (FDA) classification.[1]
  Group 1: Low water (less than 50% water content) nonionic polymers
  Group 2: High water (greater than 50% water content) nonionic polymers
  Group 3: Low water (less than 50% water content) ionic polymers
  Group 4: High water (greater than 50% water content) ionic polymers (highest affinity for tear protein deposition in group 4 lenses)
- Color.
  Clear lenses
  Light blue or green visibility tinted lenses that do not alter eye color
  Cosmetic contact lenses: principal function is to alter the color of the iris or the appearance of the cornea.
- Length of use.
  Daily use
  Extended use (worn during both waking hours and sleep)
  Sporadic use (occasional only)
  The clinician determines the wearing schedule at the time of the clinical evaluation. The wearing schedule is determined based on the patient's goals for contact lens wear.
- Lens life: disposable versus nondisposable contact lenses

3. How does one fit a hydrophilic soft contact lens?

Central Posterior Curve and Diameter

1. The central posterior curve should be approximately 0.6 to 0.8 mm flatter than the average corneal curvature measurement.[2]
2. The lens diameter should be approximately 2.0 mm larger than the horizontal visible iris diameter.[2]

The diameter is the determining factor in the centration of the contact lens. The limbus should remain covered by the lens during the blink. However, the greater the diameter, the less the movement of the lens and the greater its adherence. Ideally, the lens should move 0.5 to 1 mm with the blink.

Dioptric Power of the Contact Lens

In determining the initial power of the contact lens, one should consider the refraction, expressed in minus cylinder form. If a low degree of astigmatism is present, the spherical equivalent should be used in the determination of lens power. If the refractive error is greater than 4.00 D, a table for correction of vertex distance should be used. The central posterior curve induces little alteration in the final power of the contact lens. The use of trial lenses is highly recommended. Place the trial lens on the eye and perform a spherical overrefraction.

1. High water content and ionic contact lenses should be avoided in people whose eyes tend to form deposits.
2. The trial contact lenses should have the same characteristics as the contact lenses to be fitted.

Biomicroscopy and Overrefraction

At the slit lamp, one way to facilitate assessment of the lens–cornea relationship is to ask the patient to blink while facing forward and while looking to the side. The evaluation of the movement and over-refraction should be performed approximately 15 minutes after insertion of the lens. One should consider adequate movement as 0.5 to 1 mm of lateral movement and 0.5 to 1 mm of vertical movement with blinking.

4. What are the characteristics of a well-fitted contact lens?

- Adequate lens centration with full limbal coverage: Adequate lens diameter selection will result in approximately 1 mm of limbal coverage around the circumference of the lens.
- Movement should be assessed using the following techniques:
  Straight gaze: With the patient viewing in primary gaze, the lens should move 0.3 to 1.0 mm with the blink.
  Upgaze: When the patient is asked to look up, the lens should move 0.3 to 0.7 mm with the blink.
  Push-up test: With the patient viewing in primary gaze, gently manipulate the patient's lower lid to push the contact lens superiorly. The lens should move freely.

5. What are the signs and symptoms of a loose contact lens?

- Discomfort, even after a short period of time
- Excessive movement and displacement of the contact lens, compromising the visual acuity immediately after a blink. (Note: the view with retinoscopy and keratometry will also be distorted immediately after the blink by a loose lens.)
- Worsening visual acuity with blinking

6. What are the signs and symptoms of a tight contact lens?

- Discomfort after several hours of use
- The visual acuity, keratometric mires, and retinoscopic view in a tight-fitting contact lens may be distorted but improve immediately after the blink.
- Minimal or absent movement of the contact lens
- Perilimbal conjunctival hyperemia
- Microcystic edema
- Diffuse edema
- In severe cases of hypoxia, the following may also be noted:
  Deep corneal folds
  Blurred vision and/or halos around lights, produced by corneal hypoxia as a result of decreased diffusion of oxygen into the tear film

7. How does one follow the hydrophilic lens wearer?

The following testing should be completed at the follow-up visit for hydrophilic soft lens wearers:

1. Visual acuity measurement
2. Overrefraction
3. Assessment of the patient's contact lens–related comfort
4. Evaluation of the length of wear
5. Evaluation of lens maintenance
6. Biomicroscopy (examination for microcysts, fluorescein staining of the cornea, infiltrates, neovascularization, edema, and erosions)

The follow-up care should be ongoing. The follow-up schedule depends on the sensitivities and individual characteristics of each eye. First-time contact lens wearers should be examined 2 weeks after the initial dispensing visit and then at 3- to 6-month intervals during the first year, depending on the wearing schedule and lens type. In wearers who intend to sleep with their contact lenses, the clinician should verify that there are no contraindications to extended wear. After initial intensive follow-up care (1 day, 1 to 2 weeks), the patient should have an ocular examination every 3 to 6 months, with immediate discontinuation of use at the first signs of any adverse effects on the cornea. For those wearers who do not intend to sleep with their contact lenses, an annual examination is sufficient. In follow-up examinations, the clinician should always verify that the instructions for contact lens maintenance are being adhered to. The patient must be conscientious about mechanical cleaning, enzyme treatment and disinfection, and these must be correctly performed to minimize risks. Many eyes are very sensitive and show signs of hypoxia and overwear. In these cases, wearing time with a contact lens of low permeability should be reduced to 4 to 6 hours per day. In these circumstances, it is imperative to change the contact lens for one of higher permeability if wearing time is to be increased. For patients wearing disposable lenses, the schedule for lens disposal should be reviewed.

8. What are the signs and symptoms of a poor fit?

Some of the signs and symptoms of a poor fit have already been mentioned. They include, but are not limited to:

- Discomfort
- Blurred vision and/or variable vision with blinking
- Burning at the time of contact lens removal
- Excessive movement or immobility
- Decentration
- Perilimbal hyperemia

Close attention should be paid to complaints of halos, foreign body sensation, or itching. This may signify the presence of corneal hypoxia, epithelial erosions, or giant papillary conjunctivitis. An asymptomatic complication is corneal neovascularization, which may be observed at the biomicroscope and is caused by either a poor fit or inappropriate use of the contact lens (i.e., extended wear of a daily wear lens).

9. What is the basic trial lens set for fitting hydrophilic contact lenses?

The trial lens set should include pairs ranging from low to moderate myopic powers through +4.00-D hyperopic corrections in all available base curves. Clinicians should have an appropriate fitting set for each type of contact lens they wish to fit. Fitting sets and fitting guides are available from many contact lens companies and should be utilized whenever possible. Exceptional cases include patients with ametropias greater than ±15.00 D, which generally require special trial lenses.

References

1. Stone RP. Why contact lens groups? *Contact Lens Spectrum* 1988;3:38–41.
2. Bruce AS, Little SA. Soft lens design, fitting, and physiologic response. In: Hom MM, ed. *Manual of Contact Lens Prescribing and Fitting with CD-ROM,* 2nd ed. Boston: Butterworth-Heinemann, 2000:179–213.

Selected Readings

Mandell RB, ed. *Contact Lens Practice,* 2nd ed. Springfield, IL: Charles C. Thomas, 1974.

Ruben M, ed. *Soft Contact Lenses Clinical and Applied Technology.* London: John Wiley & Sons, 1978.

10

Disposable and Planned Replacement Contact Lenses

Nilo Holzchuh, Cleusa Coral-Ghanem, and Timothy B. Edrington

1. What is a disposable contact lens?

The disposable contact lens is the result of the development of molding-based manufacturing methods that make possible the production of uniform lenses at low cost. Clinically, they are called "disposable" because the contact lens is made of a hydrogel (soft lens) material that can be replaced after 1 day, 1 week, or 2 weeks or of a silicone hydrogel developed for extended wear and discarded monthly. Hydrogel lenses exchanged at intervals of every 3 or 6 months are often referred to as "planned or frequent replacement." Literally, all contact lenses are planned-replacement or disposable. The eye care practitioner and the patient simply choose the optimum interval at which to replace them.

2. What are the indications and contraindications for disposable contact lenses?

Disposable contact lenses are indicated for the correction of myopia, hyperopia, astigmatism, and presbyopia, as well as for cosmetic purposes. They are routinely prescribed for:

- Allergic individuals with sensitivity to chemical lens care system products
- Individuals who wish to use lenses on an extended wear basis because of difficulty with maintenance, the type of work they do, or convenience
- Patients who frequently lose contact lenses or need spare lenses
- Patients who play contact sports
- Wearers who are exposed to pollutants
- Individuals who suffer from giant papillary conjunctivitis (GPC)[1]
- Individuals with lacrimal deficiency or who form excessive deposits on the contact lenses

- Therapeutic use
- Pediatric use

Contraindications include:

- Anterior segment inflammation or infection
- Significant changes in the tear film
- Environments with chemical pollution

3. What are the basic types of disposable contact lenses?

One-Day Disposable Contact Lenses

These lenses are discarded daily or after a single use. The principal indications are for individuals who are sensitive to chemicals in their contact lens care products, who are unwilling to keep up the mainte-nance of the lenses, or who use the lenses only occasionally (part-time wear). Lens cost is generally higher for daily disposable contact lenses. However, the patient does not need to disinfect the lenses, thereby sav-ing money on lens care products.

When compared to conventional daily wear, daily disposable lens wear has been reported to provide the patient with better subjective vision and overall patient satisfaction. Also, fewer corneal complica-tions, lens deposits, and unscheduled visits have been reported.[2]

One- to Two-Week Disposable Lenses

This type of contact lens was approved by the U.S. Food and Drug Administration to be discarded after 7 days of extended wear or 14 days of daily wear. It is currently the most prescribed disposable lens option in the United States. Patients using their lenses on a daily wear basis need to disinfect their lenses between uses. It is generally not necessary to add enzyme cleaning to the lens care regimen for patients replacing their lenses every 1 to 2 weeks.

Thirty-Day Disposable Silicone Hydrogel Contact Lenses

A new generation of materials with oxygen permeability (Dk) values greater than 100 has been prescribed in parts of the world since 1999. These lenses are manufactured from a silicone hydrogel material with a treated surface that is more hydrophilic and more resistant to depos-its. In this type of material, the aqueous phase functions to promote comfort and movement, while the silicone is responsible for the high permeability to oxygen. Even though these lenses were developed for continuous use over a 30-day period, many eye care practitioners pre-scribe them for daily wear use or recommend that the lenses be removed once weekly for disinfection. Reduced lens handling should result in fewer torn and microbially contaminated lenses.

Planned Replacement Contact Lenses

Other replacement options exist for soft contact patients. Lenses marketed or prescribed for monthly and quarterly replacement are used generally to minimize lens cost for the patient. Enzymatic treatment should be added to the care regimens for patients replacing their lenses monthly or less frequently. One- to 3-month planned replacement lenses have also been shown to reduce contact lens–induced complications and to increase patient satisfaction when compared to conventional lens replacement.[3]

Disposable and Planned Replacement Toric Contact Lenses

This type of lens is an alternative for patients with significant refractive astigmatism.

Disposable Bifocal and Multifocal Lenses

Currently, aspheric and annular multifocal disposable soft contact lens designs are available. One of the advantages of fitting disposable multifocals is the availability of in-office lenses that the patient can try with minimal cost to both practitioner and patient. Before beginning the fitting, it is advisable to inform the patient that a bifocal/multifocal contact lens may not provide the same clarity as spectacles over the same range of distances and may be clearer at far than at near, or vice versa. Frequently, monovision provides better results. Monovision systems have been another factor in the development of disposable lenses because they allow trial fitting with the appropriate power for the patient and afford the opportunity to determine which eye is best corrected for near work.[4]

4. How does one fit a disposable contact lens?

The fitting of disposable contact lenses employs the same methodologies used with conventional hydrophilic lenses:

1. Perform a trial fitting with the appropriate lens for the patient. For this, it is recommended that practitioners stock different powers and curvatures that will facilitate fitting the largest number of patients.
2. Evaluate the fitting of the trial lens at the slit lamp after 15 minutes, the time usually necessary for stabilization of the contact lens on the eye. At this point, one should perform an overrefraction to determine the optimal lens power prior to dispensing the lens.

5. What are the advantages of using disposable contact lenses for therapeutic purposes?

- Frequent replacement with new, clean lenses
- Fewer lens surface deposits
- Simultaneous use with topical medication
- Reasonable cost

6. How should one follow disposable and planned replacement lens patients?

If the patient is planning extended wear, he/she should be examined:

- After overnight wear
- After 1 week of extended wear
- At the end of 1 month of extended wear
- Every 3 to 6 months

Patients who regularly sleep in their contact lenses should be examined every 6 months. In most instances, daily wearers can be examined on an annual basis. It is important to counsel a contact lens wearer about the necessity of complying with instructions regarding the length of time a contact lens is worn and its recommended disposal schedule in order to minimize complications. The responsibility of the eye care practitioner is to provide the patient with the appropriate lens and to provide appropriate follow-up care. It is extremely important that every contact lens patient with ocular complaints be reevaluated in order to avoid more serious ocular complications and the cessation of contact lens use. The patient should be counseled to regularly verify that his or her eyes are clear (not red), free from discomfort or pain, and that their lenses provide optimal vision.

7. What are the most frequent complications associated with disposable contact lens wear?

Improper or neglected instructions concerning lens replacement schedules and lens care regimens may lead to unnecessary ocular complications. Poor compliance with lens replacement instructions was demonstrated in a survey of university students; 88.5% of disposable soft contact lens wearers did not adhere to their prescribed lens replacement schedule.[5] Corneal infiltrates, contact lens–associated red eye, and giant papillary conjunctivitis are complications that may occur more frequently in patients who are not compliant with their wearing schedules, lens replacement schedules, or lens care systems.

The Dk/t of the majority of disposable contact lenses currently prescribed (excluding the silicone hydrogel lenses) is similar to that of conventional hydrophilic lenses. Therefore, hypoxia problems still exist with nonsilicone hydrogel soft contact lenses. Extended wear with conventional hydrophilic lenses can cause corneal edema, increasing the risk of infectious keratitis 10- to 15-fold when compared with daily use.[6] Alterations of the epithelium, hypoxia, and the presence of bacteria on the contact lens form a triad that predisposes the eye to the development of infectious corneal ulceration. Some studies indicated that the introduction of disposable contact lenses increased the frequency of noninfectious keratitis and may also be associated with ulcerative keratitis.[7-9] Other studies have concluded that disposable lenses worn on a daily or extended wear basis have the same or lower risk of keratitis when compared to conventional soft contact lenses worn on the same basis.[10,11] Infectious keratitis associated with the use of a hydrogel disposable lens occurs more in the periphery than in the center of the cornea, and the responsible microorganisms with the greatest frequency are gram positive, not gram negative. Moreover, the keratitis associated with disposable lenses is generally less severe than that associated with conventional hydrophilic lenses.

The incidence of giant papillary conjunctivitis is significantly less in patients who exchange their contact lenses every 3 weeks or less.[12] Continued exchange of the contact lens appears to benefit the ocular surface. There are a number of scientific studies that demonstrate that, when the contact lens material is new, there is less accumulation of deposits. Likewise, the type of material from which the disposable lens is made may influence the quantity of deposits that form on the lens.[12-15] Disposable contact lenses used in a regimen of planned replacement under the supervision of an eye care practitioner may prove to be an excellent alternative for patients who have not had success with other types of contact lenses.

References

1. Marshall EC, Begley CG, Nguyen CHD. Frequency of complications among wearers of disposable and conventional soft contact lenses. *ICLC.* 1992;19:55–59.
2. Solomon O, Freeman M, Boshnick E, et al. A 3-year prospective study of the clinical performance of daily disposable contact lenses compared with frequent-replacement and conventional daily wear contact lenses. *CLAO J.* 1996;22:250–257.
3. Pritchard N, Fonn D, Weed K. Ocular and subjective responses to frequent replacement of daily wear soft contact lenses. *CLAO J.* 1996;22:53–59.
4. Holzchuh N, Alves MR, Kara-José N. Dominância ocular e correção de presbiopia com lentes de contato através da técnica de monovisão. *Arq Bras Oftalmol.* 1997;60:184–186.
5. Coral-Ghanem C, Ghanem RC, Bortoli GW, Yamazaki ES. Comportamento e características de usuários de lentes de contato entre estudantes universitários da área de saúde. *Arq Bras Oftalmol.* 2000;63:123–127.
6. Poggio EC, Glynn RJ, Schein OD, et al. The incidence of ulcerative keratitis among users of daily-wear and extended-wear soft contact lenses. *N Engl J Med.* 1989;321:779–783.
7. Ficker L, Hunter P, Seal D, Wright P. Acanthamoeba keratitis occurring with disposable contact lens wear. *Am J Ophthalmol.* 1990;108:453.

8. Kent HD, Sanders RJ, Arentsen JJ, Cohen EJ, Laibson PR. Pseudomonas corneal ulcer associated with disposable soft contact lenses. *Contact Lens Assoc Ophthalmol J.* 1989;15:264–265.

9. Rabinowitz SM, Pflugfelder SC, Goldberg M. Disposable extended-wear contact lens-related keratitis. *Arch Ophthalmol.* 1989;107:1121.

10. Guillon M, Guillon J-P, Bansal M, Maskell R, Rees P. Incidence of ulcers with conventional and disposable daily wear soft contact lenses. *J Br Contact Lens Assoc.* 1994;17:69–76.

11. Buehler PO, Schein OD, Stamler JF, Verdier DD, Ketz J. The increased risk of ulcerative keratitis among disposable soft contact lens users. *Arch Ophthalmol.* 1992;110:1555–1558.

12. Porazinski AD, Donshik PC. Giant papillary conjunctivitis in frequent replacement contact lens wearers: a retrospective study. *CLAO J.* 1999;25: 142–147.

13. Poggio EC, Abelson M. Complications and symptoms in disposable extended-wear lenses compared with conventional soft daily-wear and soft extended-wear lenses. *Contact Lens Assoc Ophthalmol J.* 1993;19:31–39.

14. Boswall GJ, Ehlers WH, Luistro A, Worrall M, Donshik PC. A comparison of conventional and disposable extended wear contact lenses. *CLAO J.* 1993; 19:158–165.

15. Hamano HK, Watanabe K, Hamano T, et al. A study of the complications induced by conventional and disposable contact lenses. *CLAO J.* 1994;20: 103–108.

11

Astigmatism and Toric Contact Lenses

Michael Twa and Saly Moreira

1. What is astigmatism?

Astigmatism is an optical distortion that results in blur that smears the point of focus (Figure 11.1). The blur is minimum at two different focal points that are separated by the distance between their focal lengths (Figure 11.2). This optical distortion is most often caused when the cornea has a toric shape. The torus has the shape of a bicycle tire and is more curved in one meridian than the other (Figure 11.3). An optical surface with a toric shape focuses light at a short distance for the more curved meridian and at a farther distance for the less curved meridian. It is important to distinguish between astigmatism, which is an optical condition, and corneal toricity, which is a toric distortion in the shape of the cornea. Although astigmatism is most often associated with corneal toricity, one does not require the other. The correction of astigmatism is an optical problem; corneal toricity is a contact lens fit consideration.

Corneal Astigmatism

Distortion of the spherical shape of the cornea is the most common cause for astigmatism. Astigmatism results when the central cornea has a toric shape. With pure corneal astigmatism, the total power of the astigmatism is equal to the corneal toricity. This can be measured using keratometry or corneal topography and can be corrected with soft or rigid contact lenses.[1]

Residual Astigmatism

The term *residual astigmatism* has several possible meanings. In general, residual astigmatism results from causes other than the shape of the anterior corneal surface and can refer to astigmatism caused by other optical elements of the eye as well as by contact lens rotation and flexure. Residual astigmatism is most commonly caused by the optical

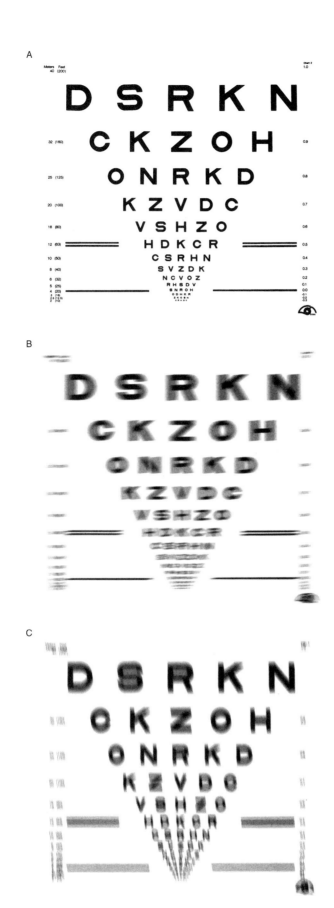

Figure 11.1. A: Normal focus. B, C: Astigmatic blur.

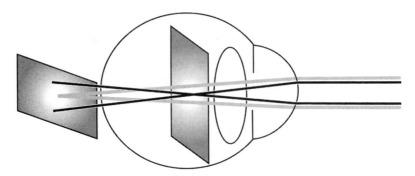

Figure 11.2. The optics of astigmatism.

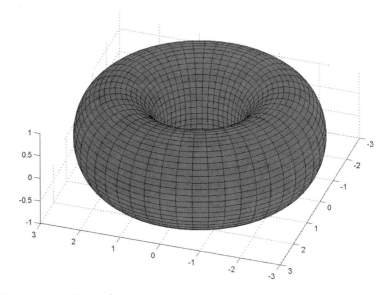

Figure 11.3. Toric shape.

power of the lens and is sometimes called *lenticular astigmatism.* Other causes for residual astigmatism include a toric posterior corneal surface and tilted or misaligned optical surfaces within the eye. Residual or internal astigmatism is commonly against-the-rule (greater refractive power in the horizontal meridian) and is not correctable using spherical contact lenses but may be treated with other lens designs.

Irregular Astigmatism

Irregular astigmatism is the name given to optical distortion that is not easily described by conventional sphero-cylindrical lenses and generally refers to optical aberrations other than defocus and regular astigmatism. Unlike regular astigmatism, which is caused by a symmetric and predictable toric corneal surface, irregular astigmatism is caused by corneal distortion that is not symmetric. Videokeratography is the best way to observe an irregular corneal surface; however, distorted keratometry mires and/or an irregular retinoscopic reflex can also reveal irregular astigmatism. Rigid contact lens designs are most useful for the correction of irregular astigmatism, where tears between the contact lens and corneal surface can compensate for mild to moderate corneal irregularity.

Total Astigmatism

Total astigmatism is measured by a standard refraction. Total astigmatism is the sum of corneal astigmatism and residual astigmatism. In some cases anterior corneal astigmatism may be balanced by internal astigmatism.

Example

Refraction   =   −2.00 sphere
Keratometry =   43.00/45.00 @ 90°

It is important to consider how much astigmatism is caused by the toricity of the anterior cornea because this will guide the selection of both optical and shape characteristics of the contact lens during the fitting process. In cases where corneal and internal astigmatism do not cancel each other, the residual astigmatism may or may not be balanced between corneal and lenticular astigmatism.

Example

Different axes:

Residual astigmatism by refraction   =   −2.00 −4.00 × 120°
Corneal astigmatism by keratometry   =   41.00/43.00 @ 90°
Calculated internal astigmatism   =   Plano −3.50 × 135

Identical axes:

Residual astigmatism by refraction   =   −2.00 −4.00 × 180°
Corneal astigmatism by keratometry   =   41.00/43.00 @ 90°
Calculated internal astigmatism   =   Plano −2.00 × 180

2. What is the best way to determine residual astigmatism?

Residual astigmatism can be determined by comparing the anterior corneal toricity with the total astigmatism determined by refraction. The residual astigmatism is the difference between these two values. This is easy to interpret when the axis of corneal astigmatism matches the axis of the astigmatism measured by refraction. However, it is more difficult to interpret when the resulting cylinder powers are crossed. Another way to determine residual astigmatism is to place a rigid spherical contact lens on the cornea and perform a sphero-cylindrical overrefraction. The quantity of astigmatism that remains uncorrected is the residual astigmatism from all other optical elements including the intraocular lens, contact lens flexure, and any tear lens formed behind the lens. Predicting residual astigmatism by calculation is not exact because the effects of eyelid pressure, lens position, lens rotation, and lens flexure are unknown. The best method to determine residual astigmatism to account for these effects is by trial fitting an approximate contact lens and performing a sphero-cylindrical overrefraction.[2]

3. What are the indications for a toric contact lens?

There are two reasons to consider a toric contact lens:

1. Spherical lenses do not provide sufficient optical correction of total astigmatism.
2. The physical fit and alignment of a spherical lens is unacceptable because of corneal toricity.

It is common to ignore small amounts of total astigmatism when fitting contact lenses. Many patients are not bothered by uncorrected refractive astigmatism less than 1.00 D. This is partly due to the correction of refractive astigmatism through tear lens effects and contact lens flexure that can reduce residual astigmatism enough to satisfy the patient. Patients with less than 2.00 D of corneal toricity and small amounts of residual astigmatism (0.50 D) by overrefraction may find that their vision is acceptable with conventional spherical lenses. When this approach is successful, it simplifies the fitting procedure for both doctor and patient and simplifies the manufacture and reproduction of future contact lens orders. However, the needs of the patient are the most important consideration. In some cases, patients with as little as 0.50 D of astigmatism will require astigmatic contact lenses to achieve satisfactory vision.

Example

A 47-year-old woman

Occupation: Chief executive officer of a computer graphics company
Goal: Wishes to wear contact lenses for presentations at business
   meetings; very demanding personality. She was a previous failure
   with contact lenses that "did not give sharp vision."
Refraction: $-3.00 -0.75 \times 090$ 20/20
Overrefraction: $-0.00 -0.75 \times 090$ 20/25 with -3.00 D sphere soft
   lens
Final lens: $-2.75 -0.25 \times 085$ 20/15

Conversely, in other cases it may appropriate to fit spherical contact lenses even for large amounts of astigmatism.

Example

A 32-year-old man

Occupation: Championship surf kayaker
Goal: Has worn lenses before that gave pretty good vision but lost

them often. Quit wearing contact lenses because they were too expensive to replace.

Refraction: $-3.75 \; -2.25 \times 167 \; 20/15$

Over-refraction: $+0.50 \; -1.25 \times 170$ with a -4.50 D sphere soft lens

Final lens: -4.50 spherical soft disposable contact lens

4. What kind of contact lenses can be used to correct astigmatism?

Astigmatism can be successfully corrected with either rigid or soft contact lens designs. Lens selection and fitting strategy are usually guided by the patient's prescription, corneal toricity, and personal concerns. A summary of lens categories follows; specific applications for each lens type are discussed in the following sections. Rigid contact lens types for the correction of astigmatism include:

1. Spherical contact lenses
2. Front toric contact lens
3. Back toric contact lens
4. Bitoric contact lens

Soft contact lenses for the correction of astigmatism include:

1. Prism ballast toric contact lenses
2. Thin zone stabilizing lens designs

5. What rigid toric contact lens materials are used for the correction of astigmatism?

Toric contact lenses can be made of rigid gas permeable or hydrophilic materials. To produce a predictable optical correction on the eye, rigid lens designs should not bend on the eye. Lens flexure on the eye can induce additional unwanted astigmatism. Lens flexure can be greater as corneal toricity increases.[2] To guard against this source of unwanted astigmatism, one can select materials with lower oxygen permeability that are generally less elastic and therefore more resistant to lens flexure on the eye. By increasing lens thickness, one can also reduce the chances of rigid lens flexure. However, this will also further reduce oxygen transmissibility of the lens.

6. How does one prescribe a spherical rigid lens for an astigmatic cornea?

Refractive astigmatism associated with corneal toricity less than 2.00 D is often successfully corrected with a spherical rigid contact lens. In this case, residual astigmatism is corrected by a tear lens formed between the contact lens and corneal surfaces. The first step is to achieve a good alignment and position of the lens on the eye. If it is not possible to achieve a good physical fit that will not compromise the health of the eye, then the quality of vision is unimportant. Trial fitting the contact lens is the best way to determine the acceptability of lens fit and vision.

The same rules for fitting spherical rigid contact lenses apply to the correction of astigmatism. First, there must be adequate tear exchange beneath the lens. This is not usually a problem with a toric corneal surface where tears can easily pool beneath a spherical lens along the steep meridian. However, in a highly toric cornea, alignment of the posterior curvature of the lens with the flat meridian can cause the lens to rock to either side of this balance point, resulting in lens displacement or even ejection. The spherical lens on a toric cornea should still center well over the pupil and move adequately with a blink. Selecting a posterior lens curvature steeper than the flattest corneal meridian can help improve lens fit and centration. An acceptable fit becomes increasingly difficult to achieve as corneal toricity increases and results in discomfort, lens decentration, lens ejection, and reduced vision. If this occurs, consider fitting a contact lens with toric surfaces.

Select the posterior curvature of the initial fitting lens from the flat keratometry value. Allow the lens several minutes to stabilize on the eye before judging alignment, positioning, and movement with a blink. Reduce excessive lens movement by reducing the posterior lens radius of curvature, increasing lens diameter, or increasing the optical zone diameter.

Fitting a Spherical Rigid Lens on a Toric Cornea

Base curve

For 2.00 D of corneal toricity, select a posterior curvature slightly greater than the flat keratometry value (e.g., 0.50 D steeper than the flat keratometric reading).

Example

Keratometry:	=	43.00/45.00 @ 90°
Refraction	=	$-2.00 -2.00 \times 180°$
Final contact lens	=	43.50 (7.7) -2.25
Diameter	=	8.8 mm

As lens diameter and corneal toricity increase, select a posterior lens curvature slightly steeper than the flattest meridian by keratometry.

7. What are the indications for a front toric rigid contact lens?

Refractive astigmatism measured in an eye with a spherical corneal surface cannot be fully corrected with a spherical rigid contact lens. Although the physical fit of the lens requires a spherical posterior lens surface, the full optical correction will not be achieved. A front toric rigid contact lens design is used in this situation. A front toric rigid contact lens is designed with an astigmatic correction on the anterior surface. To provide the correct prescription, this lens must not rotate on the eye. The lens can be stabilized by truncating the bottom edge of the lens, creating a flat surface to align against the lower eyelid margin. Another method of orienting the lens is to create ballast at the bottom and allow gravity to keep the proper lens orientation. This is done by increasing the thickness of the lower half of the lens with 0.5 to 1.50 Δ of base down prism. Sometimes these two techniques are combined to provide greater rotational stability (Figure 11.4).

8. What is the technique for fitting a front toric rigid contact lens?

Trial Fitting with a Spherical Rigid Lens

After verification of refraction and corneal curvature, place a rigid spherical lens with a base curve slightly flatter (0.25 to 0.50 D) than the flat keratometric reading on the eye. Allow the lens to stabilize on the eye for approximately 20 minutes. If the physical fit of the lens is acceptable, then perform a sphero-cylindrical overrefraction to determine the toric contact lens power. If the contact lens ordered rotates unexpectedly on the eye, then the resulting optical power of the lens will be incorrect.

Example

Spherical contact lens	=	− 3.00 D
Overrefraction	=	− 1.00 − 0.75 × 180°
Lens ordered	=	− 3.75 − 0.75 × 180°
		(corrected vertex power)
Prism ballast	=	1.25Δ

Trial Fitting with a Truncated or Prism Ballast Trial Lens

The evaluation is performed with a truncated or prism ballasted trial lens in order to establish whether the lens is rotationally stable and how the lens is oriented at rest on the eye. A dot on the lens at the

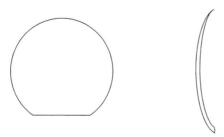

Figure 11.4. Truncated prism ballasted front-surface toric rigid contact lens design.

6 o'clock position marks the location of the prism ballast, and its rotation with blinking can be used to judge stability. These trial lenses generally have spherical optical power.

1. Select the base curve and lens diameter needed to achieve an acceptable fit. Although lens alignment should be similar to the fit of any other spherical rigid contact lens on a toric cornea, motion and position after blinking may be affected by truncation or prism ballast. Consider altering overall lens diameter, base curvature, or peripheral curves to improve the physical fit characteristics of the lens.
2. Determine the power by refraction over the trial lens. Do not forget to add the power of the trial lens to the final lens power calculation.
3. Determine the final axis of the toric contact lens power by adjusting for any rotation of the trial lens on the eye. To determine the final axis, note the location of the lens mark. From this location estimate or measure the direction and quantity of lens rotation.

For every clock-hour of rotation of the contact lens, the axis of the spectacle correction is changed by 30° (1 clock-hour of rotation = 30°). With a rotation to the left of the observer (clockwise), add the degrees of rotation to the axis of the refraction. With rotation to the right of the observer (counterclockwise), subtract the degree of rotation from the axis of the refraction (Figure 11.5).

Example

| Refraction | $= -1.50 -1.50 \times 105°$ |
| Keratometry | $=$ p 42.75/43.00 @ 100° |

Trial lens:
| Base curve | $=$ 42.50 D |

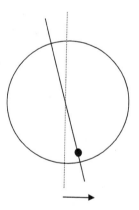

Figure 11.5. Counterclockwise rotation of toric lens. This direction of rotation would require subtracting the amount of rotation (15° in this example) from the original prescription axis to calculate the corrected axis. Clockwise rotation would be added to the original prescription axis to compensate for lens rotation.

Diameter	=	9.0 mm
Power	=	plano
Prism ballast	=	1.25 Δ
Overrefraction	=	$-1.25 - 1.00 \times 100°$

The contact lens rotates to the 5:30 clock-hour (15° rotation, counterclockwise), and in this case 15° must be subtracted from the overrefraction's axis of astigmatism. The final lens power is determined by combining the contact lens power with the results of the overrefraction. The final axis is calculated by correction for the trial lens rotation.

Example

Add the power of the trial lens	=	plano
Add the power of the overrefraction	=	$-1.25 - 1.00 \times 100°$
Corrected lens power is	=	$-1.25 - 1.00 \times 100°$
The lens rotates 15° counterclockwise		
Corrected lens axis is: (100° − 15°)	=	85°
Final lens power	=	$-1.25 - 1.00 \times 85°$

9. What is the definition of and indication for a posterior toric rigid contact lens?

A posterior toric rigid contact lens has a spherical front curvature and a toric posterior surface with toricity approximately equal to the cornea. Toricity of the posterior lens surface allows the lens to align better with the cornea, improving the physical fit characteristics of the lens. The posterior curvature of a back surface toric contact lens should align with the corneal surface but should still permit movement and tear exchange beneath the lens. There are several methods for selecting the correct amount of lens toricity to fit a toric corneal surface. Most methods allow tear exchange beneath the lens by fitting slightly flatter than alignment. A contact lens with posterior curvatures slightly flatter than the corneal toricity in each meridian orients well and aligns to the central cornea while still permitting tear exchange through the peripheral edge lift of the lens. The posterior toric contact lens is indicated for high degrees of corneal astigmatism (greater than 2.00 D of corneal toricity) especially when an acceptable fit cannot be accomplished with a spherical posterior curvature.

A toric back surface lens with a spherical front surface will induce additional astigmatism along the flat meridian of the eye due to the sphere and cylinder combination and the difference between the index of refraction of the tears and the plastic of the contact lens.[1] For this reason, this lens design has limited application and is best suited for cases where corneal toricity is flatter in the vertical meridian and residual astigmatism is against-the-rule (minus cylinder, axis 90 degrees). A compensating toric surface can be placed on the front of the contact lens to address this problem. This design is known as a bitoric contact lens and will be described in the next section.

10. How does one prescribe a rigid posterior toric contact lens?

To prescribe a contact lens with a posterior toric surface, it is necessary to know the refractive error and corneal curvature by keratometry or videokeratography. Edrington et at.[3] found that best lens stability was achieved when the base curves were nearly equal to the flat meridian with the steep meridian steeper by approximately two thirds of the total corneal toricity. One should evaluate the contact lens fit using the same criteria used for rigid spherical lenses.

Example

Lens toricity equal to two thirds of the corneal toricity

Refraction	=	$-3.00 -4.50 \times 180°$
Keratometry	=	43.00/47.00 @ 90°
		(2/3 of $-4.00 = -2.75$)
Base curve (flat meridian)	=	43.00 D
Base curve (steep meridian)	=	$43.00 + 2.75 = 45.75$ D

An alternative to the "rule of two-thirds" is to make the flat curve of the contact lens equal to or slightly different ($\pm$ 0.50 D) from the flat meridian and 0.50 D flatter than the steep meridian. This approach is also intended to provide good alignment of the posterior contact lens surface to the cornea.

The power of the contact lens is equal to the refractive sphere, taking into consideration the vertex distance when necessary. Lens diameter between 9.0 and 9.7 mm will provide better stability and centration.

Example

Refraction	=	$-4.00 -5.00 \times 180°$
Keratometry	=	41.00/46.00 @ 90°
Posterior curve (flat meridian)	=	$41.00 + 0.25 = 41.25$ D
Posterior curve (steep meridian)	=	$46.00 - 0.50 = 45.50$ D
The calculated contact lens parameters		
should be:		$(-4.25$ D: 41.25$)/(-8.50$ D: 45.50$)$

11. What are bitoric rigid gas permeable contact lenses, and how are they fitted?

Even though the calculated lens parameters for posterior toric contact lenses in the previous examples would provide good physical alignment of the lens, the optical performance would probably be poor because of residual astigmatism. A bitoric contact lens has a compensating anterior toric surface that can provide better visual acuity by compensating for any residual astigmatism induced by the toric posterior surface. It is important to understand that a contact lens with a posterior toric surface is prescribed to deal with the problem of the unstable physical fit of aspheric lens. Improved optical correction usually requires a toric anterior contact lens surface.

- The cylinder of the posterior surface coincides with the toric shape of the cornea.
- The cylinder of the anterior surface is used to correct the residual astigmatism and any astigmatism induced by the toric posterior lens surface.

A bitoric contact lens is most often used when there is more than 2.00 D of corneal toricity and a similar amount of refractive astigmatism that cannot be adequately corrected with a spherical rigid contact lens.

There are two categories of bitoric contact lenses:

1. Spherical power effect: toricity on the front surface of the lens negates the toricity of the posterior lens surface. This lens produces a constant optical correction regardless of rotational position on the eye.
2. Cylindrical power effect: toricity on the front surface of this lens is not balanced by the posterior lens toricity. As a result, this lens produces variable refractive power as it rotates on the eye.

The power of a bitoric contact lens can be calculated from the refraction and keratometry values. To simplify the process, use an optical cross diagram to calculate lens power and curvature for each meridian separately.

Example

Refraction: $-1.00 \ -4.00 \times 180°$
Keratometry: $43.00 @ 180°/47.00 @ 90°$

1. The lens power of the horizontal meridian is equal to the spherical power (-1.00 D).
2. Add the spherical and cylindrical power to determine the total lens power in the vertical meridian (-5.00 D).
3. The corneal powers from keratometry are put on the correct meridians of the optical cross.

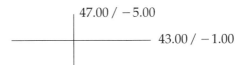

Make a vertex correction for the vertical meridian, so -5.00 D becomes -4.75 D in the contact lens plane.

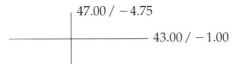

To improve the fit, the steeper meridian is flattened by 1.00 D, and the flat meridian is flattened by 0.25 D. In the steep meridian, the base curve of 47.00 D becomes 46.00 D. This will create a 1.00-D tear lens, and the lens power should be adjusted by the same amount to −3.75 D. Similarly, the base curve of the flatter meridian becomes 42.75 D, and the power adjusts to −0.75 D.

$$46.00 / -3.75$$

$$42.75 / -0.75$$

It is not necessary to specify the axis, for two reasons. First, the lens will naturally tend to align with the correct meridians. Second, if the posterior lens toricity matches the anterior lens toricity, then the lens will produce the same power on the eye regardless of lens rotation. This is called a spherical power effect lens. It is important to inform the laboratory that the power was calculated by the above methods to ensure correct fulfillment of the lens order.

The final lens base curve and power parameters are:
42.75/−0.75   46.00/−3.75

When the final lens is placed on the patient, it is possible to find significant residual astigmatism. First, confirm that the refraction and keratometry values are correct. Next, verify that the lens returned from the laboratory as ordered. Residual astigmatism that cannot be explained by adjustments to any of these measurements can be compensated by changing the lens power. After the lens has stabilized on the patient's eye, confirm that the fit is adequate or consider making adjustments to the posterior lens curvature. If the physical fit is acceptable, perform a sphero-cylindrical overrefraction and adjust the contact lens prescription based on these measurements.

12. What is the indication for a rigid gas permeable bitoric contact lens with prism ballast?

This type of lens is most commonly used when a cylindrical power effect lens is required to correct moderate residual astigmatism with moderate corneal toricity. The base curve and the power are determined as described for a bitoric contact lens. A prism ballast of 0.50 to 1.00 Δ is added to reduce rotation of the lens. It is important to communicate clearly with the contact lens laboratory about lens parameters and the correct location of the prism ballast.

13. When is a hydrophilic toric lens indicated?

Toric soft contact lenses can provide better initial comfort and less risk of lens ejection compared to rigid lenses. However, lens rotation and instability can reduce the quality of vision with these lenses compared to rigid lenses. Some common indications for soft toric contact lenses are:

1. Low to moderate corneal astigmatism
2. Intolerance of rigid contact lenses
3. Residual astigmatism

Toric hydrophilic lenses are most successful for astigmatism between −1.00 and −3.00 D when the correcting cylinder is oriented at either 90° or 180°. Conventional hydrophilic toric contact lenses for the correction of high astigmatism and disposable toric hydrophilic contact lenses for the correction of low and moderate degrees of astigmatism are available.

14. When is a toric contact lens not indicated?

Toric contact lenses may not be necessary for astigmatism less than 0.75 D. Small amounts of astigmatism can often be neutralized by spherical hydrophilic contact lenses. Thicker lenses, stiffer hydrophilic lens materials, or aspheric optic designs can mask small amounts of astigmatism.

15. For the correction of moderate astigmatism, should one choose a toric hydrophilic contact lens or a spherical rigid gas permeable lens?

Patient preference, sensitivity, and visual results obtained are important factors in the choice. Remember that a spherical rigid gas permeable contact lens provides sharp vision, is easy to handle, and is more durable. Hydrophilic toric contact lenses offer greater comfort, easier fitting, and are more appropriate for use in sports. Parameters are limited for some soft toric lens designs, and vision is usually not as sharp and consistent as with glasses or rigid contact lenses.

16. What designs are available in toric hydrophilic contact lenses?

There are many lens polymers, replacement schedules, and care systems available for soft toric contact lenses. However, there are only two general categories of hydrophilic toric contact lens designs:

1. Hydrophilic contact lens with a front toric surface
2. Hydrophilic contact lens with a back toric surface

Soft toric contact lenses are stabilized and kept from rotating on the eye by prism ballast or by tapered thin zones. The most common soft toric lens type is a back surface toric with prism ballast stabilization. Lens orientation is indicated by marks placed on the lens by the manufacturer. These marks or guides are most often located at the 6 o'clock position; however, some manufacturers place these marks in the 3 o'clock and 9 o'clock positions. The rotation of these marks quantifies the magnitude of lens rotation on the eye. Both conventional and disposable hydrophilic toric lenses are available for either daily or prolonged use. The most common markings are show below in Figure 11.6.

17. What are the techniques for stabilizing toric hydrophilic contact lenses?

Techniques are the same as those used for stabilization of rigid toric contact lenses. They maintain the cylinder axis in the necessary position and inhibit rotation of the contact lens.[4,5]

Contact Lens with Prism Ballast

As with rigid gas permeable contact lenses, prism ballast can be used as a weight to help provide rotational stability and reorientation of the lens.

Truncated Contact Lenses

Truncated hydrophilic toric contact lenses are relatively rare. The truncated edge of the lens stabilizes the lens by resting against the lower lid margin.

Beveled Contact Lenses

Contact Lenses with Tapered Superior and Inferior Peripheral Zones

Thin zones are designed to rest underneath the palpebral margin while the thicker portion of the lens fits in the interpalpebral region. Rotated lenses are reoriented as lid pressure against the lens squeezes the lens into the correct position.

Contact Lenses with a Back Toric Surface

Posterior lens toricity is less effective for providing rotational stability with hydrophilic toric contact lenses. Because the soft lens conforms to the corneal contour, a bitoric lens design is not necessary.

Combined Methods

The preceding techniques can be used in combination to maximize lens stability.

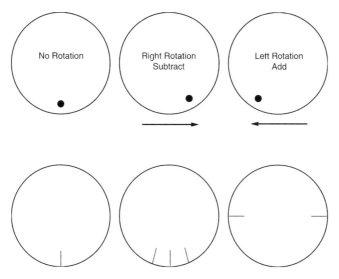

Figure 11.6. Rotational markings on contact lenses.

18. What are the methods of fitting toric hydrophilic contact lenses?

Fitting with Trial Lenses

The best method for fitting a hydrophilic toric contact lens is to use a trial lens fitting set, which minimizes the patient's fitting time by reducing the number of additional visits required for lens adjustments.[6] The most useful information that comes from trial fitting concerns lens stability.

Fitting Without a Trial Lens

1. Determine the fitting parameters from the patient's spectacle prescription.
2. Select an appropriate base curve to achieve an acceptable physical fit.
3. Round the spectacle prescription to the nearest increment available from the contact lens manufacturer. Next, account for the most likely amount and direction of lens rotation.
   OD—Subtract 5° to 10° from the cylinder axis of the glasses.
   OS—Add 5° to 10° to the cylinder of the glasses.
4. Determine the spherical contact lens power from the spherical power of the spectacle refraction. Correct for vertex distance.
5. Select a cylindrical power equal to or less than the spectacle cylinder power.

19. How is a toric hydrophilic contact lens fit using a trial set?

Trial fitting is the best approach to fitting toric soft contact lenses and greatly improves the chances for initial success.

Trial Lens Selection

1. Lenses are usually available in three base curves. Select the average base curve to begin.
2. Larger diameters help improve centration of the contact lens on the cornea. Use a lens with a diameter 2.0 to 2.5 mm greater than the diameter of the visible iris. Most lenses will range from 14.0 to 14.5 mm in diameter.
3. Use the trial lens sphere power closest to the patient's prescription.
4. The cylinder power should be equal to or less than that of the spectacle prescription.

Trial Lens Evaluation

1. Place the hydrophilic toric lens on the patient's eye and wait 15 to 20 minutes until the contact lens and tear production has stabilized.
2. Evaluate the fit using the same criteria as for spherical hydrophilic contact lenses, taking into account comfort, centration, complete coverage of the cornea, and movement (when very mobile, tighten the base curve, and when immobile, flatten the base curve).
3. The rotational stability should be verified after a good fit is obtained. Evaluate stability of the contact lens on the cornea at the slit lamp, using the guide marks. Take note of the position of the marks, the direction of rotation, and the quantity of the rotation in degrees. Remember that one clock-hour equals 30° of rotation.
   - If the lens rotates clockwise, the degree of rotation should be added to the intended cylinder axis.
   - If the lens rotates counterclockwise, the degree of rotation should be subtracted from the intended cylinder axis.
4. A spherical overrefraction determines the correct combined sphere power.
5. Consider these comments on lens stability:
   - A large diameter lens contributes to improvement of centration.
   - Toric hydrophilic lenses should be fitted slightly more tightly than spherical hydrophilic lenses.
   - A normal blink should improve stability of the lens and increase the chances of success.
   - Dry eyes and lid pathology such as giant papillary conjunctivitis may cause lenses to move excessively or rotate abnormally.

20. What is the final prescription of a toric hydrophilic contact lens?

Base Curve

The base curve is the same as the trial lens's base curve.

Power

1. The spherical power of the trial hydrophilic toric lens is added to the spherical power of the overrefraction, corrected for vertex distance if necessary.
2. The cylinder is the same as the trial lens.

Cylinder Axis

When a contact lens is not stable on the cornea, add or subtract power depending on the direction of rotation relative to the axis of cylinder of the spectacle correction.

With moderate to high cylindrical powers, lens rotation can result in a large sphero-cylindrical overrefraction. If this occurs, performing a complete sphero-cylindrical overrefraction helps determine the magnitude of any residual astigmatism. This information can be combined with the original refraction and trial contact lens powers to determine the final contact lens parameters. Calculating the resultant power of two crossed sphero-cylinder lenses requires a vector calculation. This can be programmed into a lens calculator or may be provided by the contact lens manufacturer's customer support.

References

1. Mandell RB. *Contact Lens Practice,* 4th ed. Springfield, II: Charles C. Thomas, 1988:xiii, 1025.
2. Harris MG, Gale B, Gansel K, et al. Flexure and residual astigmatism with paraperm O_2 and Boston II lenses on toric corneas. *Am J Optom Physiol Opt.* 1987;64:269–273.
3. Edrington T, Stewart B, Woodfield D. Toric base curve rotation on toric corneas. *J Am Optom Assoc.* 1989;60:162.
4. Remba MJ. Clinical evaluation of FDA approved toric hydrophilic soft contact lenses (part I). *J Am Optom Assoc.* 1979;50:289–293.
5. Remba MJ. Part II. Clinical evaluation of toric hydrophilic contact lenses. *J Am Optom Assoc.* 1981;52:211–221.
6. Szczotka LB, Roberts C, Herderick EE, et al. Quantitative descriptors of corneal topography that influence soft toric contact lens fitting. *Cornea* 2002;21: 249–255.

Selected Readings

Donshik PC, et al. Adaptação básica de lentes de contato tóricas hidrofílicas e rígidas. In *CLAO*, Nova Orleans, Luciana, 1993.

Gassett AR. *Contact Lenses and Corneal Disease: A Programmed Course.* New York: Appleton-Century-Crofts, 1976.

Kastl PR Johnson WC. Fluoropern extended wear R.G.P. contact lenses, II. Front toric fitting. *CLAO J.* 1990; 16–53.

Key JE, et al. Astigmatism and toric lenses. In: *The CLAO Pocket Guide to Contact Lens Fitting.* New York: Kellner McCaffery Associates, 1994:42–56.

Maltzman BA, Constad WH. Correction of astigmatism, with rigid lenses in contact lenses. In: Kastl PR, ed. *The CLAO Guide to Basic Science and Clinical Practice,* 2nd ed. Iowa: Kendall/Hunt Publishing, 1995:11–86.

Maltzman BA, Koeniger E, Dabezies OH Jr. Correction of astigmatism: hard lenses–soft lenses. In: Dabezies OH Jr, ed. *The CLAO Guide to Basic Science and Clinical Practice.* Orlando: Grune & Stratton, 1984:50–51.

Maltzman BA, Rengel A. Soft toric lenses: correcting cylinder greater than sphere. *CLAO J.* 1989; 15:196.

12

Presbyopia and Contact Lenses

Muriel Schornack, Cleusa Coral-Ghanem, and Ari de Souza Pena

1. Can contact lenses correct presbyopic refractive error?

Many presbyopic patients, especially those who are not accustomed to wearing spectacles, are interested in contact lens correction of their refractive error. There are a variety of ways to correct presbyopic refractive error with contact lenses. Options for contact lens correction of presbyopia can be divided into three main categories: supplemental spectacle correction over contact lenses, monovision, and multifocal contact lenses. Each of these options has advantages and disadvantages. The patient's individual priorities and visual demands can help decide which option to pursue.

Supplemental spectacle correction, in the form of either reading glasses over full distance correction in contact lenses or distance spectacles over near contact lens correction, may provide the clearest vision at all distances. However, this mode of correction requires removal and replacement of spectacles for visual tasks at various distances and may not be the most convenient for the patient. Monovision (prescription of additional plus for one eye) is very convenient but can cause a decrease in binocularity.

Multifocal lenses can be divided into two types: translating and simultaneous vision designs. Translating multifocal lenses (segmented or concentric designs) are made of rigid gas permeable materials. Though translating multifocals provide very clear distance and near vision, patients may initially notice more lid sensation with these lenses than with single vision designs. Simultaneous vision lenses (concentric, aspheric, or diffraction designs) are available in both rigid gas permeable and hydrogel materials. These lenses are as comfortable as single vision lenses, but patients may report decreased visual acuity with them. The initial interview with the patient helps determine particular visual demands and priorities, and promotes the selection of a modality that best meets the patient's needs.

The amount of add power needed by the patient is important in selecting an appropriate modality. Thus, it is useful to divide presbyopia into three stages: early, moderate, and advanced (Table 12.1).

2. What is monovision?

Monovision is the correction of one eye for distance vision and the other eye for near tasks. This method of presbyopic correction is extremely flexible and can be used with spherical or toric hydrogel lenses or rigid gas permeable lenses. The technique can even be modified to incorporate multifocal correction in one eye and single vision correction in the other. Most patients tolerate monovision reasonably well. Success rates of 70% to 80% have been reported.[12] The patient's success with monovision ultimately depends on his or her ability to suppress a central, out-of-focus image in one eye while maintaining peripheral fusion. Many patients seem to have less difficulty suppressing a blurred image from one eye than adjusting to the superimposed images created in each eye by simultaneous vision lenses.

3. How do you fit a patient with monovision contact lenses?

1. Determine the patient's balanced distance correction and an appropriate add power.
2. Determine the patient's dominant eye.
3. Fully correct the distance refractive error in the patient's dominant eye. Choose a lens that adequately corrects near vision for the non-dominant eye.
4. Adjust the power in 0.25-D increments to maximize visual performance.

Monovision is easily demonstrated. Simply hold up a loose plus lens over the nondominant eye, and allow the patient to alternately look at

Table 12.1. Options for correction of presbyopia with contact lenses

Stage of presbyopia	Technique
Early (+0.75 add)	Refractive compensation
Early and moderate (+0.75 to +1.50 add)	Monovision
Early, moderate, and advanced (any add)	Bifocal/multifocal contact lenses
Moderate and advanced (+1.50 to +2.50 add)	Modified monovision
Individuals unable to adapt to the cited techniques	Single vision contact lenses, with supplemental spectacle correction

distant and near objects. Initially, the patient may be most comfortable if the imbalance between the two eyes is minimized. Even if the refraction indicates that a patient needs a +1.25 add to achieve 20/20 acuity at near, he or she may need only +0.75 or +1.00 over the distance correction to meet the general near visual demand. Most patients can eventually tolerate a reduction in distance acuity to 20/60 or 20/70 in the near eye. This corresponds to an add of approximately +1.75 D. More than 2.00 D of undercorrection in the near eye may lead to asthenopia due to a loss of stereopsis.

Prescribe spectacles with full distance correction in both eyes and the appropriate add for prolonged, detailed visual tasks. Also consider prescribing "driving glasses" (spectacle correction to fully correct distance refractive error in the "near" eye) or an extra contact lens for the near eye that fully corrects distance refractive error, particularly if the patient's distance acuity is less than 20/40 in the "near" eye. Most contact lenses are very stable on the surface of the eye, but a monovision patient could have difficulty if the lens that corrects distance refractive error becomes dislodged for any reason while driving. Warn beginning monovision wearers that their depth perception may initially be reduced and instruct them to take extra care when driving.[3]

In general, a patient is most comfortable when his or her dominant eye is corrected for distant visual tasks.[2] However, there are some exceptions to this rule. If patients spend a majority of their time on detailed near tasks, they may prefer to use the dominant eye for near work. Individuals who have better visual acuity in one eye generally prefer this eye for the distance correction. For example, a spherical hydrogel contact wearer with unilateral astigmatism will probably prefer to use the eye without astigmatic refractive error for distance tasks.

4. What are the advantages and disadvantages of monovision correction?

Advantages

1. Easily demonstrated.
   - To show a patient how monovision works, simply hold a plus lens over one eye while the patient is wearing full distance correction and allow him to look at both distant and near objects binocularly.
2. Considerable flexibility.
   - Any single vision lenses can be used in monovision correction. If the patient finds the distance acuity compromise with single vision lenses unacceptable, a multifocal lens can be used for the "near" eye.
3. Relatively low cost.
   - Because single vision lenses are most frequently used, this method of correction costs no more than wearing full distance correction.

Disadvantages

1. Loss of stereopsis. Monovision decreases fine stereoacuity.[45] Patients are most aware of this loss of depth perception immediately after

beginning monovision contact lens wear. This discomfort generally subsides as the patient's ability to preferentially suppress the image from one eye improves. Nevertheless, it is best to avoid monovision correction in individuals whose daily tasks require excellent stereoscopic vision.

2. Reduction in distance acuity. Most individuals see better when using both eyes than when using just one eye.[6] Thus, when we intentionally decrease the distance acuity in one eye, patients frequently report that their vision does not seem as clear as it was with full distance correction in both eyes. Again, most patients adjust to this within a few weeks of monovision wear. Because of this, however, monovision should be avoided in individuals who require excellent distance acuity in both eyes, such as professional drivers and aviators.

3. Difficulty with night driving. In low ambient illumination, the pupils dilate. This increases spherical aberration. Lack of visual contrast can increase image confusion, especially when one eye is not corrected accurately for distance. As discussed above, patients may benefit from a pair of glasses that brings the undercorrected eye to 20/20 distance acuity, or by having a third contact lens (or lenses) with full distance correction for the habitual near eye.

4. Reduction of contrast sensitivity. The decrease in contrast sensitivity is similar to that encountered in bifocal contact lens users with bilateral simultaneous vision.[7]

5. What are the favorable and unfavorable factors for success in monovision contact lens correction?

Favorable Factors

- Patients who have historically accepted less-than-optimal distance correction typically have little difficulty adjusting to monovision's compromise in acuity. For example, if patients have been satisfied with 20/25 spectacle acuity in each eye, they may not even notice the slight decrease in acuity caused by monovision correction.

- Emerging presbyopes are good candidates for monovision. Because the difference between their distance and near correction is small, the disparity between the two eyes is minimized. The near visual complaints can often be addressed with as little as +0.75 over the "near" eye. This would minimally impact distance acuity and stereopsis.

- Individuals whose near visual demands are not primarily in downgaze, such as computer users, will appreciate the clear vision in any field of gaze with monovision contact lenses.

- Patients with well-developed suppression patterns are good candidates for monovision. For example, an asymptomatic intermittent alternating exotrope's visual system has already developed the ability to suppress one eye's image to avoid diplopia. It would not be difficult for this individual to learn to suppress the out-of-focus image.

Unfavorable Factors

- Patients who demand superb distance acuity are not ideal monovision candidates. Spectacle correction over contact lenses may be a better option for the patient who has historically been very sensitive to minimal changes in contact lens or spectacle correction.
- Mature presbyopes who have not previously worn monovision may not do well with this form of correction. If a 65-year-old spectacle-corrected myope decides that he would like to try monovision contact lenses for the first time, the disparity between the two images may be overwhelming. On the other hand, a mature presbyope who began wearing monovision correction early in the process of presbyopic development may be able to tolerate gradual increases in image disparity with increasing add powers.
- Some patients are able to demonstrate significantly better acuity binocularly compared to monocularly. These individuals may struggle with the 20/20 line during monocular testing and easily read the 20/15 line when allowed to use both eyes. Because of the strength of their binocular visual system, they are not ideal candidates for monovision.

6. What types of bifocal/multifocal contact lenses are available?

Bifocal/multifocal contact lenses are available in both rigid gas permeable and hydrogel designs. Several hydrogel multifocal lenses are now available as frequent replacement lenses, and a number of additional disposable hydrogel designs are currently in development. Bifocal/multifocal lenses fall into two broad categories:

1. Translating designs, by means of either segmented (Figure 12.1) or concentric (Figure 12.2) lenses.

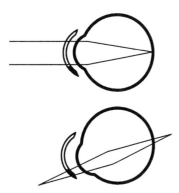

Figure 12.1. Bifocal contact lens with segmented design.

2. Simultaneous image, by means of concentric (Figure 12.2 and 12.3), aspheric (Figure 12.4A and B), or diffraction-based (Figure 12.5A and B) designs.

7. How do "simultaneous image" contact lenses work?

Simultaneous image bifocal contact lenses focus images of both far and near objects on the retina at the same time. When the patient looks at

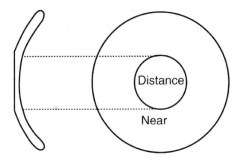

Figure 12.2. Bifocal contact lens with concentric design.

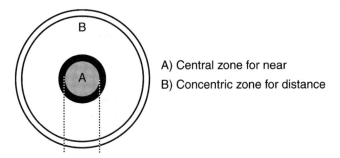

A) Central zone for near
B) Concentric zone for distance

Figure 12.3. Bifocal contact lens with concentric design for simultaneous images.

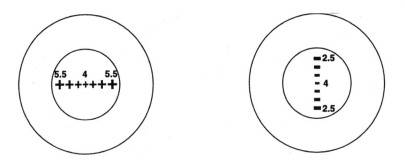

Figure 12.4. A: Multifocal contact lens with an aspheric design and positive power. B: Multifocal contact lens with an aspheric design and negative power.

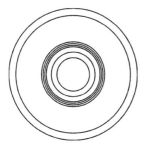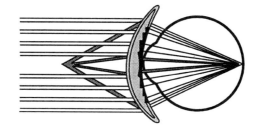

Figure 12.5. A: Bifocal contact lens with diffraction design (frontal). B: Bifocal contact lens with diffraction design (profile).

a distant object, light from that object passing through the distance portion of the contact lens focuses a clear image on the macula. Light from the distant object also passes through the near correction zone and forms an image in front of the retina. This image appears blurred and is superimposed on the clear image. When the patient focuses on near objects, light that passes through the near correction zone of the lens is focused on the retina, and light rays passing through the distance correction focus behind the retina. The contact lens wearer may be bothered by the "shadows" or "ghost images" (superimposed blurred images) around clear central images when looking at both distant and near visual targets. As in monovision, visual adaptation occurs with time. Patients who continue to wear the lenses in spite of the initial visual disturbance report a decrease in visual symptoms within the first several weeks.

8. What are the major categories of simultaneous image contact lens designs?

Simultaneous image lenses can be categorized into three basic types: concentric design, aspheric design, and diffraction-based design. Each design uses a different method of providing both distance and near correction, but all three simultaneously focus light entering the eye at various points in relation to the retina. Simultaneous image designs are available in both rigid gas permeable and hydrogel materials.

9. What are the defining characteristics of concentric simultaneous vision lenses?

Concentric simultaneous vision lenses have well-defined zones of correction for various distances arranged in a bull's-eye pattern. The lenses can have either the distance or near correction in the center of the lens. Some lenses also incorporate zones of correction for intermediate distances. The presence of distinct zones of correction for various distances is the defining characteristic of lenses with this design.

The AcuVue Bifocal™ (Vistakon), a lens designed for 1- to 2-week replacement, incorporates this design. AcuVue Bifocal™ lenses feature distance correction in the central zone with four additional alternating concentric rings of near and distance correction. The design, with its multiple correction zones for both distant and near tasks, attempts to minimize visual compromise in dim illumination. The Horizon 55 Bi-Con™ (Westcon) is a conventional (annual replacement) hydrogel lens with a central near zone with a peripheral distance correction zone. The Lifestyle MV2™ (Lifestyle Company) is a monthly replacement hydrogel lens. This lens incorporates a concentric design with a central zone for intermediate vision combined with either peripheral distance correction or peripheral near correction. Generally, a lens with peripheral distance correction is placed on the patient's dominant eye, while a lens with peripheral near correction is placed on the nondominant eye. Computer users and others who have specific intermediate visual demands may appreciate the central zone of correction for their primary visual tasks.

10. What factors must be considered when fitting concentric bifocal lenses?

Adequate pupil size is essential for success in fitting any lens with a concentric design. If the pupil is too small, light passing through more peripheral correction zones may not be able to enter the eye. If the pupil is too large, the patient may notice more ghosting as light passing through the peripheral zones of the lens focuses in front of or behind the retina. Consider a patient with 3-mm pupils. The patient should be able to read well with a concentric design with central near correction. However, the patient would probably report unsatisfactory distance vision with this lens, because the small pupil size would keep light from passing through the peripheral distance correction zone from entering the eye. If we fit a lens with a central distance correction zone, the patient's distance vision would improve, but he or she would not be able read comfortably. A patient with 7-mm pupils will experience more image confusion with either distance center or near center designs because the large pupil will continuously allow light from both zones to enter the eye.

The lenses also need to center well and move minimally to avoid fluctuations in vision. Some concentric designs allow the contact lens fitter to specify the size of the central zone to maximize visual acuity and minimize ghosting.

11. What are the defining characteristics of aspheric simultaneous vision lenses?

Contact lenses with an aspheric design are also called multifocals. The gradual flattening of curvature from the center to the periphery of the lens accompanies progressive power change. This progressive power change resembles the power change present in progressive addition spectacle lenses. Aspheric lenses with both distance and near central zones of correction are available.

Focus Progressives™ (CIBA) are aspheric lenses and are available as either 2- to 4-week replacement or single use disposable lenses. These lenses have a concentrated central zone of near correction surrounded by progressively increasing distance correction. SofLens Multifocals (Bausch and Lomb) are also aspheric lenses with near central correction. These lenses are available as 2- to 4-week replacement lenses, and they allow the clinician to specify either low or high add power. Frequency 55 Multifocals™ (CooperVision) are available as monthly replacement lenses. Like the MV2™, this lens system features two designs: one with central distance correction and the other with central near correction. Rigid gas permeable aspheric multifocals are also available. Examples include the Unilens™ (Unilens Corp.) and the Essential RGP Multifocal™ (Blanchard Contact Lens).

12. What factors must be considered when fitting aspheric simultaneous image contact lenses?

Concentric and aspheric multifocal contact lenses all use the same basic optical principles; light is focused differently through central and peripheral zones of the lens. Thus, pupil size and lens centration are very important factors to consider when fitting aspheric simultaneous image lenses.

Because aspheric lenses flatten toward the periphery, the proper fit for a back-surface aspheric rigid gas permeable lens requires a base curve that is steeper than one would expect based on keratometry readings. It is possible to order these lenses based on the patient's refractive error and keratometry readings, but the evaluation of the performance of trial lenses enhances success. Most trial sets include fitting guidelines for the specific designs, and these guidelines provide an excellent starting point for the contact lens fit.

Aspheric lenses correct vision at a range of working distances, just like progressive addition spectacle lenses. Patients with a fair amount of intermediate work may therefore prefer aspheric lenses to concentric designs.

13. What are the defining characteristics of diffractive simultaneous vision lenses?

Diffraction of light occurs when light waves interact with obstacles. This interaction changes the trajectory of the light rays. Diffraction bifocal contact lenses utilize this optical principle by incorporating a diffraction plate (a series of concentric ridges) into the center of the lens. Differences between the curvature of the front and back of the contact lens correct distance refractive error, and the plate diffracts light to provide the additional correction necessary for near tasks. Thus, these lenses use both refraction and diffraction to provide good vision at all distances.

The Hydron Echelon™ (Ocular Sciences, Inc.) is the only hydrogel lens that uses this design. Unfortunately, the lens is not available as a planned replacement lens. Patients also report "ghosting" of images with this lens. Furthermore, clear vision heavily depends on excellent illumination, because much light is diffused as it passes through the diffraction plate. Good vision is not as dependent on pupil size as in other simultaneous vision lenses because all light passing through the diffraction plate contributes to images of both distant and near objects. The lenses have not been widely used because of the limited range of parameters available, conventional (annual replacement) use, and patient reports of poor contrast sensitivity in anything but perfect illumination.

14. What is modified monovision?

There are two types of modified monovision:

1. Modified monovision I utilizes bifocal or multifocal contact lenses for both eyes. The dominant eye is more fully corrected for distance, and the nondominant eye is more fully corrected for near tasks.
2. Modified monovision II utilizes a single vision lens that fully corrects distance refractive error in the dominant eye, and a simultaneous vision bifocal contact lens in the nondominant eye.

15. What are the advantages and disadvantages of simultaneous image lenses?

Advantages

- Ease in fitting. Each brand of hydrogel simultaneous image lenses has a specified range of parameters. With available diagnostic trial lens sets, it is easy to see whether the lenses will work for a given patient. For example, if a patient is interested in AcuVue Bifocals™, trial lenses can be inserted. Because AcuVue Bifocals are available in a single base curve, whether the lenses will provide an adequate fit can be determined quickly. If the lenses move, cover, and center well, the power can be adjusted. If the fit is not acceptable, another option can be considered.
- Good comfort. Patients who have worn single vision contact lenses (either hydrogel or rigid gas permeable) will notice little difference between the comfort of their single vision lenses and simultaneous vision lenses. With the introduction of the frequent replacement hydrogel bifocal lenses, hydrogel wearers can continue to enjoy the comfort and health benefits of disposable lenses.
- Acceptable intermediate vision. Aspheric lenses provide some correction for intermediate visual tasks. Some concentric designs, such as the MV2™, also provide intermediate correction. Simultaneous vision lenses can be used in modified monovision to provide even better intermediate clarity.

Disadvantages

- "Ghost" images. All simultaneous vision lenses work by focusing light in various planes parallel to the retina. Therefore, it is impossible to completely eliminate the blurred image that is perceived along with the clear image of the object of regard. Reassure patients that their awareness of the "ghost" images will fade with time.
- Dependence on pupil size. As discussed above, the quality of the patient's vision will be reduced if pupils are either too large or too small. Simultaneous vision lenses may not be the best choice for the blue-eyed patient with 7-mm pupils in normal room illumination or for the 68-year-old with 3-mm pupils in a dark room.
- Fitting requirements. Because good vision depends on excellent centration and little movement, these lenses are frequently fitted rather tightly. Undesirable physiologic effects, such as limbal vascular congestion or edema, may ensue.
- Limited add power available. As with monovision, visual disturbances (halos, glare, ghost images) increase as add power increases. Mature presbyopes may have difficulty adjusting to these symptoms.

16. What are the favorable and unfavorable factors for success in simultaneous image contact lens wear?

Favorable factors

- Patients with realistic visual expectations are more likely to wear simultaneous vision lenses successfully. Before beginning the fitting process, make sure that the patient understands that contact lenses cannot restore pre-presbyopic vision. A successful bifocal contact lens fit is one in which the visual needs of the patient are met. This may mean that distance vision is not as clear as with single vision distance correction. A successful bifocal contact lens fit may not provide equal acuity in both eyes; in some cases, a modified monovision technique must be employed.
- Patients who are highly motivated to wear contact lenses are more likely to succeed with simultaneous vision lenses. Adjusting the design and power of the lenses to maximize visual performance takes more time than fitting single vision lenses. Motivated patients are more likely to complete the process.
- Spherical hydrogel multifocals work best for patients with minimal astigmatic refractive error. Patients with more than 0.75 D of astigmatism should consider rigid gas permeable lenses, multifocal toric hydrogels, or monovision.
- The use of diagnostic trial lenses during the initial fitting visit allows the contact lens fitter to observe the performance of the contact lens on the eye and the visual response of the patient. Diagnostic lenses also allow the patient to experience the vision provided by these lenses and to develop realistic expectations for final visual acuity.

- Spending a few minutes educating the patient on what to expect with initial simultaneous vision lens wear will assure the patient that the novel ocular and visual sensations experienced are normal and may encourage wearing the lenses throughout the adaptation period.

Unfavorable Factors

- As in monovision, patients need to be willing to accept an incremental decrease in distance acuity. Patients who demand excellent vision at all distances will not do well with simultaneous vision lenses.
- Patients with unusually large or small pupils may find that simultaneous lenses do not meet their visual needs. Those with large pupils are likely to notice more image confusion, while those with small pupils may not be able to utilize all correction zones within the lens.
- Patients who have tried unsuccessfully to wear single vision contact lenses in the past are generally not good candidates for simultaneous vision lenses. These lenses are no more comfortable than single vision lenses; they require the same amount of care, and they do not provide perfectly clear vision at all distances.
- Mature presbyopes may find that simultaneous vision lenses do not adequately correct for near visual demands without reducing distance acuity to an unacceptable level.

17. How do translating bifocal contact lenses work?

Alternating contact lens designs provide better acuity at both distance and near than either monovision or simultaneous designs. Most patients are familiar with lined bifocal or trifocal spectacle lenses and can easily understand how alternating designs work.

In the segmented bifocal contact lens, the superior portion of the lens corrects the patient's distance refractive error, while the inferior segment corrects the patient's near vision. Ideally, the lenses rest on the patient's lower lids. When the patient looks straight ahead, the distance correction is positioned in front of the pupil. When the patient looks down, the lower lids push the contact lens upward and the near correction is aligned with the pupil.

Most alternating bifocals are made of rigid gas permeable materials. Rigid lenses are designed to move up to several millimeters with each blink, so translation of the lens with changes in position of gaze is easy to achieve with these lenses. A variety of rigid gas permeable designs are available, including the Tangent Streak Bifocal™ (Fused Contacts of Missouri), Presbylite Translating Bifocal™ (Lens Dynamics), Bi-Seg™ (Precision Optics), and X-Cel Solution™ (X-Cel Contacts). Hydrophilic alternating bifocal contact lenses are available but have not been widely used. Because hydrogel lenses move much less than rigid gas permeable lenses, contact lens manufacturers have had difficulty designing a soft lens that translates adequately when the patient looks down to read. Examples of hydrogel alternating bifocal lenses include the

CoSoft 55 Crescent Bifocal™ (California Optics) and the UCL Bifocal™ (United Contact Lenses).

18. How do you fit a patient with translating bifocal contact lenses?

Translating bifocal contact lenses have a reputation of being difficult to fit. Certainly there are a number of parameters that need to be determined during a translating bifocal fit. Physiologic factors, such as tear film quantity and quality, lid tension, lower lid position, and corneal astigmatism, must be considered during the fitting process.

The goal in translating bifocal fitting is to find a lens that provides clear distance and near vision, demonstrates rapid and predictable vertical translation with changes in eye position and with blinking, and maintains good corneal health. Trial lens fitting is strongly recommended. Choose a trial lens with a slightly flatter base curve and larger diameter than would be selected if fitting a single vision lens. Perform a spherical overrefraction with loose lenses for both distance and near power. Evaluate the lens's movement: the lens should move up with each blink but should drop rapidly back into position following the blink. Lens position is also important. The segment for reading correction should consistently position inferiorly. Some nasal rotation of the segment may be acceptable, but temporal rotation may move the segment away from the pupil in downgaze. The upper edge of the segment should be located near the pupillary margin in primary gaze. At follow-up examinations, check for nasal and temporal corneal epithelial compromise. If staining is noted, the edge design of the lens may need to be altered.

19. What are the advantages and disadvantages of translating bifocal contact lenses?

Advantages

- Clear distance and near vision. When appropriately fitted, translating bifocal contact lenses provide exceptional clarity for distant and near tasks.
- No disruption of binocular vision. Because the upper portions of both lenses correct the patient for distant tasks and the lower portions of both lenses provide correction for near tasks, stereopsis is not compromised.
- Availability of high add powers. The amount of add power incorporated into the lower portion of the lens can be exactly specified. Because the lens does not attempt to correct distance and near vision simultaneously, high add powers do not negatively affect distance vision.
- Visual and physiologic benefits of rigid gas permeable lenses. Rigid gas permeable lenses provide accurate and stable correction of re-

fractive error. Properly prescribed rigid gas permeable lenses produce little or no corneal pathology.

Disadvantages

- Initial lid sensation. Even established rigid gas permeable lens wearers may notice some additional lid sensation when first wearing translating multifocals, particularly if their single vision lenses are normally positioned under the upper lid. Prism ballast and truncation, the stabilization systems that keep the segment near the bottom of the lens, make the lower edges of the lenses thicker. Patients can be assured that this sensation abates with time.
- More complicated fitting process. Many beginning practitioners are somewhat intimidated by translating bifocal contact lens fitting. Although translating bifocals are more challenging to fit than monovision or simultaneous vision lens, one can become proficient quite quickly. Most contact lens laboratories are more than happy to help providers design translating bifocals for individual patients.

20. What are the favorable and unfavorable factors for success in translating bifocal contact lens wear?

Favorable Factors

- Current rigid gas permeable lens wearers already appreciate its crisp vision and know that the initial lens awareness is temporary.
- Patients who intend to wear the contact lenses full-time are better candidates for translating bifocals than those who intend to wear lenses infrequently. Lens awareness may be more bothersome in part-time wearers.
- Individuals who demand perfectly clear distance and near vision will appreciate the clarity provided by these lenses.
- Patience is a virtue, especially when participating in a translating bifocal contact lens fit. Both patient and practitioner should acknowledge that a number of parameters must be specified in order to provide clear vision and a good fit. The chances of ordering a lens with exactly the right parameters on the first try are small.

Unfavorable Factors

- Former rigid lens wearers who discontinued single vision contact lens use due to discomfort will find these lenses even less comfortable than their single vision lenses. Hydrogel lens wearers who flatly refuse to allow you to place a hard lens on their eyes are also poor candidates for translating bifocal contact lenses.
- Individuals with near visual demands in positions of gaze other than

downgaze will not be able to use the segment effectively. Simultaneous vision lenses or monovision would work better for such patients.

21. How should a new practitioner begin to develop presbyopic contact lens fitting skills?

The number and variety of options for presbyopic contact lens fitting can seem daunting to the new practitioner. However, the field of potential options can be narrowed by paying close attention to the patient's visual needs and priorities during the initial interview. Remember that a successful presbyopic contact lens fit is one in which patient's visual needs are met with minimal visual compromise. If a patient is satisfied with 20/40 near vision, 20/20 may not be necessary.

Creativity is essential. Sometimes, a single patient may require several different modes of correction for different visual tasks. For example, a computer programmer who enjoys trapshooting may need simultaneous vision lenses at work and distance correction with supplemental spectacles for his hobby.

Supplemental spectacle correction and monovision contact lenses require no special fitting expertise. Simultaneous vision lenses and translating multifocals are more challenging to fit, but fitting these lenses can be much more rewarding than prescribing the simpler designs. Rather than attempting to master each individual lens design, new practitioners should choose one or two lenses from each category and master those designs. Most trial lens sets include fitting suggestions, and a local optical laboratory can provide more specific fitting tips.

References

1. Gauthier CA, Holden BA, Grant T, Chong MS. Interest of presbyopes in contact lens correction and their success with monovision. *Optom Vis Sci.* 1992;69:858–862.
2. Jain S, Arora I, Azar DT. Success of monovision in presbyopies: review of the literature and potential applications to refractive surgery. *Surv Ophthalmol.* 1996;40:491–499.
3. Harris MG, Classe JG. Clinicolegal considerations of monovision. *J Am Optom Assoc.* 1988;59:491–495.
4. McGill E, Erickson P. Stereopsis in presbyopes wearing monovision and simultaneous vision bifocal contact lenses. *Am J Optom Physiol Opt.* 1988;65:619–626.
5. Back A, Grant T, Hine N. Comparative visual performance of three presbyopic contact lens corrections. *Optom Vis Sci.* 1992;69:474–480.
6. Campbell FW, Green DG. Monocular vs. binocular visual acuity. *Nature.* 1965;208:191–192.
7. Collins MJ, Brown B, Bowman KJ. Contrast sensitivity with contact lens corrections for presbyopia. *Ophthalmic Physiol Opt.* 1989;9:133–138.

Selected Readings

Bennett ES, Allee HB, eds. *Clinical Manual of Contact Lenses*. Philadelphia: JB Lippincott, 19xx.

Schwartz CA. *Specialty Contact Lenses: A Fitter's Guide*. Philadelphia: WB Saunders, 19xx.

Tyler's Quarterly Soft Contact Lens Parameter Guide, P.O. Box 250406, Little Rock, Arkansas 72225-0406. (Updated quarterly)

Color Plates

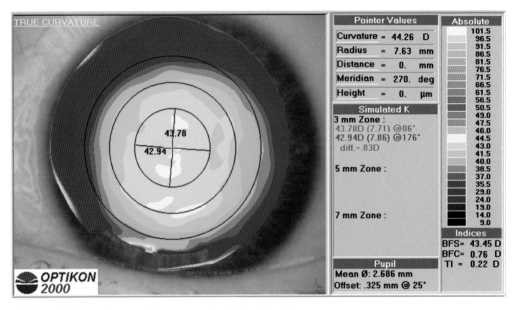

Plate 1 Normal corneal topography (Chapter 6).

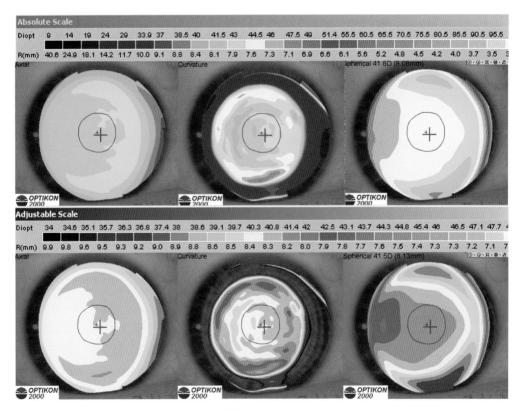

Plate 2 Corneal topography maps (Chapter 6).

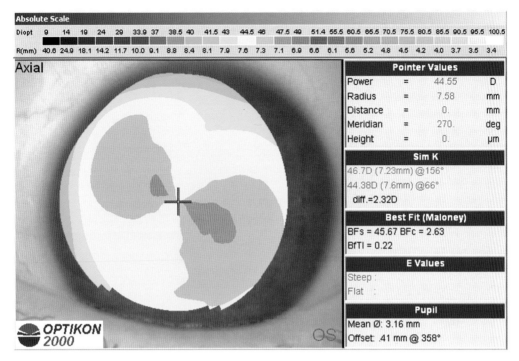

Plate 3 Bow-tie pattern of corneal astigmatism (Chapter 6).

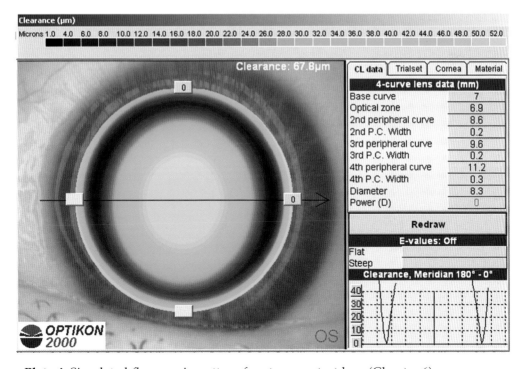

Plate 4 Simulated fluorescein pattern for steep contact lens (Chapter 6).

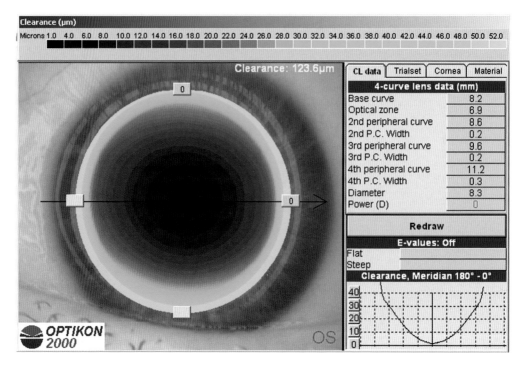

Plate 5 Simulated fluorescein pattern for flat contact lens (Chapter 6).

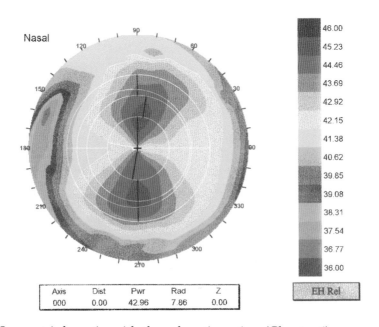

Plate 6 Symmetric bow tie, with-the-rule astigmatism (Chapter 6).

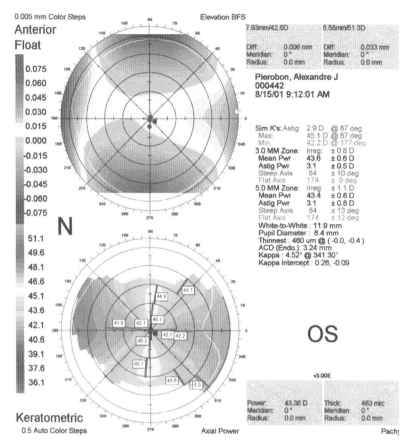

Anterior Float and Keratometric color scales with the elevation/axial power maps

Plate 7 Elevation map for with-the-rule astigmatism (Chapter 6).

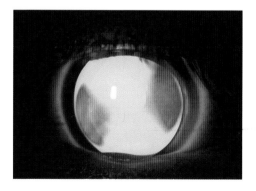

Plate 8 Fluorescein pattern in with-the-rule astigmatism demonstrating pooling of fluorescein in the vertical meridian (Chapter 6).

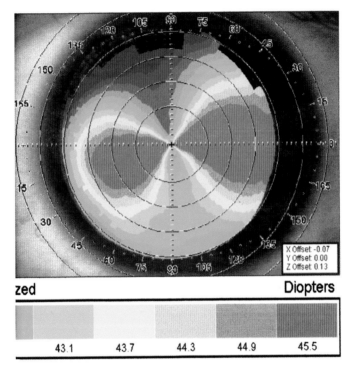

zed   Diopters

| 43.1 | 43.7 | 44.3 | 44.9 | 45.5 |

Plate 9 Bow tie, against-the-rule astigmatism (Chapter 6).

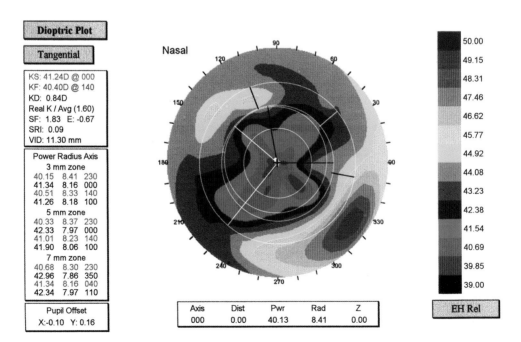

Plate 10 Curvature map, post-RK cornea (Chapter 6).

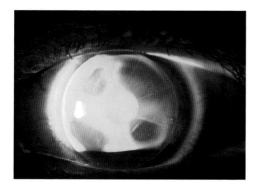

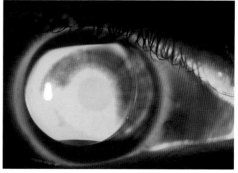

Plate 11 Fluorescein pattern in a post-RK cornea demonstrating apical pooling and mid-peripheral touch (Chapter 6).

Plate 13 Fluorescein pattern in a post-LASIK cornea demonstrating apical pooling, mid-peripheral touch, and, in this case, lens decentration with edge lift (Chapter 6).

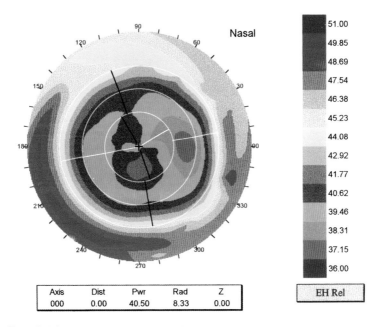

Axis	Dist	Pwr	Rad	Z
000	0.00	40.50	8.33	0.00

Plate 12 Post-LASIK curvature map demonstrating an oblate corneal curvature (Chapter 6).

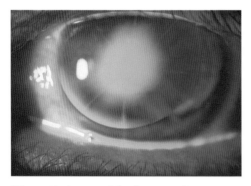

Plate 14 Acceptable fluorescein pattern of a spherical contact lens fitted on a cornea after radial keratotomy.

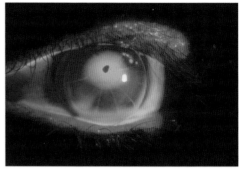

Plate 15 A central bubble is a result of a contact lens with a steep base curve and/or large optical zone. Excessive pressure in the mid-peripheral zone causes small epithelial erosions along the corneal incision lines.

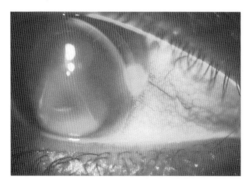

Plate 16 Inferior decentration of a contact lens (off the limbus), causing lens adhesion.

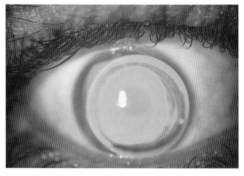

Plate 17 Acceptable fit of contact lens with a keratoconic design on an eye with corneal ectasia after LASIK. A mild three-point touch fluorescein pattern is demonstrated.

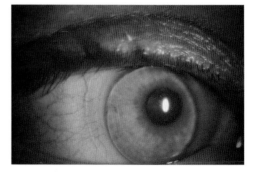

Plate 18 Piggyback system showing the combination of a high Dk RGP lens over a well-centered silicone hydrogel lens.

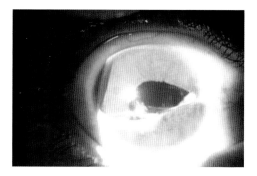

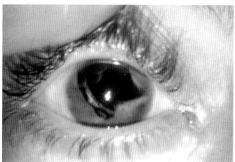

Plate 19 Healed corneal laceration and traumatic aphakia with paracentral scar across the optical axis.

Plate 20 Post-traumatic aphakia corrected with a hydrophilic aphakic contact lens.

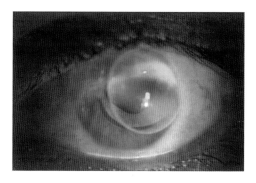

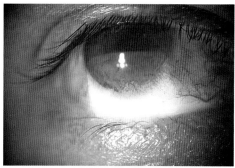

Plate 21 Post-traumatic cornea and anterior segment fit with rigid gas permeable lens. Although the lens may not have the fitting appearance customary with RGPCL fitting, comfort and function determine the adequacy of the fit.

Plate 22 Epithelial changes caused by drying of a hydrophilic lens.

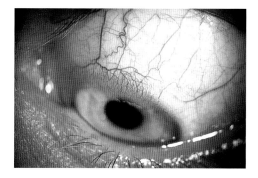

Plate 23 Superior arcuate epithelial lesion induced by a hydrophilic lens.

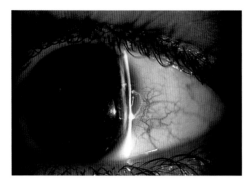

Plate 24 Dellen with use of a rigid contact lens.

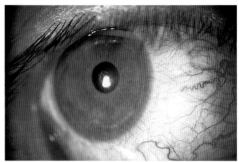

Plate 25 Neovascularization of the cornea (>2mm) from use of a hydrophilic lens.

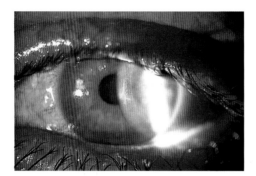

Plate 26 Pseudodendritic keratitis secondary to thimerosal and chlorhexidine.

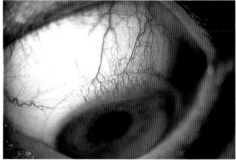

Plate 27 Soft-contact-lens-induced superior limbic keratoconjunctivitis.

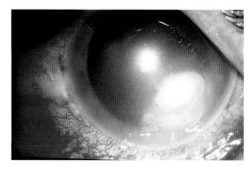

Plate 28 Pseudomonas corneal ulcer in a soft contact lens user.

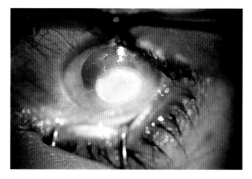

Plate 29 *Acanthamoeba* corneal ulcer.

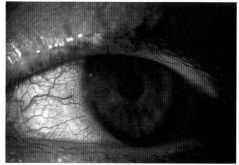

Plate 30 Subepithelial infiltrates in an acute early morning red eye.

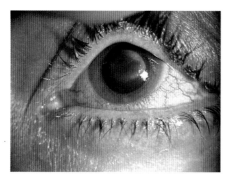

Plate 31 Ring infiltrate in a patient with an *Acanthamoeba* ulcer.

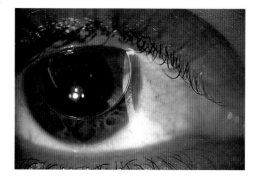

Plate 32 Peripheral corneal drying (3 and 9 syndrome, 2 +).

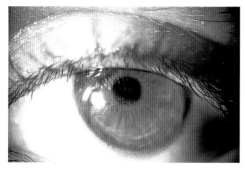

Plate 33 RGP lens adhesion with trapped debris under the lens (fixed lens syndrome).

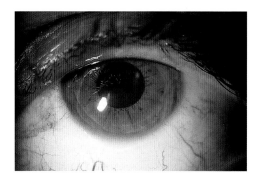

Plate 34 Corneal molding. Indentation in the cornea and conjunctiva after removal of a "stuck" lens.

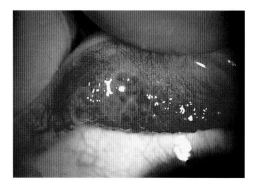

Plate 35 Soft-contact-lens-induced giant papillary conjunctivitis (GPC) with giant papillae in zones 1 and 2 of the conjunctiva.

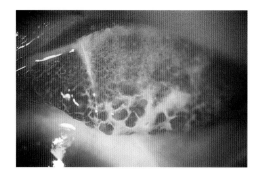

Plate 36 Giant papillary conjunctivitis (GPC). Giant papillae stained with fluorescein in zones 1 and 2 of the superior tarsal conjunctiva.

13

Contact Lens Fitting in Aphakia

Adamo Lui Netto and Jeffrey J. Walline

1. When should one fit a contact lens in aphakia and what are the advantages?

Since the advent of cataract surgery with intraocular lens implantation, the indication for contact lens fitting in aphakia occurs significantly less frequently. A contact lens is indicated when an intraocular lens implant cannot be placed in the eye. The contact lens reduces the retinal image size, diminishes the aberrations,[1] and lessens the peripheral distortion produced by glasses. This causes significantly less visual distortion and improves the quality of vision. Aphakic contact lenses are particularly indicated in monocular aphakia, due to aniseikonic symptoms experienced with spectacle wear. Due to new materials, better lens designs, and improved contact lens care solutions, aphakic patients have much more success in contact lens fitting.

Due to the improved intraocular lens designs and surgical techniques, adults are rarely fitted with contact lenses for aphakia. The primary contraindications to intraocular lenses are aniridia, chronic uveitis, endothelial compromise, and glaucoma. Aphakic children are typically fitted with contact lenses because during development their refractive error changes quickly and the visual correction may need to be changed regularly.[2]

2. When should one fit a hydrophilic lens versus a rigid gas permeable lens?

Infantile aphakia should be corrected immediately after the cataract surgery has been performed due to the high potential for amblyopia during the child's critical period of visual development. Adults do not need to be fitted as soon as infants because their visual development is complete and amblyopia will not result. In the adult, it is generally recommended to wait two months after surgery, prior to fitting, in order to achieve corneal topographic and refractive stability. Children and adults can be fitted with either hydrophilic or rigid gas permeable contact lenses,[3] so the timing of the contact lens fitting is dependent primarily on the age of the person being fitted with contact lenses.

Rigid gas permeable contact lenses allow more oxygen to reach the cornea, so they should be considered, especially if the patient is going to wear the contact lenses on an extended wear basis. Adult patients' ability to handle the contact lenses should be considered when choosing the contact lens type. Some adults prefer a large contact lens (hydrophilic), and some prefer a rigid gas permeable contact lens.

3. When is a daily wear versus an extended wear aphakic lens indicated?

Due to increased risks of serious complications such as neovascularization and infection with extended wear contact lenses, ideally every person should be fitted with daily wear contact lenses. Occasionally, patients may be incapable of contact lens insertion due to physical or mental barriers. These patients may be fitted with extended wear contact lenses. Children whose parents are not experienced contact lens wearers may also benefit from extended wear contact lenses. Infants fitted with daily wear contact lenses are more likely to be successful contact lens wearers as toddlers because they are used to contact lens insertion and removal. Patients who remove the contact lenses daily are also more capable of dealing with acute onset problems because they are able to remove the contact lenses when necessary.

4. What is the technique for fitting a rigid gas permeable aphakic contact lens?

Aphakic contact lenses can be designed with a single cut design or a lenticular design. The single cut contact lens has a more curved anterior surface and an anteriorly displaced center of gravity, which may cause the lens to displace inferiorly. Single cut rigid contact lenses should be attempted only when lenticular contact lenses do not work. A contact lens with a lenticular design has a flatter anterior curvature and a peripheral flange to facilitate better lens centration. The most commonly used design is the lenticular design with a minus carrier. The minus carrier facilitates lid attachment, which centers the contact lens better. Lenticular contact lenses can be used for all aphakic patients, but they are particularly indicated for corneas flatter than 43.00 D.

The base curve of the contact lens is selected based on the keratometry readings of the cornea (Table 13.1). The power of the contact lens should be determined by performing an overrefraction with a trial lens power close to the patient's refraction. If the power of the trial refractive lens is greater than ± 4 D, the additional power in the overrefraction is added to the contact lens, taking into account vertex distance. The diameter of a rigid gas permeable aphakic contact lens typically ranges from 8.5 to 9.5 mm. The choice of a final contact lens should be based on the centration, movement, fluorescein pattern of the contact lens, as well as the vision and ocular health of the eye.

Table 13.1. Rigid contact lens base curve selection based on
keratometry readings

Corneal toricity	Base curve*
Spherical	0.50 D flatter than flat keratometry reading
0.12–0.62 D	0.25 D flatter than flat keratometry reading
0.75–1.37 D	Same as flat keratometry reading
1.50 D or more	Flat keratometry reading + (1/3 times difference between steep and flat keratometry reading)

*Final base curves may be slightly steeper than indicated by this table in order to improve stability of the contact lens on the eye.

5. What is the technique of fitting a hydrophilic aphakic contact lens?

Most aphakic soft contact lenses are made of silicone elastomer material. High-water-content contact lenses may be more comfortable, and they provide better oxygen permeability. Low-water-content contact lenses are more durable, but they transmit less oxygen to the cornea. The keratometry readings are of little use in a hydrophilic contact lens fitting.[4] An 8.4-mm base curve in one brand of hydrophilic contact lens may yield a tight fit, whereas the same base curve in another brand may provide a loose fit. The best method of fitting a soft contact lens is to examine the fit of a trial lens on the eye. The trial lens used for fitting an aphakic patient should be close to the power required by the patient because a high plus-powered contact lens fits differently than a low-powered contact lens, and the overrefraction will be more accurate. Place the lens on the eye and let it settle for at least 10 minutes prior to evaluating the fit of the lens and conducting an overrefraction. The final lens choice should center well with complete limbal coverage and should move 0.50 to 1.25 mm. An overrefraction should be performed. The vertex distance of the trial lens should be considered if the overrefraction is 4 D or greater.

6. What are the principal characteristics of fitting aphakic lenses?

In children under six months of age, children with congenital aphakes, or young children with unilateral trauma, early fitting is essential in order for vision to develop normally without the development of amblyopia. In older children and adults, the importance of fitting is to develop more visual comfort for near and distance, eliminating the visual distortion, improving the visual field, and improving the chances of good vision in the operated eye of monocular aphakia.

The contact lens position, the pupillary size, the corneal curvature, the lid tension and position, the refractive error, and any preexisting diseases are factors that influence the design of the contact lens. Each individual will require unique contact lens parameters. Fitting guidelines are written to approximate the initial contact lens design, but trial fittings and careful follow-up are necessary for attaining the final contact lens prescription.

7. What are the disadvantages of aphakic contact lenses and the alternatives for aphakia?

The principal disadvantages of contact lens correction of aphakia are the diminished oxygen transmission to the cornea, the increased risk of infection and corneal vascularization, and the higher cost and limited availability of contact lens options.

The primary alternatives to contact lenses are spectacles and intraocular lens implants. Young patients with growing eyes may not be ideal candidates for intraocular implants because the optics of an intraocular lens implant cannot compensate for the changing power of the growing eye. Patients with trauma, in whom a standard posterior chamber lens is not possible, can be implanted with either an anterior chamber lens or a transscleral fixated posterior chamber lens.

High plus spectacles are cosmetically unappealing and uncomfortable, and they cause visual distortion. Spectacles are very difficult for unilateral aphakic patients to wear because of aniseikonia and prismatic effects of high plus spectacle lenses. Epikeratophakia is a treatment option for patients with aphakia, but it is rarely performed today due to relatively poor predictability of the refractive error result.

8. What are the contraindications to contact lenses in the correction of aphakia?

The most frequent contraindications to contact lens wear for aphakic patients are ocular health-related issues such as Fuchs' endothelial dystrophy, persistent corneal inflammation, chronic uveitis, pterygium, and ptosis. Contact lens intolerance due to dry eye syndrome or discomfort are also strong indicators of potential contact lens failures.

9. What is the fitting procedure for fitting aphakic infants?

Contact lenses should be dispensed as soon after the cataract surgery as the contact lens fitter and the surgeon feel comfortable. Fitting the contact lenses on the day of the cataract surgery decreases the time that the child's vision is not corrected and eliminates an unnecessary administration of general anesthesia solely for the contact lens fitting. When fitting the contact lenses in the operating room, the priority is to determine the appropriate power of the contact lens. The best method to determine the power is to place a contact lens on the eye that approximates the resulting refractive error of the child (approximately +35 D). Retinoscopy should be performed over this contact lens using trial lenses to determine the most appropriate power. Placing a high plus contact lens on the eye reduces the error potentially induced by the variable working distance of a high plus refractive trial lens. It may be necessary to stand on a stool or a short ladder in order to achieve the appropriate working distance on a child lying on an operating room table.

An infant's visual world is very close; therefore, prescribing approximately +3.00 D greater than the child's refractive error may enhance the child's visual experience. The power of the contact lens should be reduced to correct the child to emmetropia as the child begins to walk.

Over the first 1 to 2 years, the hyperopic refractive error decreases rapidly as the eye grows. The child should be examined every week for the first month or two of contact lens wear then every 1 to 3 months until the child reaches school age. The power of the contact lenses should be checked at each visit, and a new power should be provided as needed. The fit of the contact lens may also change as the eye continues to grow, so the diameter and base curve may need to be adjusted accordingly. A smaller diameter contact lens may be necessary for infants, but the size of the contact lens should increase to approximately adult size by the time the child is two years old. Larger contact lenses are less likely to become displaced when children rub their eyes.

Most children, especially those with unilateral aphakia, require vision therapy to treat amblyopia. Vision therapy should begin at as early an age as possible and continue until about age 8 years. Patching can be performed with an occluder contact lens.[5]

Although continuous wear contact lenses are available and routinely prescribed,[6] nightly removal and cleaning should be recommended except in rare cases. Daily wear contact lenses decrease the potential for serious complications of contact lens wear, such as neovascularization or infection, and parents and children are better able to adapt to the routine care of contact lenses if they perform it daily, which will be a great benefit when the infant becomes a toddler.

References

1. Collins MJ, Franklin R, Davis BA. Optical considerations in the contact lens correction of infant aphakia. *Optom Vis Sci.* 2002;79:234–240.
2. Hutchinson AK, Wilson ME, Saunders RA. Outcomes and ocular growth rates after intraocular lens implantation in the first 2 years of life. *J Cataract Refract Surg.* 1998;24:846–852.
3. Shaughnessy MP, Ellis F, Jeffery AR, Szczotka L. Rigid gas-permeable contact lenses are a safe and effective means of treating refractive abnormalities in the pediatric population. *CLAO J* 2001;27:195–201.
4. de Brabander J, Kok JH, Nuijts RM, Wenniger-Prick LJ. A practical approach to and long-term results of fitting silicone contact lenses in aphakic children after congenital cataract. *CLAO J* 2002;28:31–35.
5. Joslin CE, McMahon TT, Kaufman LM. The effectiveness of occluder contact lenses in improving occlusion compliance in patients that have failed traditional occlusion therapy. *Optom Vis Sci.* 2002;79:376–380.
6. Ozbek Z, Durak I, Berk TA. Contact lenses in the correction of childhood aphakia. *CLAO J* 2002;28:28–30.

14

Pediatric Contact Lenses

Cleusa Coral-Ghanem and
Jeffrey J. Walline

1. What are the indications for contact lens fitting in the child?

Children may benefit from contact lens wear for a variety of reasons, ranging from correction of refractive error to vision therapy. The most frequent indication for fitting children with contact lenses is the correction of refractive error. Glasses worn to correct high refractive error may result in image magnification or minification, peripheral distortion, prismatic distortion, and a reduced field of view. The spectacles worn to correct high refractive error may also be uncomfortable and cosmetically unappealing, and children can easily remove spectacles that are uncomfortable, unappealing, or provide poor vision. Contact lenses may decrease many of the symptoms suffered by children who wear spectacles for high refractive error, and they are more difficult for young children to remove.

The purpose of contact lens wear in young children is generally to optimize visual input so that the child does not develop amblyopia, but contact lenses may also be fitted to improve the child's appearance or to enhance amblyopia therapy routines. Disfigured eyes or unappealing spectacles may be very traumatic for a young child, so contact lenses may be used to mask disfigured eyes.

Contact lenses may also be used to decrease the amount of light that reaches the retina in photophobic children, to patch an eye for children who do not like to wear adhesive patches for amblyopia therapy, or to decrease the magnitude of nystagmus, thereby improving the vision and the appearance of children who exhibit nystagmus.

2. Is there a difference between the fitting of contact lenses in a child compared to an adult?

A child's eye is adult sized by 2 years of age. Few contact lenses are manufactured to fit children's eyes, specifically so much of the fitting process is similar to adults. The primary challenge in fitting a child is not due to physical differences. The most difficult aspects of fitting a child are overcoming the child's stress, communicating with the child, and accommodating the rapid development of a young eye.

Despite many similarities between a child's and an adult's eye, a child's palpebral fissure is generally smaller, which makes it more difficult to insert and remove contact lenses. This difficulty is exacerbated when the child is crying. The aqueous component of the tear film is generally increased in children. Since the concentration of lipids and proteins in the tears are reduced in children, they rarely have problems with contact lens deposits, except with contact lenses made of silicone elastomers, on which lipid deposits may accumulate quickly. The curvature of the cornea decreases over the first 2 years of age from approximately 45 D to 43 D, and the corneal diameter increases from approximately 10 mm at birth to 11.5 mm by 3 or 4 years of age.

3. What contact lenses are utilized in children?

Children can wear rigid gas permeable contact lenses or soft contact lenses. The indication for contact lens wear and the parents' experience with contact lenses should be considered when determining the most appropriate type of contact lens.

Soft contact lenses are most commonly fitted in children. Parents are more likely to have experience with soft contact lenses than with rigid contact lenses, and soft contact lenses may be prescribed in a frequent replacement program so that spare lenses are readily available. However, it is difficult to find soft contact lenses with pediatric parameters. They require more dexterity in handling than rigid gas permeable contact lenses, and they pose a greater risk of infection than rigid contact lenses, especially with extended wear.

Rigid gas permeable contact lenses are frequently well tolerated by children, and they are more practical in terms of maintenance and care. These lenses have excellent oxygen permeability, they correct irregular astigmatism, and they can be custom made to fit children's eyes. However, rigid contact lenses may be less comfortable initially, they are more likely to dislocate or be lost than soft contact lenses, and they are not available in multipacks.

4. How does one fit the child?

Some professionals use general anesthesia to fit a contact lens in an infant. This will certainly facilitate the measurement of the ocular parameters, refractive power, and evaluation of the contact lens on the eye, but there are serious potential risks associated with general anesthesia. Contact lens fitting under general anesthesia should be restricted to those children who are impossible to examine and fit appropriately in the office. When fitting the contact lenses in the operating room, the main priority is to determine the appropriate power of the contact lens. The best method to determine the power is to place a contact lens on the eye that approximates the resulting refractive error of the child (approximately +35 D). Retinoscopy should be performed over this contact lens using refractive trial lenses to determine the most appropriate power. Placing a high plus contact lens on the eye reduces the error potentially induced by the variable working distance of a high plus refractive trial lens. It may be necessary to stand on a stool or a short ladder in order to achieve the appropriate working distance for a child lying on an operating room table.

A toddler fitted in the office may need to be restrained, which can be accomplished by having the parent hold the child, by wrapping a sheet around the child, or by straddling the child while he or she is lying on the floor. At least one extra pair of hands is necessary to conduct the fitting.

An eye care practitioner may consider having an office assistant insert the contact lens in the child's eye. Children may not trust the person who inserts the first contact lens for some time thereafter, so evaluation of the contact lens prescription may become very difficult. Once the child calms down, the eye care practitioner should evaluate the prescription and fit of the contact lens.

5. How does one examine the lens–cornea relationship in a child?

Children 5 years and older can typically be examined using a slit-lamp biomicroscope with fluorescein and a cobalt blue filter. Small children may need to sit on their knees and hold the slit lamp "like a motorcycle" in order for them to reach the chin rest and for them to be interested enough to sit still for 1 to 2 minutes. If a child cannot be examined with a slit lamp in the office, then a hand-hold Burton lamp with fluorescein can be used. Portable slit lamps and a direct ophthalmoscope/20 D lens combination works when other methods are not available.

When evaluating a contact lens fit, the key fitting criteria are similar to those looked for in the adult. One should check the movement, centration, and fluorescein pattern of a rigid contact lens, and the movement and centration of a soft contact lens. Determination of whether the power of the contact lens is appropriate is also necessary in all contact lens fittings.

6. When should contact lenses be fitted in an aphakic child, and what is the visual prognosis?

The developing visual system of an infant requires clear vision in order to achieve maximum visual potential. As little as 1 to 2 weeks of constant visual deprivation can result in amblyopia. When possible, a contact lens should be fitted immediately after surgery or within 1 week. Fitting the child with a contact lens while he or she is still on the operating table eliminates the potential need for a second dose of general anesthesia, and it decreases the time until the dispensing of the contact lens.

Contact lens correction is more important and urgent for a unilateral aphakic child than a bilateral aphakic child. The aphakic eye requires high plus correction, which results in image size magnification. The images of the two eyes are not equal in size, so they cannot be fused. This can lead to symptoms and poor binocular vision development. Fitting the unilateral aphake with contact lenses minimizes the image size difference and allows for proper visual input for both eyes.

With careful monitoring and diligent care, an aphakic child can achieve excellent visual acuity. The parents must be educated about the continued care and therapy that is necessary to avoid amblyopia, and the child must be examined regularly. The longer a child has good vision before a cataract develops, the better the prognosis. The visual prognosis of an aphakic child following congenital cataracts is worse than the visual prognosis of an aphakic child following trauma. The child who experienced ocular trauma is more likely to have had a period of normal visual development than a child with congenital cataracts.

7. What is the best contact lens for fitting the aphakic child?

Rigid gas permeable contact lenses for aphakia are available in nearly any material because they are custom designed for individual patients. Two soft contact lenses specifically designed for pediatric aphakia are available (Table 14.1).

8. How should one follow up the aphakic infant in a contact lens?

An aphakic infant should be examined every week for the first 2 months. If the lens fits well and the health of the eye is maintained, visits may be reduced to every 2 to 4 weeks for several months. When the refractive error begins to stabilize (at approximately 6 months of age), the child may be examined every 3 months. This schedule should continue until the child enters school. At each visit, the child's vision should be evaluated, the fit and power of the contact lens should be evaluated, and the ocular health should be assessed.

Glaucoma may occur in about 10% of children following cataract removal; therefore, follow-up examinations should consist of routine glaucoma checks as well. The child should be dilated every 6 to 12 months to evaluate the eye's posterior segment.

9. What are the complications encountered in pediatric contact lenses?

The most commonly encountered ocular complications are deposits, tight contact lenses, and signs of hypoxia. Children may also encounter

Table 14.1. Soft contact lenses specifically indicated for pediatric aphakia.

Manufacturer	Series	Material	Base curve	Diameter	Power
Flexlens Products	Pediatric	Hefilcon A	6.0 to 10.8 mm (0.3-mm steps)	10.0 to 16.0 mm (0.5-mm steps)	+10.50 to +30.00 D (0.50-D steps)
Bausch & Lomb	Silsoft Super Plus (Pediatric)	Elastofilcon A	7.5, 7.7, 7.9	11.3	+23.00 to +32.00 D (3.00-D steps)

corneal abrasions and ulcers, but these are more rare. By far, the most commonly encountered complication is contact lens loss or breakage.

10. What is the social responsibility of the eye doctor?

In the case of a child with a congenital cataract, if surgery is indicated, the eye care practitioner must be concerned that the family's socioeconomic and psychological condition can support the long treatment that will be necessary. On the other hand, it is possible to create false expectations and anxiety in the family that has already been assaulted by the child's disease. It is necessary that the parents understand the proposed objectives for treatment and the potential benefits and risks. They must be aware of the duration of the treatment as well as the expenses that will be incurred. On the other hand, they must also understand that only their initiative will allow the child to develop better vision.

Selected References

Donzis PB, Weissman BA, Demer JL. Pediatric contact lens care. In: Bennett ES, Weissman BA, eds. *Clinical Contact Lens Practice,* Philadelphia: JB Lippincott, 1994: Chapter 51, pp. 1–8.

Matsumoto ER, Murphree L. The use of silicone elastomer lenses in aphakic pediatric patients. *Int Eyecare.* 1986; 2:214–217.

Moore B. Managing young children in contact lens. *Contact Lens Spectrum.* 1996; 34–38.

Pe'er J, Rose L, Cohen E, Benezra D. Hard and soft contact lens fitting in infants. *CLAO J.* 1987; 13:46–49.

Stenson SM. Pediatric contact lens fitting. In: Kastl PR, ed. *Contact Lenses—The CLAO Guide to Basic Science and Clinical Practice,* Vol 3. Iowa: Kendall/Hunt Publishing, 1995:179–195.

15

Fitting Contact Lenses After Refractive Surgery

Kaaryn Pederson and Cleusa Coral-Ghanem

The fitting of contact lenses after refractive surgery is a challenge for the majority of eye care professionals. Not only are there problems because of limited designs for oblate corneas but in addition many patients opt for refractive surgery in the first place due to contact lens intolerance. In such cases, patients require encouragement and psychological support during the process of fitting.[1]

Incisional techniques such as radial and astigmatic keratotomy cause corneal alterations that are different from those techniques in which tissue is removed, such as photorefractive keratectomy (PRK) and laser in situ keratomeleusis (LASIK). For this reason, the fitting of contact lenses in each of these classes of surgery is detailed separately.

1. What are the indications for fitting contact lenses after radial keratotomy?

- Undercorrection
- Overcorrection
- Irregular astigmatism
- Anisometropia
- Progressive hyperopic shift
- Glare
- Fluctuating vision

The optical complications most commonly encountered after radial keratotomy are undercorrection, overcorrection and induced astigmatism (regular or irregular) that can result in anisometropia and subsequent aniseikonia. The results of the Prospective Evaluation of Radial Keratotomy (PERK) Study[2] showed that 28% of subjects were undercorrected by more than 1.00 D and 17% were overcorrected by more than 1.00 D after 4 years.[3,4] After 10 years, the PERK Study Group found that 26% of subjects were more than -0.50 D undercorrected and 36%

were more than $+0.50$ D overcorrected, indicating the need for optical correction after many years.[5] Other problems after radial keratotomy (RK) include disabling glare, difficulty with vision in low illumination, monocular diplopia, and fluctuating vision.[2–9]

Irregular astigmatism is caused by differential scarring of the various incisions, inadvertent placement of an incision in the visual axis, a decentered optical zone, and micro- or macroperforations. Anisometropia, which may be the result of residual refractive error, results in retinal images of different sizes and may necessitate contact lenses, since glasses are intolerable.[2–9]

Glare may be caused from aberrations induced by incisions in the visual axis, scarring, or irregular astigmatism. Although most wavefront aberrations are a result of astigmatism or defocus, significant higher order aberrations have been found after radial keratotomy.[8] Glare, light sensitivity, and poor vision in low illumination appear to be related to a small optical zone, a large pupillary diameter, and wide corneal scars. Symptoms are generally more intense in the first postoperative months and diminish proportionally with the decrease in the density of the scars. However, when persistent, glare can be made less problematic with a contact lens.[9]

Fluctuating vision is a problem secondary to incomplete healing of the corneal incisions. The cornea remains flexible after radial keratotomy, and abnormal collagen fibers are found within the incisions on histopathologic examination.[2,10] The clinical manifestation of a flexible cornea is a diurnal variation in refraction. Some authors have suggested a relationship between this refractive instability and the alteration in corneal curvature. The corneal radius steepens throughout the day, resulting in a gradual myopic shift in power.[11–15] Others suggest that the diurnal fluctuation is the result of stromal hydration and lid pressure. After RK, corneal thickness swells 4% to 5% more than the normal cornea after overnight lid closure, leading to a different refractive error in the morning for these patients.[4,14–16] Lastly, others have found that intraocular pressure contributes to the diurnal change in visual acuity after RK. Higher intraocular pressures in the morning exert force on the cornea, allowing peripheral corneal steepening with central flattening as compared to the reduced intraocular pressures in the afternoon.[7,17] Nonetheless, it is well known that, after RK, eyes measured in the morning show a flatter overall corneal shape, a more hyperopic refractive error, higher intraocular pressure, and increased corneal thickness compared to the same measures in the afternoon. In a study of 20 patients post-RK, two-thirds experienced fluctuating vision not related to the size of the optical zone. The refractive changes were present in 40% of patients two years after surgery. Fourteen percent of these required contact lens correction for part of the day, and 26% required lens wear all of the time.[1] The most recent results from the PERK Study Group showed that diurnal fluctuation in refraction and visual acuity persists for at least 11 years after surgery.[15] In practice, a significant number of patients after radial keratotomy demonstrate progressive hyperopia, and in many cases anisometropia and irregular astigmatism that are not amenable to spectacle correction.

2. When can a contact lens be fitted after radial keratotomy?

Ideally, contact lens fitting can be undertaken when topography and refraction appear stable. For this reason, one should wait at least 3 months, the minimal time necessary for the disappearance of peripheral corneal edema, stabilization of the scarring, and, as such, a decrease in the likelihood of contact lens–related complications.[18–21] Extended wear and long wearing hours are discouraged to reduce contact lens–related diurnal fluctuation in vision and the risk of edema.

3. What are the contact lens options after radial keratotomy?

- Spherical rigid gas permeable contact lenses with high oxygen permeability (Dk).
- Hydrophilic contact lenses
- Special designs (both hydrophilic and rigid gas permeable lenses)
- Piggyback systems
- Hybrid contact lenses (Softperm™)

The first choice of treatment should be a rigid gas permeable (RGP) contact lens. This lens, supported on the mid-peripheral cornea, stabilizes vision by creating a smooth and consistent optical surface. An ideal lens of this type is one made of fluorosilicone acrylate because of its high oxygen permeability. It permits better oxygen transmission to the cornea with less risk of complications compared to polymethylmethacrylate (PMMA), RGP lenses with a lower Dk, and hydrophilic lenses.

Soft hydrophilic contact lenses do not offer the benefit of stable and clear visual acuity because of the flexible nature of the material. In addition, because of lower oxygen permeability, they may increase the risk of corneal neovascularization to the incision scars.

A piggyback system—the combination of a soft lens under an RGP lens—is an option for patients with RGP intolerance. However, even with the advent of silicone extended wear disposable soft lenses, this system has the disadvantage of being more expensive, less convenient, and less healthy for the cornea than a RGP lens alone.

A hybrid lens offers greater convenience than piggyback systems but is more expensive and offers less oxygen transmissibility to the cornea. Both the rigid center and the soft skirt have a low Dk, which may lead to hypoxic conditions. This is complicated by the fact that these lenses tend to tighten on the eye, further increasing the risk of neovascularization and corneal edema. Both piggyback and hybrid options should therefore be avoided unless no other successful alternatives are available.

4. What rigid gas permeable lens specifications are recommended for post–radial keratotomy fits?

Due to the flattening and dislocation of the corneal apex to the mid-periphery after radial keratotomy,[22] it is typical for RGP lenses to decenter on the cornea. Large-diameter lenses are used in order to improve centration. Average diameters range between 9.6 and 11.0 mm.[20,23] In addition, the optic zone diameter should be significantly less than the optical zone of a traditional lens. We recommend an optic zone diameter 2.5 mm less than the total diameter, in order to avoid retention of the tear film and debris over the flat cornea. Although larger optical zone diameters help decrease the amount of flare and glare from the contact lens, they result in significant central pooling and air bubbles, leading to unacceptable fits.

5. What are the types and methods of fitting rigid gas permeable contact lenses used after radial keratotomy?

- Spheric and aspheric lenses (Figure 15.1)
- Inverse geometry (reverse curve) contact lenses (Figure 15.2)
- Other specialized designs

Techniques of Fitting Spherical or Aspheric Contact Lens after Radial Keratotomy

Standard designs should be tried first for simplicity. If these trial lenses exhibit a poor fit or visual outcome, specialty designs are then recommended. To select a trial lens, one can use several different parameters based on preoperative or postoperative readings or computed tomographic analysis.

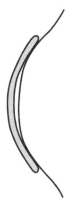

Figure 15.1. Profile of the relationship of a spherical or aspheric contact lens on an oblate cornea after radial keratotomy.

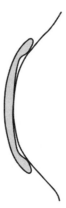

Figure 15.2. Profile of the lens–cornea relationship when a reverse-curve contact lens is used after radial keratotomy.

Preoperative Keratometry

Begin with a base curve equal to the mean preoperative keratometry reading. Note that larger overall diameters (9.8 to 10.0 mm) often require a base curve up to 1.00 D flatter than the flatter preoperative keratometry value. If only one eye received surgical treatment, use the keratometry readings of the unoperated eye as the starting point.[19,21,24]

Postoperative Keratometry

If preoperative keratometry readings are not available, begin with a base curve approximately 2.00 D steeper than the postoperative keratometry reading. Then proceed with an empirical fit.[20]

Measurement of the Mid-Peripheral Zone

One can use computed topographic analysis to evaluate the corneal curvature of the steeper mid-peripheral "knee" or "bend." In many cases, this "bend" in the cornea produced by surgery is a measurement that will determine the initial base curve. McDonnell et al.[25] suggested using the corneal measurement 3.5 mm above the visual axis to select an initial base curve. They had success in achieving lid attachment fitting relationships when using the superior reading. If corneal topography is not available, have the patient look 3 mm off-axis in each of the four quadrants while in the keratometer. The average of these readings gives a good basis of the mid-peripheral corneal curvature.[26]

Whatever the point of departure, a good fit depends on the experience of the professional in evaluating the fluorescein pattern. The goal is to fit a contact lens that is decentered slightly superiorly as a result of support from the superior lid or which is perfectly centered over the optical zone. Frequently, centration is difficult to achieve because the contact lens tends to decenter to the steepest area of the cornea.

The typical fluorescein pattern of a spherical or aspheric contact lens that is fitted adequately is demonstrated in Color Plate 14. An adequate pattern includes apical pooling of fluorescein, pressure on the midperipheral zone of the cornea (which is slightly less with an aspheric as opposed to a spherical lens), and peripheral alignment with very slight edge lift. The power is determined by overrefraction of the trial contact lens. The tear film forms a positive lens between the posterior surface of the contact lens and the flat central cornea, leading to power values similar to the preoperative refractive spherical equivalent.

6. What problems are most often encountered in fitting spherical or aspheric rigid gas permeable lenses in these patients?

- Excessive pressure on the mid-peripheral zone
- Decentration
- Excessive movement
- Fluctuating vision
- Flare and Glare

The contact lens may be well designed but still may not exhibit an optimal fluorescein pattern compared with a contact lens fit on a normal cornea. However, if the patient is comfortable, the lens is well tolerated by the cornea, and vision is satisfactory, this type of fit is acceptable with appropriate monitoring by the practitioner.

Troubleshooting for high-riding lenses can involve changing designs to that of a reverse geometry or an aspheric style or adding lens mass or prism ballast to help get the lens to drop to an inferior position. If the lens decenters too far inferiorly, one can try increasing or adding lenticulation to the lens edge, decreasing the lens mass, or changing to a specialty design to help keep the lens under the upper lid. If vision fluctuates with the contact lens on the eye, this may be a result of lens flexure. This is usually the result of a lens that is too steep, too thin, or both. To eliminate flexure, try a flatter base curve or increase the center thickness of the lens. Flare and glare symptoms with contact lens wear are generally associated with an optic zone diameter or total diameter that is too small. Increasing the diameter allows better pupillary coverage; changing to an aspheric design eliminates the sharp demarcation between the optic zone and peripheral curves.

7. What complications and causes of contact lens intolerance are most often encountered in rigid gas permeable contact lens fitting after radial keratotomy?

Complications include the following:

- Epithelial defects
- Air bubbles (Color Plate 15) and debris
- Contact lens decentration/adhesion (Color Plate 16)
- Epithelial erosions along incision lines (Color Plate 15)

Causes of lens intolerance include the following:
- Gross decentration
- Significant changes in the tear film
- Persistent discomfort

8. What are the special rigid gas permeable contact lens designs utilized in the post-radial keratotomy patient?

There are special multicurve lenses and designs with reverse-curve geometry that can be used in place of traditional lens designs. The designs with reverse-curve geometry (Figure 15.3), that is, with a secondary curve steeper than the base curve, are designed to fit the topographically altered post-RK cornea. These contact lenses tend to center better than standard aspheric or spherical contact lenses but may be less mobile. Each of the lenses is constructed slightly differently, and for this reason fitting should be done according to the recommendation of the manufacturer. Secondary curves range from 2 to 6 D steeper than the base curve and are available in spherical and aspheric designs. Optical zones typically vary from 6.0 to 8.0 mm in size, depending on the design and manufacturer (Table 15.1).[23,27,28]

An initial base curve selection for reverse geometry contact lenses should be approximately 1.00 D steeper than the postoperative central keratometry reading or the measurement midway between the flat center and the steepest mid-peripheral bend on corneal topography. Secondary curves should align with the steepest curvature in the mid-

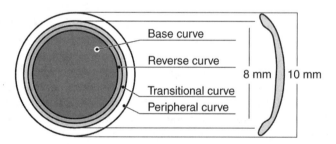

Figure 15.3. Design of the Plateau™ contact lens (Menicon) with a reverse secondary curve.

Table 15.1. Contact lenses with a secondary inverse curve (reverse-curve design)

Name	Manufacturer
OK Lens	Contex, Inc., Sherman Oaks, CA
RK Bridge Lens	Conforma Lab., Norfolk, VA
Plateau Lens (Figure 15.3)	Menicon, Clovis, CA
Metro Optics RA	Metro Optics, Austin, TX

peripheral zone, while peripheral curves should flatten and provide adequate lift for tear exchange.[29,30] A recommended optic zone diameter is one that correlates with the size of the central flat zone, measured from the middle of the transition area on one side to that on the other as seen in the topography map. The fluorescein pattern of the trial lens should be evaluated, and further adjustments should be made accordingly.[31]

As the secondary curves are made steeper or wider in a reverse geometry designed lens, the overall fit of the lens steepens. In addition, the larger the optic zone diameter, the looser the fit. Large differences between the base and secondary curves (a tighter periphery) decrease lens movement, increase peripheral bearing, and decrease the amount of tear flow under the lens. Smaller differences between the base and secondary curves (a looser periphery) reduce peripheral bearing, allowing more lens movement and tear flow.[30–32]

Another special multicurve design is that of the Lexington-RK Splint Aero GBF Contact Lens, formerly known as the Quintasphere-PRK. It has a large central base curve with four peripheral curves. Its peripheral design mathematically approximates the aspheric shape of the normal peripheral cornea. The progressive rate of flattening (or asphericity) of the peripheral curves has been shown to perform well on eyes after surgery.[33]

9. What are the indications and types of hydrophilic contact lenses for fitting post–radial keratotomy?

The indications for fitting hydrophilic contact lenses post-RK include:

- Rigid gas permeable lens intolerance
- Recurrent epithelial erosion
- Glare

Before a hydrophilic contact lens is fitted, it is necessary to wait for stabilization of the cornea. The advantages of a hydrophilic lens as opposed to an RGP lens are comfort and good centration. The disadvantages are poorer acuity and a much greater frequency of complications.

Hydrophilic Lenses Indicated for Use After Radial Keratotomy

- Silicone hydrogel disposable lenses with daily removal (PureVision, Bausch & Lomb; Focus Night & Day™, CIBAVision)
- One-day disposable lenses
- Toric lenses for daily use
- Special-design lenses (e.g., Flexlens Harrison Post–Refractive Surgery Lens™; Paragon Vision Sciences)
- Opaque or colored imprinted lens in order to reduce glare[34]

Hydrophilic Contact Lenses Contraindicated After Radial Keratotomy

Thick and low-water-content contact lenses are contraindicated because they cause edema much more rapidly after RK as compared to a normal cornea, especially when endothelial function is compromised.[35]

10. What is the technique for fitting a spherical hydrophilic contact lens?

The principles of fitting are the same as those utilized in a normal cornea. The diameter of the first lens should be 1 to 2 mm greater than the horizontal diameter of the visible iris. For a thin and high-water-content contact lens, the radius of curvature of the posterior optical zone should be 0.2 to 0.4 mm flatter than K. One should wait 20 to 30 minutes before performing biomicroscopy. A contact lens should be correctly centered and should move 1 to 2 mm with blinking without compression of the perilimbal vasculature. It is important to ensure adequate tear exchange under the soft lens to prevent corneal hypoxia. If the patient reports symptoms of fluctuating vision with the soft lens, it may be a result of the base curve being too steep. Steep central curvatures change shape after each blink, distorting the vision. A flatter base curve should be tried in these cases. If flatter base curves are too loose on the eye, the Harrison™ post–refractive surgery lens (Paragon Vision Sciences) may be tried. This soft lens has a flatter central curve and steeper mid-periphery, which allows it to function like a reverse geometry lens.

If residual astigmatism is an issue after RK, soft toric lenses may be an option. With the advent of disposable and higher water content soft toric lenses, many adverse reactions have been reduced. However, secondary to the unevenness of the corneal shape, it is often difficult to achieve rotational stability and consistent vision with these lenses. In addition, soft toric lenses are thicker by design and therefore pose a more significant health risk on postsurgical eyes.

11. What are the complications of using hydrophilic lenses after radial keratotomy?

The complications of using hydrophilic lenses after radial keratotomy include corneal neovascularization, corneal edema, and infectious keratitis.

Corneal Neovascularization

Various studies have demonstrated that the use of conventional hydrophilic contact lenses after RK may facilitate or induce corneal neovascularization. The incidence of neovascularization varied from 33% to 50% when the user removed the contact lenses for sleeping and was much greater in those who wore the lenses continuously. It should be noted that neovascularization developed almost exclusively along the radial incisions.[2–7,20,23]

It is possible that the surgery alters the oxygen demand of the cornea or the manner in which the oxygen reaches the stroma, stimulating neovascularization. Another factor that may increase neovascularization is the absence of proper scarring. Even a lens with high oxygen permeability may compress the limbus, affecting both corneal curvature and epithelial physiology. In addition to this, a hydrophilic contact lens facilitates deposit formation, increasing the risk of epithelial erosion and infection. For these reasons, prolonged use should be avoided.[36]

The development of disposable contact lenses, especially those of a silicone hydrogel material, has permitted the use of lenses post-RK with a decreased risk of neovascularization.

Corneal Edema

The hydrophilic lens, even one with high water content, stands as a barrier to oxygen permeability and may cause transient edema in normal corneas. The potential for corneal edema is much greater in post-RK patients, especially if endothelial function has been compromised. Certainly, silicone hydrogel contact lenses of silicone hydrogel provide oxygenation in these corneas, decreasing the incidence of edema.[35]

Infectious Keratitis

Even though bacterial contamination can occur during surgery, it can also be problematic months or years after RK, primarily related to problems with the scarring of the incisions.[36–38] Histopathologic studies have demonstrated that there is an abnormal organization of endothelial cells in the region of the incisions that persists years after RK. Minor epithelial trauma in the corneas of these patients may result in erosions or disruption of the epithelial layer, creating circumstances that favor bacterial adherence and development of infectious keratitis.[39,40]

The user must be informed of the importance of compliance with proper hygiene of contact lenses and the importance of looking for any adverse symptoms. A cornea after RK is predisposed to epithelial erosion, and a soft contact lens is susceptible to the formation of deposits and bacterial contamination, presenting a constant risk of infectious keratitis.

12. What are the principal indications for fitting contact lenses after photorefractive keratectomy (PRK)?

- Undercorrection/regression
- Overcorrection
- Residual and induced astigmatism

- Decentered treatment zone
- Central island
- Central stromal haze
- Presbyopia
- Anisometropia

Between 9% and 30% of patients who undergo PRK will not end up with uncorrected visual acuity of 20/40 or better, or a refractive error within 1.00 D of the intended refraction.[41-46] In part, this is secondary to regression, which typically occurs over the first 4 to 6 months after surgery. The amount of regression has been shown to be related to the amount of refractive error treated; the higher the amount of preoperative myopia treated, the greater the magnitude of regression. Specifically, corrections over −5.00 or −6.00 D have been shown to have low reliability and predictability of surgical outcome secondary to regression.[41,43,44,46] For this reason, it is common practice to intentionally overcorrect myopic patients and use a postoperative course of topical steroids to help achieve a better surgical outcome.[43,45,46]

Anterior stromal haze is a complication of surgery that is most prevalent 6 months after surgery and gradually diminishes. However, in some patients this stromal haze persists, causing a decrease in visual acuity and contrast sensitivity. Other problems, although rare, are central scarring, central islands, and eccentric ablations.[41,42,47,48]

13. What types of contact lenses are recommended for fitting after photorefractive keratectomy?

- Hydrophilic lenses (spherical, toric, and specialized designs)
- RGP (spheric and aspheric lenses)
- Piggyback systems
- Hybrid lenses

The majority of patients who have PRK undergo ablation of the central zone of the cornea, approximately 6 mm in diameter. Corneal topography typically shows a flattened uniform power within the optical zone, accompanied by a smooth power transition at the margin of the ablation zone and normal peripheral regions.[49-51] The technique of PRK, in addition to preserving the mid-peripheral and peripheral zones, does not produce endothelial dysfunction.[52] For these reasons, patients who require contact lenses do not have a propensity for neovascularization, edema, or infectious keratitis, as do RK patients. In addition, contact lenses tend to center better after PRK, making fitting much easier in post-RK patients.[53]

Patients requiring simple over- and undercorrections or the correction of presbyopia will generally perform well with a soft lens. If visual acuity cannot be adequately corrected with a soft contact lens, then RGP lenses are recommended. Lim et al.[54] compared soft and RGP lenses and found that more patients were successful with soft lens wear after PRK because of better centration, stability, and comfort. Only 25% of patients fitted with RGP lenses were able to tolerate and wear them all day. Both types of lenses showed no significant complications.

It should be noted that RGP contact lenses with a reverse secondary curve are rarely necessary for fitting post-PRK patients because the transition from the central operated zone to the normal cornea is not abrupt. In addition, hybrid and piggyback systems should be saved for rare patient cases.

14. How much time should one wait after photorefractive keratotomy before fitting a contact lens?

Generally, one waits a minimum of 3 months after surgery to fit a contact lens. However, waiting between 6 and 12 months in order for the corneal shape and refraction to stabilize is advisable.[53–58] Ideally, the patient will have discontinued the use of any medication, and corneal haze will have diminished before contact lenses are fit. Although bandage soft contact lenses can be fitted successfully immediately after surgery to help epithelial healing, soft lenses needed for optical corrections should be deferred for at least 3 to 6 months.

15. When are rigid gas permeable lenses indicated after photorefractive keratotomy?

Rigid gas permeable lenses are indicated particularly in:

- Irregular astigmatism
- Decentered ablation zones
- Central islands
- Significant haze

These conditions typically cause an irregular corneal surface and, therefore, require a rigid and uniform refracting surface to improve visual acuity. In most cases, post-PRK haze gradually decreases, disappearing by 6 months. However, if there is residual haze, the use of an RGP lens generally provides the patient with vision comparable to the presurgical acuity.

16. What are the techniques for fitting a rigid gas permeable lens after photorefractive keratotomy?

Base Curve Determination

If the individual used RGP lenses before surgery, the same contact lens can serve as a point of departure for analysis at the slit lamp, especially if it was an aspheric lens design. Or one can use one of following options:

1. If the preoperative keratometric measurements are known, start with a base curve 0.50 or 1.00 D flatter than the keratometry reading.
2. Use a base curve equal to the measurement of the mid-peripheral curve.
3. Measure the postoperative keratometry readings, then choose a base curve 0.50 D steeper than the mean K.

The base curve of the final contact lens is generally 0.50 to 1.00 D flatter than the flat preoperative K reading, and the power approximates the presurgical measurement because the tear film forms a positive lens between the contact lens and the flattened cornea.[55-58]

Diameter/Optic Zone Diameter

A large lens (9 to 10.5 mm) with an optical zone of 2.5 mm less than the diameter of the lens is preferable to avoid central bubbles and adhesion of the lens. One should attempt to fit a lens that has vertical movement with each blink to ensure good tear exchange and removal of debris, which tends to collect in the center of the flattened cornea. The typical fluorescein pattern demonstrates apical pooling and alignment in the mid-periphery.

Design

One should begin with a spherical contact lens with a standard peripheral design. The slit-lamp examination will indicate the necessity for aspheric lenses or special designs.

17. What are the bandage contact lens options after photorefractive keratotomy?

Therapeutic contact lenses provide pain relief, corneal protection, and facilitation of corneal wound healing after surgery. Although there are many conventional therapeutic soft lenses on the market, disposable contact lenses have become very popular bandage lenses, although their use is considered "off-label." The advantages of disposable lenses include less expense, less risk of corneal infection, and less risk of toxic complications with concurrent use of topical medications. They are also easy to replace if a contact lens is accidentally dislodged or lost. Standard hydrophilic disposable lenses (e.g., Acuvue™, Vistakon) approved for extended wear have shown good clinical efficacy, but silicone hydrogel disposable lenses (PureVision™, B&L; or Focus Night & Day™, CIBAVision) also offer the advantage of decreasing the risk of hypoxic complications with continuous wear.[59-61]

Although the risk of infectious keratitis with the use of therapeutic contact lenses after PRK is low, bacterial contamination has been found on the bandage contact lenses after removal. Microorganisms found on the lenses typically represent the bacteria found in the normal ocular flora, indicating the need for careful monitoring and follow-up. Topical antibiotics combined with no handling of the lenses by the patient reduce the risk of bacterial infection.[62,63]

18. What should one look for in fitting a therapeutic hydrophilic lens after photorefractive keratotomy?

At the conclusion of the PRK procedure, the surgeon generally places a disposable contact lens on the eye. The contact lens should be chosen based on the preoperative measurements. The patient should be examined at the slit lamp approximately 30 minutes later to determine the contact lens–cornea relationship.

If the contact lens movement is great (the ideal movement is approximately 0.5 mm with a blink), there may be both patient discomfort as well as interference with reepithelialization. Check to be sure the contact lens is not inverted before changing base curves.

If the contact lens does not have movement, the causes may be:

1. A steep base curve, which may produce corneal edema. In this case, try a flatter curve.
2. Edema of the conjunctiva produced by the use of a device such as a suction ring. In this case, the contact lens should not be disturbed.

If there is foreign material, rolled epithelial edges, and/or significant debris under the contact lens, it should be exchanged. On the other hand, if the quantity of debris is very small, one should avoid disturbing the lens. Its removal, aside from producing discomfort, may actually increase the size of the epithelial defect.

19. What recommendations should be given to the patient with a therapeutic lens after photorefractive keratotomy?

1. Avoid removing the lens at home, especially if the patient has no experience with contact lenses. Removal will typically be done at an office visit, once the epithelium is intact. Manipulation of the contact lens by the patient could increase the risk of infection.
2. Avoid environmental pollutants and activities that significantly reduce the blink rate, which may cause dehydration of the contact lens. A dried contact lens produces discomfort, facilitates deposit formation, diminishes oxygenation of the cornea, and increases the risk of infection.
3. Avoid cosmetics around the eyes until the contact lens has been removed.
4. Use lubricants, preferably nonpreserved, between administration of other topical medications in order to lubricate and clean the contact lens.
5. Discard the contact lens if it comes out of the eye.

20. What are the concerns that one should have in the office in removing a therapeutic contact lens post–photorefractive keratotomy?

The following steps are recommended:

1. Wet the contact lens and wait 2 to 5 minutes before removing it.
2. Use a drop of anesthetic if necessary to reduce trauma.
3. Ask the patient to look up.
4. Pull the contact lens inferiorly and remove it with fingers or with a fine, nontoothed forceps at the slit lamp.

21. What are the primary indications for fitting contact lenses after LASIK?

- Overcorrection
- Undercorrection
- Perforation, dehiscence, decentration, or loss of the flap
- Irregular astigmatism or surface irregularities
- Stromal haze or scarring
- Corneal ectasia

LASIK has become the most commonly performed refractive surgery procedure around the world. It involves the passage of a microkeratome to create a corneal flap, followed by a laser ablation of the stromal bed and replacement of the corneal flap. Although it is technically riskier than PRK, it produces more predictable results in high myopes and is less painful for patients. In addition, there is less ocular inflammation and therefore quicker recovery and less need for topical medications after surgery. However, every surgical procedure runs the risk of complications. LASIK has been reported to have an overall complication rate varying from 3.4% to 11.8%.[64] Complication rates are thought to be inversely related to surgeon experience.

It is estimated that of the patients who have myopic astigmatism and undergo LASIK, approximately 5% experience overcorrection and 15% experience undercorrection.[65] In addition, roughly 9% of patients experience intraoperative or postoperative complications related to the corneal flap.[66] Intraoperative complications include incomplete or irregular keratectomies such as a buttonhole and free cap. Postoperative conditions include displaced flaps, flap folds, epithelial ingrowth, and diffuse lamellar keratitis. Epithelial ingrowth occurs in 1% to 20% of treated eyes, depending on the study,[64,67] whereas diffuse lamellar keratitis has an incidence of 0.9% to 1.4%.[68,69] Other common complications after LASIK are decentered ablations,[70] central islands (roughly 6% of treated eyes),[71,72] and corneal ectasia (less than 1% of eyes treated).[72,73]

22. How does corneal topography change after LASIK?

Corneal topography after LASIK reveals central flattening with a steeper periphery, similar to that seen in PRK. However, because LASIK can treat greater amounts of myopia, the oblate corneal contour may be more pronounced.[74] The topographic map will typically not appear as altered as in RK, though, because the corneal periphery is left intact. Studies have also shown that the hinge of the flap affects corneal topography. The area closest to the hinge is generally a flatter curvature than the opposing side and is also slightly elevated secondary to flap retraction.[75]

23. What types of contact lenses are used in fitting post-LASIK patients?

- Hydrophilic contact lenses (spherical or special designs)
- RGP lenses (spherical, aspheric, and reverse geometry designs)
- Piggyback systems
- Hybrid lenses

24. When is a soft lens indicated after LASIK, and what period of time is recommended after surgery before proceeding with the fitting?

Unlike with RK, soft lenses are not contraindicated in LASIK patients. Studies have shown that LASIK does not have a negative effect on the corneal endothelium,[76] and because the flap incision is only superficial and paracentral, the risk of neovascularization is similar to that of an untreated eye.[77] In fact, patients with simple over- and undercorrections may request a hydrophilic contact lens for comfort. If the patient is complaining of night vision problems, an aspheric lens (such as Specialty Choice A.B.™, Specialty Ultravision) is the best option.[78] These lenses help create an aspheric optical surface and decrease spherical aberrations induced after surgery. Soft lenses may be fitted as early as 1 to 3 months after surgery, as soon as the refraction has stabilized.[79]

It should be noted that although bandage soft lenses are not typically used after LASIK, they might be needed in cases of flap loss or disruption to promote proper healing and decrease epithelial ingrowth at the flap edge. Although bandage lenses have been shown to cause corneal edema and delayed corneal healing after LASIK,[80] if warranted, the fitting guidelines and advice as described in the PRK section would apply.

Some doctors may also use a soft contact lens with the concurrent use of ketorolac tromethamine (AcularTM; Allergan) to reduce small amounts of overcorrection after laser surgery. This technique has been described by Augustine and Gonzalez[81] and named "contact lens-assisted, pharmacologically induced keratosteepening." One side effect of topical ketorolac (typically used to decrease ocular inflammation and pain) is corneal epithelial thickening. The soft contact lens is used to promote corneal hypoxia and increase contact time of the medication, which allows the cornea to thicken. This technique results in an average of $+0.50$ D regression after a few weeks and should be discontinued after 1 month.[81]

25. When is a rigid gas permeable contact lens indicated after LASIK, and what period of time is recommended after surgery before proceeding with a fitting?

The RGP lenses should be the primary choice for visual correction after surgery. They offer the best optics and visual acuity, while also providing adequate oxygen transmissibility for proper corneal health, and are always indicated in cases of irregular astigmatism. Surface irregularities, such as those resulting from decentered ablations, central islands, and corneal ectasia, reduce best-corrected visual acuity and cause symptoms of diplopia, decreased contrast sensitivity, shadowing, and glare. The RGP lenses are the best treatment option to improve symptoms. It is advised to wait at least 3 months before fitting an RGP lens.[79,81]

26. What techniques are utilized for fitting rigid gas permeable lenses after LASIK?

Base Curve Determination

It is not advised to use postoperative keratometry readings to select an initial base curve, because this results in an excessively flat fitting contact lens. Instead, use one of the following options:

Measurement of the Mid-Peripheral Cornea

Szczotka[82] recommends using an axial map (rather than a tangential one) in determining the base curve with corneal topography. The "averaged" plot used in axial maps will more closely reflect the base curve needed.[81] The power at the inflection point of the mid-peripheral cornea, as well as the value at 3.5 mm superior to the visual axis should be used as the starting point.[81-83]

Preoperative K Readings

Use the flatter preoperative keratometric reading minus one third of the reduction of the refractive error.[84]

Example: a patient with preoperative keratometry readings of 45.00/46.00 D who undergoes a myopic reduction of 4.50 D by LASIK may be fitted by choosing a base curve of $45.00 - 1/3 \times 4.5 = 43.50$ D.

Postoperative K Readings

Steepen the mean K by 1.5 to 2.0 diopters.[78,85]

Diameter

In general, one should use an optical zone diameter approximately 2.5 mm smaller than the total diameter to avoid bubbles, retention of debris, and contact lens adhesion. When possible, a contact lens with a diameter of 9.5 to 11.5 mm should be employed to avoid glare. Nonetheless, smaller diameter lenses are preferred in cases of plus-power contact lenses in order to reduce weight and improve centration.

Design

One should begin with a spherical contact lens. One can modify the periphery or try an aspheric trial lens, depending on the appearance at the slit lamp. The transition from the central zone of the cornea to the mid-periphery is less dramatic than that seen in the post-RK patient, and for this reason it is rarely necessary to use a contact lens with a reverse-curve design, a hybrid contact lens, or a piggyback lens. In cases of ectasia after LASIK, one should consider a fitting similar to the type performed in keratoconus: a minimal central apical clearance fluorescein pattern or one that exhibits a slight three-point touch pattern (Color Plate 17).[86]

27. Will ocular dryness after LASIK affect contact lens wear?

Many patients experience dry eye symptoms after LASIK. In fact, 1 month postoperatively, patients demonstrate a significant reduction in tear flow[87] and tear breakup time.[88] This is thought to be, in part, secondary to decreased corneal sensation and a reduced blink reflex rate after surgery.[87,88] Dry eye symptoms, although typically transient, can last for up to 1 year.[89] For this reason and because many refractive surgery patients were originally contact lens intolerant, LASIK can exacerbate symptoms of dryness with contact lens wear. Therefore, it is important to stress the need for tear supplements and use punctual plugs when indicated. In addition, regular contact lens follow-up appointments are necessary to check for punctate epithelial keratopathy.

28. When is a piggyback system indicated after refractive surgery?

After refractive surgery, a piggyback system is indicated for the following conditions:

- Difficulty with epithelialization
- Persistent epithelial staining caused by mechanical trauma from an RGP lens
- Persistent discomfort with an RGP lens

29. What is the technique for fitting a piggyback system?

The piggyback system traditionally consists of fitting a high DK, RGP lens over a disposable hydrogel lens (Color Plate 18). At times, it is necessary to use a hydrophilic contact lens with positive power to aid centration of the RGP lens. After fitting the hydrophilic lens, one performs keratometry over the lens and begins the fitting with an RGP with a base curve 0.1 mm steeper than that keratometric reading. A tight RGP contact lens is certainly acceptable, as long as there is reasonably good tear exchange under the soft lens.

The Flexlens™ piggyback system consists of a hydrophilic lens 14.5 mm in diameter with a central depression 10.2 mm in diameter in which one can place an RGP lens 9.2 mm in diameter. This system helps center the RGP lens within the inset of the lens, if standard disposable or silicone lenses were unsuccessful.

The patient with a piggyback system needs to be followed more frequently because of the less favorable levels of oxygenation produced by the double barrier of two lenses on the eye.

30. When does one fit a hybrid contact lens (e.g., Softperm™) after refractive surgery?

A hybrid contact lens is indicated to neutralize an irregular corneal surface and to provide better visual acuity in cases in which an RGP lens is not tolerated because of discomfort or decentration. The hybrid contact lens made by CIBAVision (SoftPerm™) has a rigid center 8 mm in diameter with a 7-mm optical zone. The peripheral curve is made of butyl styrene, silicone/methacrylate, and a wetting agent. The hydrophilic skirt is of HEMA (2-hydroxyethyl methacrylate) with a water content of 25%. The diameter of the lens is 14.3 mm. Due to the low Dk and the tendency of the lens to adhere tightly to the eye, the daily hours of use of this lens may be limited. In addition, patients must be followed by the practitioner very closely, particularly after RK surgery, due to the strong propensity for corneal neovascularization.

31. Can the range of the keratometer be extended?

After refractive surgery, keratometry readings may be flatter than 36.00 D, the flattest keratometry reading on Bausch and Lomb keratometers. If this is the case, the range can be extended by placing a −1.00 D trial lens on the side of the keratometer closest to the patient's eye and subtracting 6.00 D from the reading. Likewise, if the patient has corneal ectasia after surgery and the range needs to be extended steeper than 52.00 D, place a +1.25 D trial lens on the front of the keratometer and add 8.00 D to the reading.

32. How does hyperopic photoreactive keratotomy or LASIK differ from myopic treatments?

To achieve a hyperopic correction, the central cornea must be steepened with respect to the periphery. By using diverging lenses, erodible disks, or a circular pattern of treatment, the excimer laser ablates tissue in the mid-peripheral zone and spares the central cornea. This is a more difficult procedure, and, although it is becoming more popular, the success of hyperopic treatments has been limited by the lack of predictable results.[90] The best surgical outcomes have been on patients with refractions of +5.00 D or less and expected postoperative corneal curvatures of less than 49 D.[91] In addition, studies have found that larger optical zones and corneal flaps produce greater stability and safety profiles than smaller optical zones.[92]

Corneal topography after hyperopic laser surgery shows a steep central region, surrounded by an annular flat "gully" and a steepening of tissue in the corneal periphery. A properly fitted RGP contact lens shows mild central bearing surrounded by a ring of fluorescein pooling and adequate peripheral edge lift. Central keratometry readings after a hyperopic treatment are steep and misleading, so preoperative keratometry readings are recommended for selecting an initial base curve. If only one eye received treatment, the keratometry readings from the unoperated eye should be used as a starting point. If postoperative keratometry readings are all that is available, subtract 1.00 D for each diopter of refractive error treated and then proceed with a diagnostic fit. Because a negative tear lens is created under the contact lens, lens powers often resemble the original hyperopic prescription.

Large lens diameters (10 mm or bigger) are recommended to distribute the weight of the contact lens between the central and peripheral regions of the cornea and to cover the large ablation and corneal flap diameters. Optical zone diameters need to be small to reduce the number of bubbles in the mid-peripheral "gully." Because of the contour of the cornea, tears accumulate in the ablated mid-peripheral region and often do not adequately cover the central corneal apex. For this reason, contact lens fitting is difficult, and patients should be monitored closely.

References

1. Powers MK, Meyerowitz BE, Arrowsmith PN, et al. Psychosocial findings in radial keratotomy patients 2 years after surgery. *Ophthalmology.* 1984;91:1193–1198.
2. Waring GO III, Lynn MJ, Gelender H, et al. Results of the prospective evaluation of radial keratotomy (PERK) study one year after surgery. *Ophthalmology.* 1985;92:177–198.
3. Waring GO, Lynn MJ, Fielding B, et al. Results of the PERK Study 4 years after surgery for myopia. *JAMA* 1990;263(8):1127.
4. Waring GO, Lynn MJ, Nizam A, et al. Results of the prospective evaluation of radial keratotomy (PERK) study five years after surgery. *Ophthalmology.* 1991;98:1164–1176.

5. Waring GO, Lynn MJ, McDonnell PJ. Results of the PERK study 10 years after surgery. *Arch Ophthalmol.* 1995;113:1225–1226.

6. Ajamian PC. Radial keratotomy: an overview. *J Am Optom Assoc.* 1986;57:580–582.

7. Werner DL. Refractive surgery: radial keratotomy. *J Am Optom Assoc.* 1986;57:584–588.

8. Hjortdal JO, Olsen H, Ehlers N. Prospective randomized study of corneal aberrations 1 year after radial keratotomy or photorefractive keratectomy. *J Refract Surg.* 2002;18:23–29.

9. Tomlinson A, Caroline P. Effect of radial keratotomy on the contrast sensitivity function. *Am J Optom Physiol Opt.* 1988;65:803–808.

10. Binder PS, Nayak SK, Deg JK, et al. An ultrastructural and histochemical study of long-term wound healing after radial keratotomy. *Am J Ophthalmol.* 1987;103:432–440.

11. Schanzlin DJ, Santos VR, Waring GO III, et al. Diurnal change in refraction, corneal curvature, visual acuity, and intraocular pressure after radial keratotomy in the PERK study. *Ophthalmology.* 1986;93:167–175.

12. Kwitko S, Gritz DC, Garbus JJ, et al. Diurnal variation of corneal topography after radial keratotomy. *Arch Ophthalmol.* 1992;110:351–356.

13. McDonnell PJ, Fish LA, Garbus J. Persistence of diurnal fluctuation after radial keratotomy. *Refract Corneal Surg.* 1989;5:89–93.

14. Kiely PM, Carney LG, Smith G. Diurnal variations of corneal topography and thickness. *Am J Optom Physiol Opt.* 1982;59:976–982.

15. McDonnell PJ, Nizam A, Lynn MJ, et al. Morning-to-evening change in refraction, corneal curvature, and visual acuity 11 years after radial keratotomy in the PERK study. *Ophthalmology.* 1996;103:233–239.

16. MacRae S, Rich L, Phillips D, et al. Diurnal variation in vision after radial keratotomy. *Am J Ophthalmol.* 1989;107:262–267.

17. Kemp JR, Martinez CE, Klyce SD, et al. Diurnal fluctuations in corneal topography 10 years after radial keratotomy in the PERK study. *J Cataract Refract Surg.* 1999;25:904–910.

18. Salz JJ, Salz JM, Salz M, Jones D. Ten years' experience with a conservative approach to radial keratotomy. *Refract Cataract Surg.* 1991;7:12–22.

19. DePaolis MD. The role of contact lenses in the management of the radial keratotomy patient. *Optom Clin.* 1994;4:25–34.

20. Lee A, Kastl P. Rigid gas permeable contact lens fitting after radial keratotomy. *CLAO J* 1998;24:33–35.

21. Shivitz IA, Russell BM, Arrowsmith PN, et al. Optical correction of postoperative radial keratotomy patients with contact lenses. *CLAO J* 1986;12:59–62.

22. McDonnell PJ, Garbus J. Corneal topographic changes after radial keratotomy. *Ophthalmology.* 1989;96:45–49.

23. Shin J, Ackley K, Caroline P. Use of "plateau" designed lenses to improve corneal health in a post-operative radial keratotomy patient. *Optom Vis Sci.* 1993;72:82–83.

24. Shivitz IA, Arrowsmith PN, Russell BM. Contact lenses in the treatment of patients with overcorrected radial keratotomy. *Ophthalmology.* 1987;94:899–903.

25. McDonnell PJ, Garbus JJ, Caroline P, et al. Computerized analysis of corneal topography as an aid in fitting contact lenses after radial keratotomy. *Ophthalmic Surg.* 1992;23:55–59.

26. Chan J, Burger D. The use of peripheral corneal measurements for fitting a PK/PRK patient. *Optom Vis Sci.* 1996;73:235.

27. Szczotka L. Contact lenses for the irregular cornea. *Contact Lens Spectrum.* 1998;13:21–27.

28. Shovlin J. What lenses are OK after RK? *Rev Optom.* 1999;136:105.

29. Mathur A, Jones L, Sorbara L. Use of reverse geometry rigid gas permeable contact lenses in the management of the postradial keratotomy patient: review and case report. *ICLC* 1999;26:121–127.

30. Minucci G, Scheid T. "Bridge" contact lens improves post-RK acuity. *Contact Lens Spectrum.* 1994;9:64.

31. Lim L, Siow K, Sakamoto R, et al. Reverse geometry contact lens wear after photorefractive keratectomy, radial keratotomy, or penetrating keratoplasty. *Cornea.* 2000;19:320–324.

32. Scheid T. *Clinical Manual of Specialized Contact Lens Prescribing.* Boston: Butterworth-Heineman, 2002.

33. Koffler BH, Smith VM, Clements LD. Achieving additional myopic correction in undercorrected radial keratotomy eyes using the Lexington RK splint design. *CLAO J* 1999;25:21–27.

34. Estrada LN, Rosenstiel CE. Prosthetic contact lenses: a role in the treatment of ruptured RK incision with iris damage. *CLAO J* 2002;28:107–108.

35. Inoue T, Maeda N, Inoue Y, et al. Minimizing radial-keratotomy-induced diurnal variation in vision using contact lenses. *J Cataract Refract Surg.* 2000; 26:1680–1683.

36. Schivitz IA, Arrowsmith PN. Delayed keratitis after radial keratitis. *Arch Ophthalmol.* 1986;104:1153.

37. Mandelbaum S, Waring GO, Forster RK, et al. Late development of ulcerative keratitis in radial keratotomy scars. *Arch Ophthalmol.* 1986;104:1156.

38. Panda A, Das GK, Vanathi M, et al. Corneal infection after radial keratotomy. *J Cataract Refract Surg.* 1998;24:331–334.

39. Karr DJ, Grutzmacher RD, Reeh MJ. Radial keratotomy complicated by sterile keratitis and corneal perforation. *Ophthalmology.* 1985;92:1244.

40. Deg JK, Zavalla EY, Blinder OS. Delayed corneal wound healing following radial keratotomy. *Ophthalmology.* 1985;92:734.

41. Gartry DS, Kerr, Muir MG, Marshall J. Excimer laser photorefractive keratectomy. 18-month follow-up. *Ophthalmology.* 1992;99:1209–1219.

42. Maguen E, Salz JJ, Nesburn AB, et al. Results of excimer laser photorefractive keratectomy for the correction of myopia. *Ophthalmology.* 1994; 101:1548–1556.

43. Tengroth B, Eptstein D, Fagerholm P, et al. Excimer laser photorefractive keratectomy for myopia. Clinical results in sighted eyes. *Ophthalmology.* 1993;100:739–745.

44. Piovella M, Camesasca FI, Fattori C. Excimer laser photorefractive keratectomy for high myopia. *Ophthalmology.* 1997;104:1554–1565.

45. Gartry DS, Larkin DF, Hill AR, et al. Retreatment for significant regression after excimer laser photorefractive keratectomy. A prospective, randomized, masked trial. *Ophthalmology.* 1998;105:131–41.

46. Chatterjee A, Shah S, Bessant DA, et al. Results of excimer laser retreatment of residual myopia after previous photorefractive keratectomy. *Ophthalmology.* 1997;104:1321–1326.

47. Seiler T, Holschbach A, Derse M, et al. Complications of myopic photorefractive keratectomy with the excimer laser. *Ophthalmology.* 1994; 101:153–160.

48. Seiler T, McDonnell PJ. Excimer laser photorefractive keratectomy. *Surv Ophthalmol.* 1995;40:89–118.

49. Wilson SE, Klyce SD, McDonald MB, et al. Changes in corneal topography after eximer laser photorefractive keratectomy for myopia. *Ophthalmology.* 1991;98:1338–1347.

50. Maloney RK. Corneal topography and optical zone location in photorefractive keratectomy. *Refract Corneal Surg.* 1990;6:363–371.

51. Klyce SD, Smolek MK. Corneal topography of excimer laser photorefractive keratectomy. *J Cataract Refract Surg.* 1993;19(suppl):122–30.

52. Stulting RD, Thompson KP, Waring GO. The effect of photorefractive keratectomy on the corneal endothelium. *Ophthalmology.* 1996;103:1357–1365.

53. Shovlin JP. A comparison between patients wearing contact lenses following radial keratotomy and myopic photorefractive keratectomy with the eximer laser. *ICLC* 1992;19:141–142.

54. Lim L, Siow K, Chong JS, et al. Contact lens wear after photorefractive keratectomy: comparison between rigid gas permeable and soft contact lenses. *CLAO J* 1999;25:222–227.

55. Schipper I, Businger U, Pfarrer, R. Fitting contact lenses after excimer laser photorefractive keratectomy for myopia. *CLAO J* 1995;21:281–284.

56. Astin CL, Gartry GS, McG Steele AD. Contact lens fitting after photorefractive keratectomy. *Br J Ophthalmol.* 1996;80:597–603.

57. Bufidis T, Konstas A, Pllikaris I, et al. Contact lens fitting difficulties following refractive surgery for high myopia. *CLAO J* 2000;26:106–110.

58. Astin CL. Contact lens fitting after photorefractive keratectomy: a comparison of two groups of patients. *Ophthalmic Physiol Opt.* 1995;15(5):371–374.

59. Lim L, Tan DT, Chan WK. Therapeutic use of Bausch & Lomb PureVision contact lenses. *CLAO J* 2001;27:179–185.

60. Bouchard CS, Trimble SN. Indications and complications of therapeutic disposable Acuvue contact lenses. *CLAO J* 1996;22:106–108.

61. Lindahl KJ, DePaolis MD, Aquavella JV, et al. Applications of hydrophilic disposable contact lenses as therapeutic bandages. *CLAO J* 1991;17:241–243.

62. Dantas PE, Nishiwaki-Dantas MC, Ojeda VH, et al. Microbiological study of disposable soft contact lenses after photorefractive keratectomy. *CLAO J* 2000;26:26–29.

63. Detorakis ET, Siganos DS, Houlakis VM, et al. Microbiological examination of bandage soft contact lens used in laser refractive surgery. *J Refract Surg.* 1998;14:631–635.

64. Stulting RD, Carr JD, Thompson KP, et al. Complications of laser in situ keratomileusis for the correction of myopia. *Ophthalmology.* 1999;106:13–20.

65. Perez-Santoja JJ, Bellot J, Calaramonte P, Ismail MM, Alio J. Laser *in situ* keratomileusis to correct high myopia. *J Cataract Refract Surg.* 1997;23:372–385.

66. Lin RT, Maloney RK. Flap complications associated with lamellar refractive surgery. *Am J Ophthalmol.* 1999;127:129–136.

67. Wang MY, Maloney RK. Epithelial ingrowth after laser in situ keratomileusis. *Am J Ophthalmol.* 2000;129:746–751.

68. Johnson JD, Harissi-Dagher M. Pineda R, et al. Diffuse lamellar keratitis: incidence, associations, outcomes, and a new classification system. *J Cataract Refract Surg.* 2001;27:1560–1566.

69. Wilson SE, Ambrosio R Jr. Sporadic diffuse lamellar keratitis (DLK) after LASIK. *Cornea.* 2002;21:560–563.

70. Wilson SE LASIK: management of common complications. *Cornea.* 1998; 17:459–467.

71. Duffey RJ. Central islands and decentered ablations after LASIK. *Int Ophthalmol Clin.* 2000;40:93–10.

72. Johnson JD, Azar DT. Surgically induced topographical abnormalities after LASIK: management of central islands, corneal ectasia, decentration, and irregular astigmatism. *Curr Opin Ophthalmol.* 2001;12:309–317.

73. Pallikaris IG, Kymionis GD, Astyrakakis NI. Corneal ectasia induced by laser in situ keratomileusis. *J Cataract Refract Surg.* 2001;27:1796–802.
74. Barker NH, Couper TA, Taylor HR. Changes in corneal topography after laser in situ keratomileusis for myopia. *J Refract Surg.* 1999;15:46–52.
75. Ginsberg NE, Hersh PS. Effect of lamellar flap location on corneal topography after laser in situ keratomileusis. *J Cataract Refract Surg.* 2000;26:992–1000.
76. Kent DG, Solomon KD, Peng, Q, et al. Effect of surface photorefractive keratectomy and laser in situ keratomileusis on the corneal endothelium. *J Cataract Refract Surg.* 1997;23:386–397.
77. Szczotka LB, Aronsky M. Contact lenses after LASIK. *JAMA.* 1998;69: 775–784.
78. Ward MA. Solving refractive surgery problems with contact lenses. *Review of Contact Lenses.* 2002;30–31.
79. Zadnik K. Contact lens management of patients who have had unsuccessful refractive surgery. *Curr Opin Ophthalmol.* 1999;10:260–263.
80. Kanellopoulos AJ, Pallikaris IG, Donnenfeld ED, et al. Comparison of corneal sensation following photorefractive keratectomy and laser in situ keratomileusis. *J Cataract Refract Surg.* 1997;23:34–38.
81. Augustine JM, Gonzalez K. Manage overcorrected LASIK with CLAPNIKS. *Prim Care Optometry News.* 2001;6:34.
82. Szczotka LB. Contact lenses for the irregular cornea. *Contact Lens Spectrum.* 1998;13:21–27.
83. Egglink FA, Beekhuis WH, Nuijts RM. Rigid gas-permeable contact lens fitting in LASIK patients for the correction of multifocal corneas. *Graefes Arch Clin Exp Ophthalmol.* 2001;239:361–366.
84. Bennett ES, Depaolis MD, Henry VA, Barr JT. RGP lens management of the irregular cornea patient. *Contact Lens Spectrum.* 1999;21–25.
85. Ward MA. Visual rehabilitation with contact lenses after laser in situ keratomileusis. *J Refract Surg* 2001;17:433–440.
86. Eggink FA, Beekjuis WH. Contact lens fitting in a patient with keratectasia after laser in situ keratomileusis. *J Cataract Refract Surg.* 2001;27:1119–1123.
87. Yu EW, Leung A, Rao S, et al. Effect of laser in situ keratomileusis on tear stability. *Ophthalmology.* 2000;107:2131–2135.
88. Toda I, Asano-Kato N, Komai-Hori TK. Dry eye after laser in situ keratomileusis. *Am J Ophthalmol.* 2001;132:1–7.
89. Ang RT, Dartt DA, Tsubota K. Dry eye after refractive surgery. *Curr Opin Ophthalmol.* 2001;12:318–322.
90. Sher NA. Hyperopic refractive surgery. *Curr Opin Ophthalmol.* 2001;12:304–308.
91. Choi RY, Wilson SE. Hyperopic laser in situ keratomileusis: primary and secondary treatments are safe and effective. *Cornea.* 2001;20:388–393.
92. Argento CJ, Cosentino MJ. Comparison of optical zones in hyperopic laser in situ keratomileusis: 5.9 mm versus smaller optical zones. *J Cataract Refract Surg.* 2000;26:1137–1146.

16

Contact Lens Fitting After Corneal Transplantation

Loretta B. Szczotka, Paulo Ricardo de Oliveira, and Newton Kara-José

1. What are the principal indications for contact lens fitting after corneal transplantation?

The principal indications are high, regular, or irregular astigmatism, anisometropia, poor vision with glasses, poor surface healing requiring bandage lens therapy, or residual refractive error with the patient's preference for contact lens use. Considering that there is a greater risk of complications with contact lenses than with glasses, the vision with contact lenses must be superior to spectacle-corrected vision. Spectacles are often of limited value postoperatively, especially in the presence of preoperative corneal pathology. The limitations are based on the optical shortfalls of spectacles, including (1) the inability to correct significant irregular astigmatism; (2) aniseikonia induced by spectacle-corrected anisometropia; (3) barrel and pin cushion distortions in highly myopic and hyperopic prescriptions, respectively; (4) visual distortion in high astigmatic corrections; (5) induced prism in peripheral gaze; and (6) image minification in high minus prescriptions. Contact lenses not only minimize the limitations induced by spectacles but also can stabilize fluctuating visual acuity. They have been known to augment or intentionally mold the cornea for an intensified surgical effect, and they are useful in decreasing relative spectacle magnification that may be induced in refractive anisometropia.

2. When should contact lenses be fitted after a corneal transplant?

Some eye care practitioners feel that, in general, contact lens fitting should not be performed until 6 months or more after the removal of sutures. Others will fit contact lenses as early as 3 months after surgery with the sutures in place.[1] Many surgeons believe that sutures are not a contraindication to contact lens fitting unless suture removal is going to be performed soon. Contact lenses can be safely fitted over sutures as long as the sutures are completely covered by epithelium and all knots are buried. The fitter should be aware, however, that the presence of sutures increases the possibility of epithelial erosion and, therefore, infection. To diminish the risk of complications and to increase the success of fitting, it is best to fit the contact lens when the donor tissue is completely healed and when the keratometric measurements and refraction results are stable. Contact lens fitting can and should be performed earlier in children in whom amblyopia may develop without adequate optical correction.

3. What types of contact lenses can be used?

All contact lens types have been fitted postoperatively including soft, rigid gas permeable (RGP), piggyback, or hybrid lens designs. Hydrophilic lenses are indicated in cases in which the cornea is relatively regular only when there is absolute intolerance of rigid contact lenses. Because they may cause corneal edema and neovascularization, hydrophilic lenses are less desirable than RGP lenses for daily wear and should be avoided in patients with sutures in place. Hydrophilic contact lenses worn for extended wear have been directly implicated in the neovascularization and possible rejection of the donor tissue.[2-4] However, others have documented safe contact lens wear postoperatively with soft contact lenses.[5] The transplanted eye is an avascular, immunologically privileged area, which limits the immune host mechanisms from entering the tissue. If neovascularization develops secondary to contact lens wear, the cornea's immuno-privileged status is removed.

Considering that contact lenses are primarily indicated when spectacle-corrected acuity is poor because of astigmatism or an irregular corneal surface, RGP lenses are most appropriate. They provide better optics and oxygenation for the cornea, and there is less risk of corneal edema and vascularization. In cases where the cornea is highly irregular, a larger diameter can be used with highly oxygen permeable materials, which facilitates positioning over the cornea.

Another indication for posttransplant contact lens use is wound dehiscence that does not lend itself well to a surgical repair. The placement of a medium water content, relatively stiff hydrogel contact lens worn on an extended wear basis for weeks to months can facilitate healing of the wound without the need for resuturing.[6]

4. What are the criteria for choosing the initial rigid gas permeable trial lens?

There is no strict rule, and it is always recommended that one begin with the simplest option; for example, first trying a standard spherical lens with a base curve equal to or slightly steeper than the flatter meridian of the cornea. Another option is to begin with a lens design suggested by corneal topography. Because of the limitations and lack of validation of software programs for contact lens fitting that are currently available, in most cases corneal topography provides only the design options and parameter suggestions for the first trial lens.

Corneal topography should guide the contact lens fitter in selecting the best posterior surface RGP design. Five classic corneal shapes have been described following keratoplasty[7]: (1) prolate shape: regular astigmatism with a central red bow-tie pattern that denotes a steeper center and flatter periphery; (2) oblate shape: regular astigmatism with a central blue bow tie that denotes a flatter center and steeper periphery; (3) mixed shape: regular astigmatism that extends through the topographic map; (4) asymmetrical pattern with the two steepest hemimeridians not symmetric and not 180 degrees apart; and (5) steep-to-flat pattern where the cornea is steepest on one side and becomes progressively flatter toward the other.

The thought process supporting RGP design selection based on the topography follows physical, mechanical, and centration considerations. Visually, most eyes do well with spherical rigid lenses for optical purposes. Rarely will residual astigmatism be present over a standard RGP design because most of the astigmatism in surgically induced and is, therefore, predominantly refractive corneal cylinder. The design options listed in Table 16.1 address the physical fitting characteristics of an RGP lens to the front of an irregular corneal surface.

The prolate shape can be fitted with standard lens designs including spherical, aspheric, or bi-aspheric, because this shape may closely resemble the normal corneal asphericity. If the degree of central corneal steepening is excessive, a keratoconic design may be indicated to vault the central steep area and to limit apical bearing.

The oblate shape is best fitted with one of the reverse geometry lens

Table 16.1. Design options for rigid gas permeable lenses

Shape	Designs
Prolate	Aspheric
	Bi-aspheric
	Bitoric
	Keratoconic
	Stanndard spherical posterior curves
Oblate	Reverse geometry lens
Mixed	Bitoric
Asymmetric	Aspheric
	Bi-aspheric
	Keratoconic
	Standard spherical posterior curves
Steep to flat	Large diameter and optic zone
	Standard spherical posterior curves

designs that feature a plateau shape with secondary curves 2 to 5 D steeper than central posterior curve of the optic zone. These lenses were initially designed for use in orthokeratology, but they have found increased use in postoperative transplant and refractive surgery patients as well. The lenses provide flatter base curves and steeper intermediate curves to better align with the oblate corneal contour.

If significant corneal toricity extends throughout the entire graft, the cornea may be classified as a mixed prolate and oblate shape factor. A bitoric lens design is then indicated to ensure comfort and centration and to prevent excessive impingement that would occur from a spherical lens.

Due to the asymmetry of the steep-to-flat pattern as well as the asymmetric pattern, it may be very difficult to center an RGP lens on the cornea. These patterns account for an estimated 22% of the penetrating keratoplasty (PK) topographies and often require acceptance of suboptimal cornea-to-lens fitting relationships. The fitting of both the asymmetric and steep-to-flat patterns depends on the location of the steep hemimeridian and the direction of lens decentration. The incorporation of RGP fitting techniques to limit decentration is an important part of the fitting process.

5. How does one evaluate the fitting?

To evaluate the fitting of any type of rigid contact lens, the position, mobility, and fluorescein pattern must be observed. The power is determined by subjective overrefraction. The objective is to obtain a lens that provides good visual acuity and comfort for at least 8 to 10 hours of use per day, that is well centered, and that covers the entire graft. However, if it is not possible to achieve perfect centration, it is acceptable to have slight decentration superiorly, inferiorly, nasally, or temporally. The fitter should not expect the same fluorescein pattern as one would see on a normal cornea because frequently these corneas are deformed and irregular. The difficulty of fitting is greater than in eyes that have never had a surgical procedure. In view of the fact that the corneal surface is generally irregular in these cases, there is no optimal fluorescein pattern. It is important, however, to avoid both excessive touch as well as excessive pooling under the contact lens.

6. Should rigid lenses be larger or smaller in diameter than the graft?

Ideally, the RGP lens should be well centered and should cover the entire graft. However, in many cases this is not possible. The majority of lenses that are fitted have diameters between 8.5 and 9.8 mm. However, when the fitter is not able to obtain good centration, lenses with diameters greater than 10.5 mm may be used. In these cases, the fitter needs to pay special attention to corneal oxygenation and utilize materials with a oxygen permeability (Dk) value of at least 60.

7. When it is not possible to obtain a satisfactory fit with rigid gas permeable lenses alone, what other options are available?

Among less commonly used options are piggyback systems employing a hydrophilic carrier beneath an RGP optical lens or, alternatively, a hybrid lens such as the Softperm lens by CIBA Vision.

8. How does one fit a piggyback system?

Used more commonly for keratoconus, the piggyback system is also sometimes useful after corneal transplant in cases in which it is not possible to obtain adequate centration, when the patient cannot tolerate a rigid contact lens, or for persistent epithelial staining secondary to mechanical trauma after RGP wear. However, this system should be used with caution, because the use of a soft hydrophilic lens beneath an RGP significantly limits corneal oxygenation. The rigid contact lens is fitted over the hydrophilic lens. The patient generally tolerates this type of fitting despite the need for the use of two lenses in each eye. The ophthalmologist or optometrist must watch closely for the development of hypoxia and corneal edema. A combination of a disposable soft contact lens and a high-Dk gas permeable lens can be employed. Some fitters prefer the hydrophilic lens to be positive to effectively steepen the cornea and provide a central carrier that the RGP lens may position over. The power of the disposable lens might be, for example, $+2.00$ D; the power of the gas permeable lens is determined by overrefraction. Others prefer to use a minus power hydrophilic lens to flatten effectively a steep cornea or to provide a thinner center for better oxygen flux. High Dk, soft silicone-hydrogel lenses have been used more recently as carriers to promote maximum corneal oxygenation.

Currently in the United States, there is a piggyback lens system (Flexlens) that is designed with a central depression into which a rigid lens can be fitted. The diameter of the rigid lens is 1 mm smaller than the diameter of the depression. The fitting is performed based on keratometry obtained over the area of the lens depression, with a piggyback lens carrier placed in the patient's eye.

9. What are the advantages and disadvantages of the hybrid (e.g., Softperm) lens?

The hybrid lens, in the same manner as the piggyback system, is indicated in cases of rigid contact lens intolerance and poor centration. The system consists of a rigid center with a Dk of 14 and a peripheral hydrophilic skirt with a water content of 28%. These lenses, therefore, have low oxygen permeability. Their primary advantage is comfort and good centration. The disadvantages are difficulty with insertion and removal, separation of the rigid and soft portions of the lens, low Dk, and high cost. In addition, the hydrophilic portion of the lens can dehydrate, causing tightening of the lens, hypoxia, and consequent corneal edema. This has been termed *steep lens syndrome*. The fitting technique of the Softperm lens involves choosing a base curve slightly steeper than the mean keratometric cylinder and analyzing the fluorescein pattern with high molecular weight fluorescein (Fluoresoft).[8,9]

10. What are the principal characteristics of the quintisphere penetrating keratoplasty?

The quintisphere PK has five curvatures—a central curve and four peripheral curves. This lens was designed for fitting on a corneal graft. The central curve remains supported on the donor cornea and the four peripheral curves on the recipient cornea. This design facilitates good positioning of the lens and provides greater comfort to the wearer.

11. What precautions should be taken by patients who wear contact lenses after corneal transplantation?

Special attention should be paid to contact lens users after corneal transplant because between 30% and 39% of patients who have a corneal graft develop glaucoma, 4% to 6% develop an infection, 21% to 24% experience a graft rejection, and 9% to 35% have a graft failure. The most common causes of failure are epithelial failure, infection, edema, and graft rejection. The risk of infection is particularly important because these corneas, besides having areas that are dry or poorly hydrated, also have diminished corneal sensation, which impairs their capacity for self-defense. The endothelium of any contact lens user may develop pleomorphism and polymegethism. Donor corneas utilized for transplantation often demonstrate an endothelial cell loss of 4.5% to 7.8% during surgery, with an additional 0.6% cell loss each year thereafter. Although studies of the corneal endothelium in patients who have undergone corneal transplantation and who use contact lenses show no loss of endothelial cells secondary to contact lens use, it is prudent to prevent chronic hypoxia and, even with a good fitting pattern, to perform cell counts at regular intervals.[10] It is important that the ophthalmologist or optometrist follow the patient for the possibility of epithelial erosion, infiltrates, infection, vascularization, rejection, and endothelial alterations. Lastly, long-term graft stability after contact lens wear has been documented with consistent corneal topography 3 years after contact lens fitting.[11]

12. What are the most common causes for failure of contact lens fitting after corneal transplantation?

Instability of the lens or decentration because of the presence of a step-off in the junction between donor and recipient, high astigmatism, and other irregularities of the corneal surface are the principal causes of contact lens failure. Contact lens–corrected visual acuity or the acuity with the correction of anisometropia should be equal or better than the acuity obtained with spectacles. Failure to provide a higher quality of vision with contact lenses is a common cause for a return to spectacle wear. Another cause of failure is contact lens intolerance.

13. When should a post–corneal transplant contact lens fit be considered successful?

The success rate in the literature of fitting contact lenses after PK is as high as 84%.[12] When one obtains a well-centered contact lens fit, or even a slightly decentered one, with visual acuity results better than with spectacles and sufficient for the patient's visual needs, and when the patient is able to use the lens for the majority of waking hours without risk of damage to the cornea, the fit is considered successful.

References

1. Wilson SE, Friedman RS, Klyce SD. Contact lens manipulation of corneal topography after penetrating keratoplasty: a preliminary study. *CLAO J.* 1992;18:177–182.
2. Beekhuis WH, Van Rij G, Eggink S, Vreugdenhil W, Schoevaart CE. Contact lenses following keratoplasty. *CLAO J.* 1991;17:27–29.
3. Mannis MJ, Matsumoto ER. Extended wear aphakic soft contact lenses after penetrating keratoplasty. *Arch Ophthalmol.* 1983;101:1225–1228.
4. Lemp MA. The effect of extended wear aphakic hydrophilic contact lenses after penetrating keratoplasty. *Am J Ophthalmol.* 1980;93:331–335.
5. Dangle ME, Kracher GP, Stark WJ, Maumenee AE, Martin NF. Aphakic extended wear contact lenses after penetrating keratoplasty. *Am J Ophthalmol.* 1983;95:156–160.
6. Mannis MJ, Zadnik K. Hydrophilic contact lenses for wound stabilization in keratoplasty. *CLAO J.* 1988;14:199–202.
7. Schanzlin DJ, Robin JB. *Corneal Topography—Measuring and Modifying the Cornea.* New York: Springer-Verlag, 1992:70–72.
8. Binder PS, Kopecky L. Fitting the Softperm contact lens after keratoplasty. *CLAO J.* 1992;8:170–172.
9. Maguen E, Caroline P, Rosner I, Macey J, Nesburn A. The use of the soft-perm lens for the correction of irregular astigmatis. *CLAO J.* 1992;18:173–176.
10. Bourne WM, Shearer DR. Effects of long term rigid contact lens wear on the endothelium of corneal transplants for keratoconus 10 years after penetrating keratoplasty. *CLAO J.* 1995;21:265–267.
11. Gomes JA, Rapuano CJ, Cohen EJ. Topographic stability and safety of contact lens use after penetrating keratoplasty. *CLAO J.* 1996;22:64–69.
12. Mannis MJ, Zadnik K, Deutsch D. Rigid contact lens wear in the corneal transplant patient *CLAO J.* 1986;12:39–42.

Selected Readings

Baucher JA. Long-term use of Saturn II and SoftPerm contact lenses for keratoplasty and keratoconus: a case report. *ICLC.* 1992;19:35–38.

Koffler BH, Clements LD, Litteral GL, Smith UM. A new contact lens design for post-keratoplasty patients. *CLAO J.* 1994;20: 170–175.

Lopatynsky MO, Cohen EJ. Post keratoplasty fitting for visual rehabilitation. In: Kastl PR, ed. *Contact Lens—The CLAO Guide to Basic Science and Clinical Practice.* Iowa: Kendall/Hunt, 1995:79–89.

Moreira SMB, Moreira H. Adaptacao de lentes de contato apos ceratoplastia penetrante para reabilitacao visual. In: Moreira SMB, Moreira H, ed. *Lentes de Contato.* Rio de Janeiro: Cultura Medica, 1993:204–206.

Netto AL. Adaptacoes pos–transplante de cornea, pos-ceratotomia e pos-ceratectomia foto-refrativa. In: Coral-Ghanem, C, Kara-Jose N, eds. *Lentes de Contat na Clinica Oftalmologica.* Rio de Janeiro: Cultura Medica, 1998:71–77.

17

Contact Lens Fitting After Ocular Trauma

Adamo Lui Netto and Eric Ritchey

1. What are the principal causes of ocular trauma?

Corneal opacity due to trauma is a common cause of ocular morbidity throughout the world. These types of trauma result from accidents: workplace accidents (where projectiles are the most common causes), automobile injuries, domestic injuries (principally in children, caused by sharp or pointed objects), chemical or thermal burns, assaults, sports injuries, and electrical injuries. Contact lenses are also responsible for one of the three most frequent types of ocular trauma, metal foreign bodies and automobile accidents being the other two most common.[1,2]

2. What is the prevalence of ocular trauma?

Ocular trauma is common. In the United States, it is estimated that there are approximately 1 million to 2.4 million new ocular traumas occur per year, which lead to approximately 40,000 cases of blindness per year.[3] In India, trauma is the fifth most common cause of visual loss, with a prevalence of 7.3/1000 inhabitants, and trauma constitutes 1.52% of causes of blindness. This large variation in the number of reported cases is largely related to regional differences. Additionally, many ocular traumas, particularly minor ones, are treated in private clinics and are not registered. In the United States, 20,000 to 68,000 patients are hospitalized per year with serious ocular trauma that may compromise vision (Color Plate 19). Admission of male patients for ocular trauma exceeds that of females by three times, and young adults are the most common patients sustaining ocular trauma.[1,4,5]

In the United States, the National Society to Prevent Blindness reports that trauma is the second most common cause of ocular damage in the population, second only to cataract. In 1997, approximately 938,000 patients presented with visual deficits caused by trauma that occurred at some point in life; 7% had severe loss of visual acuity; 79% were blind in one eye; 75% of these patients were below age 65, 78% were men.[5]

3. How can contact lenses traumatize the eye?

The contact lens is a modality commonly used to correct refractive errors, providing an improvement in visual acuity in millions of individuals throughout the world. In the United States an estimated 30 million individuals wear contact lenses and in Europe, 15 million.[6] Perhaps 75 million patients wear contact lenses worldwide, 80% of whom are hydrogel lens wearers.[7]

Trauma can occur in contact lens users, but the contact lens may also be the cause of injury.[6] Ocular lesions caused by contact lenses include corneal abrasions, foreign body tracks caused by material under the contact lens, and chemical cleaning and disinfection products that cause ocular irritation and keratitis. Typically trauma induced by the use of contact lenses is minor and self-limiting. It typically resolves with discontinuation of lens wear for 24 to 48 hours. Corneal ulcers in contact lens users may produce serious visual loss, necessitating corneal transplant for visual rehabilitation.[5,6,8] Incidence of corneal microbial infection is 1/1000 users per year. The incidence of infectious keratitis with daily wear hydrogel contact lenses ranges from 2.2 to 5.3 cases per 10,000 users per year. This increases to 20.9/10,000 patients/year when this modality is used on an extended wear basis.[9]

4. What are the principal indications for contact lenses after ocular trauma?

The principal indications for a contact lens after ocular trauma are: anisometropia; aphakia; irregular pupils or iridodialysis; aniseikonia; the need for a corneal bandage; regular or irregular corneal astigmatism; an inability to wear spectacles secondary to craniofacial abnormality/ trauma; and opacities that are thin and in the superficial cornea, limited to the subepithelial layers or the anterior stroma. The fine, diffuse regular opacity involving the pupillary axis more commonly interferes with vision than the localized, dense cicatricial lesion outside of the visual axis. These opacities irregularly refract light and blur the retinal image.[8,10]

The blurring caused by irregular astigmatism from opacities is difficult to correct with spherical, cylindrical, or spherocylindrical spectacle lenses, because these lenses do not correct the irregularities of the corneal surface. Rigid gas permeable lenses or corneal transplantation are options. Due to the inherent complications of corneal transplantation, that option is less desirable. Rigid gas permeable lenses improve visual acuity by masking the irregular astigmatism from these corneal opacities[8,10] through the creation of a tear lens using the precorneal tear film.

In cases of a denser lesion that present as a corneal leukoma in the central and paracentral regions of the pupillary axis, rigid gas permeable contact lenses can be tried to determine if visual rehabilitation with contact lenses is indeed possible. In cases of deep lesions that produce scars and localized iridocorneal adhesions outside the visual axis, visual rehabilitation is more feasible than for scars localized in the optical zone. In addition, contact lenses are indicated in patients with ocular trauma and in patients with disfigured pupils or eyes that are cosmetically deformed for the prevention of amblyopia and for stabilization of the traumatized eye.[8,10]

Patients with herpetic keratitis, dry eye, lid abnormalities, changes in the posterior segment of the eye, and amblyopia need to be carefully evaluated before they are excluded from contact lens use.[8,10]

5. How soon after trauma can contact lenses be fitted?

The waiting period prior to contact lens fitting after trauma requires a careful ophthalmic examination and varies with each individual. Visual acuity without correction and best-corrected vision with spectacles should be noted. A detailed ophthalmologic examination should be performed, including examination of the lids and the ocular adnexa. The tear meniscus should be examined, and a Schirmer test and evaluation of the tear breakup time should be performed. Measurement of the size of the corneal opacity should be noted as well as its relationship to the pupillary axis. The cornea should be carefully examined for signs that contraindicate lens wear such as herpetic eye infection, loss of corneal sensitivity, pleomorphism and polymegethism of the corneal endothelium, severe dry eye, and active ocular inflammation. Careful biomicroscopic examination, fundus evaluation, tonometry, keratometry, and/or video keratoscopy should also be performed.[11]

If there is traumatic aphakia without opacities in the pupillary axis, a hydrophilic contact lens can be fitted early after surgery (Color Plate 20).[11]

Rigid gas permeable lenses should be fitted after suture removal in some cases. To achieve visual rehabilitation early, rigid gas permeable lenses can be fitted prior to removing sutures. However, the patient must be advised of the risks and potential complications. Corneal sutures should be rigorously examined. Staining in the area of a suture may indicate a potentially loose suture that should be removed. The patient must contact the fitter with any decrease in visual acuity, increase in redness/photophobia/pain, or discharge (particularly mucopurulent discharge) or if there is inflammation or discomfort with the contact lens.[8,10,11]

6. What type of contact lens is best for fitting after ocular trauma?

Rigid gas permeable (RGP) lenses have a number of advantages over hydrogels for postsurgical contact lens fits. Oxygen permeability (Dk) values tend to be higher in RGP materials than in traditional hydrogel materials. Practitioners can also set the center thickness of the lens to get an estimate of the oxygen transmissibility of the lens (Dk/t values are based on t equal to the average lens thickness). The RGP parameters can be customized by the doctor for each individual patient and are not limited to the manufacturers' stock designs. The RGP lenses are easier to handle, insert, and remove and more durable for the patient with reduced acuity. Cleaning RGP lenses is easier, and they are less prone to damage from the cleaning process. The RGP lenses can correct irregular astigmatism through the use of a tear lens formed by the precorneal tear film underneath the rigid lens.

There are disadvantages to the use of RGP lenses following surgery. High Dk lenses tend to be less durable than low Dk lenses. Thus, high Dk materials are more prone to warpage and instability. High Dk materials are more prone to lens deposits and may not wet well. A stable precorneal tear film is helpful in the fitting of post-trauma patients.

The use of hydrogel and silicone hydrogel lenses can be beneficial to the patients. Hydrogel and silicone hydrogel lenses can be used as a bandage as an alternative to pressure patches for corneal abrasions. High-water-content hydrogel lenses may help protect the epithelium and allow for proper healing. Low-water-content hydrogel lenses are beneficial for people with dry eye disorders and provide a tighter fit in cases where excessive lens movement is not desirable.

Theoretically, RGP lenses with high Dk provide better fitting characteristics with excellent oxygen transmissibility, movement, tear exchange, and visual acuity.[9] High-Dk RGP materials can be less stable and more prone to damage and warpage. Theses materials should be replaced on a more regular basis. High-Dk RGP materials also tend to have poorer wettability compared to lower Dk lenses. These materials have an affinity for binding lipid deposits. Proper cleaning and care techniques are critical for long-term success with these lens materials.

7. What are the criteria for choosing between hydrophilic or rigid gas permeable lenses?

The fitting of a hydrophilic contact lens post-trauma is indicated primarily when there is ametropia from traumatic aphakia. It is also indicated when the corneal scars are outside the optical zone. After removal of the sutures, RGP lenses may be a better choice because they are less likely to induce inflammation or corneal neovascularization.[1,2,4,5,6,8,11] The hydrophilic contact lens should be of high Dk and for prolonged use; however, it should be removed on a daily basis. After suture removal, this can be switched to an RGP lens.[1,2,5,6,8,10,11]

8. What hydrophilic lenses are indicated after ocular trauma?

In general, we recommend high-Dk, extended-wear lenses or disposable lenses that are removed on a daily basis. When the trauma has resulted in aphakia, the hydrophilic lens may offer good visual acuity, either with regular or irregular astigmatism because these lenses are so thick in the center that they provide good visual correction.[5,6,8]

9. Which rigid gas permeable lenses are most commonly indicated after ocular trauma?

High-Dk RGP lenses, preferably with a Dk of 92 to 100 or more, provide good oxygen transmissibility. Because these lenses are more flexible, they may not correct higher degrees of regular or irregular astigmatism and are more prone to lens warpage. In such cases, one should fit with less flexible lenses with a lower Dk (35, 56, etc.), to improve the quality of vision.[1,2,5,6,8,10,11]

10. What is the function of the contact lens for visual rehabilitation after trauma with loss of the crystalline lens?

Aphakia can result from severe penetrating ocular trauma. The lens may be perforated, subluxated, or completely dislocated, and it may be necessary to remove it during the rehabilitation process. Alternatively, it may become opacified later, requiring surgical removal and intraocular lens implantation. If the anatomy of the eye is significantly altered by trauma and intraocular lens implantation is not an option, the eye remains aphakic. For children during the amblyogenic years, aphakia requires special care. Combined with corneal laceration, the optical management and the treatment of amblyopia requires significant attention. In such cases, lenses are indicated, especially in monocular aphakia, which will accentuate the anisometropia and enhance the amblyopia.[1,2,5,6,8,10,11]

In case of a perforation only, the practitioner can opt for either a hydrophilic contact lens or an RGP lens, depending on the total amount of corneal and refractive astigmatism. The hydrophilic lens is better tolerated from the standpoint of comfort and serves to protect the traumatized eye. In the case of myopia, hyperopia, or moderate residual astigmatism, glasses can be used to effect the correction.[1,2,5,6,8,10,11]

An RGP contact lens may be indicated when the principal objective is to improve vision in cases of irregular astigmatism. Irregular astigmatism in various forms is common after ocular trauma, especially soon after the trauma. If the astigmatism persists, localization of and assessment of the extent of the irregularity determine the best form of correction. Irregular astigmatism occurs in chemical injuries, severe corneal abrasions, nonpenetrating trauma from blunt objects, and other types of lacerations. Irregular corneal astigmatism exists when the eye cannot be corrected to 20/20 and when the irregularity is evident on corneal topography. Certain more superficial injuries improve with time; others require contact lens correction.[1,2,5,6,8,10,11] Gross trauma, penetrating or nonpenetrating, commonly leads to disruption of a large portion of the anterior segment of the eye, including the iris and lens. Iris injuries may also produce optical problems as well as cosmetic disfiguration.[6,10,11]

When damage to the iris produces visual symptoms, these can be corrected with hydrophilic contact lenses or RGP lenses, depending on whether or not there is regular or irregular astigmatism that will affect the spectacle correction, to provide better visual acuity.[1,2,5,6,8,10,11] Trauma can induce iris abnormalities by injury to the second cranial nerve or by paralytic mydriasis from a lesion to the sphincter muscle. It may induce rupture of the sphincter muscle or traumatic iridectomy, or even loss of a section or all of the iris. The restoration of the physical appearance is just as important as reestablishment of visual function. Abnormalities of pupil shape, or polycoria, aside from the cosmetic problems, may also induce significant optical problems. It is more common in the aphakic and pseudophakic patient but may be present even in phakic patients. Multiple images and photophobia are associated. In such cases, the contact lens serves as a new "optical diaphragm," creating an artificial pupil and appropriately limiting the entry of light into the eye through the contact lens.[1,2,5,6,8,10,11]

Trauma may disfigure the eye from corneal opacities, iris damage, cataract, or scleral, conjunctival, and palpebral lesions. Cosmetic lenses, prostheses, or scleral shells can be fitted, depending on the extent of the abnormalities. Therapeutic lenses are indicated primarily in cases that require protection of the corneal epithelium from trauma by the lids or in cases of abrasions or lacerations of the superficial cornea, as well as in small perforating lesions or descemetoceles. A disposable hydrophilic lens can be used. Collagen lenses are less useful because they dissolve so rapidly,[1,2,5,6,8,10,11] usually within 24 to 72 hours.

11. When should a contact lens be fitted after trauma?

It is important in fitting a contact lens post-trauma to take a complete history of the patient. It is important to check whether the patient has had previous experience with optical correction, including any problems experienced with glasses or contact lenses.

One should verify the nature of the ocular trauma and examine the eye, ocular adnexa, face, head, neurologic function (cranial nerves III, IV, VI, V_1, and VII), and extremities to evaluate the capacity for insertion and removal of the contact lens.[6,10,11]

One should ask about allergies, diabetes, neurologic abnormalities, or musculoskeletal problems that might affect the function of the lids, altering the blink. Allergies to storage products as well as contact lens cleaners are one of the most common problems. Patient motivation should be moderate to high so that the patient can accept the fitting problems that will undoubtedly be part of visual rehabilitation. It is important for the patient to understand the problems that will be part of the initial fitting process and to emphasize the importance of following instructions precisely to avoid contact lens complications.[1,2,5,6,8,10,11]

A detailed physical examination for evaluation of the structures that are affected by the trauma should include inspection of the structural and functional aspects of the visual system, assessment of any anatomic or neurologic deficits, careful inspection of ocular anatomy and the corneal surface, assessment of visual acuity, refraction, and assessment of ocular motility and tear function.[5,6,8]

12. How should visual acuity be evaluated and refraction performed?

Visual acuity without correction and with correction should be measured to serve as references for future comparisons. Moreover, such comparisons and visual acuity measurements, pre- and postfit, may help serve to motivate the patient.[10] Measurement of refraction is as important as the visual acuity measurement. In infants, children, and phakic, pre-presbyopic adults, cycloplegia is indicated. If the corneal surface is irregular, an RGP lens may be used to perform refraction.[10]

13. What are the corneal topographic changes that occur after ocular trauma?

A traumatic corneal laceration can be associated with significant regular or irregular astigmatism, even after a meticulous surgical procedure. Familiarity with corneal topography after trauma is essential for choosing a hydrophilic or RGP contact lens.[1,2,5,6,8,10–12] In general, the cornea flattens at the incision and 90 degrees away. The effect of this flattening is greater when the incision or laceration is near the visual axis. When there is a nonperforating laceration, the flattening is accentuated in the area of the laceration. This flattening is secondary to the margin of the wound and the subsequent additional tissue, beginning with the formation of an epithelial block. This block is subsequently replaced by stromal collagen (scar tissue), and the addition of this tissue creates corneal flattening.

A laceration that penetrates into the anterior chamber results in accentuated flattening due of movement of the anterior stroma of the edematous cornea and the wound dehiscence.[8] A laceration that requires suturing results in corneal flattening due to the compression of the cornea, which occurs with closure of the laceration. While the compression suture flattens the cornea directly at the suture, it induces steepening in that suture meridian.

The post-traumatic cornea frequently maintains sphericity or near-sphericity in the periphery. It is fundamental for fitting an RGP lens that one has touch in the midcorneal periphery, approximately 4 mm from the geometric center, typically in the 3 and 9 o'clock positions. Studies demonstrate that a large part of ocular traumas occur below the midline of the cornea. Maintaining normal superior corneal topography after trauma is the optimal condition for a successful fitting of an RGP contact lens. It permits the lens to maintain a large area of superior alignment, aided by the upper lid, which helps to keep it in position. The cornea traumatized inferiorly can either flatten or steepen. The inferior elevation creates little or no difficulty for contact lens visual rehabilitation. There is significant difficulty in fitting contact lenses after trauma occurs in the superior corneal region. This situation makes maintenance of lens alignment very difficult.[1,2,5,6,8,12] It is important to remember that corneal flattening and induced astigmatism are much greater when the laceration approximates the central cornea. Keratometric measurements may produce an error that is used as a parameter for the trial lens. The definitive lens is the one that most normally aligns on the superior cornea; this is easiest when the superior cornea is not substantially involved in the lesion.[1,2,5,6,8,12]

In summary, the major effect of corneal laceration on vision is due to surface irregularity. The resulting scar may have a significant effect on the vision if it is in the visual axis or occludes a major part of this area. Scars outside the visual axis often affect vision by altering corneal topography and creating irregular astigmatism.[1,2,5,6,8,12]

14. Why check the tear film in contact lens fitting after trauma?

The quality and volume of the tear film are equally important in the fitting of a contact lens after trauma, just as it is in all patients fitted with contact lenses.[5,6,8] Lacrimal insufficiency in eyes with irregular topography accentuates epithelial problems induced by the contact lens. Testing for tear breakup time may indicate a significant meibomian gland dysfunction if the breakup time is less than 10 seconds.[5,6,8] Tear breakup time can be measured invasively through the use of sodium fluorescein or noninvasively by using the keratometric mires or a placido disk system. The inferior lacrimal lake should be evaluated. A lacrimal lake of less than 0.3 mm should be considered suspicious for lacrimal insufficiency. If, because of tear abnormalities, corneal deepithelialization is accelerated, there may be an increased number of desquamated cells under the contact lens, increasing the complications and worsening tolerance of the lens. The Schirmer test has limited value but may be useful if other tests are inconclusive. This test in traumatized eyes can lead to a false negative finding.[5,6,8]

15. How does one select a contact lens for fitting after trauma?

A spherical RGP contact lens is the first choice for patients with corneal laceration and represents the "gold standard" for visual rehabilitation after such injuries. The rigid lens optically corrects the corneal deformities by neutralizing both regular and irregular astigmatism.[5,6,8]

There is no fixed, established rule for fitting RGP contact lenses in patients with ocular trauma, but the initial trial lens may be based on videokeratoscopy. Likewise, the assessment of the relationship between the lens and cornea is based on the biomicroscopic findings (Color Plate 21). Normally, the base curve of the lens is selected based on the midperipheral zone of the cornea; this should be approximately 3 mm superior to visual axis. For the first trial lens, one selects a base curve flatter than the flat keratometric reading. For astigmatism less than 1

D, one fits with a base curve equal to the flat keratometric reading on K. For astigmatism between 1 and 2 D, one adds 0.5 D to the flat keratometric reading. For astigmatism greater than 2 D, one adds 25% to the flat keratometric reading.[5,6,8,12]

To maintain stability of the lens, the diameter should be large; between 9 and 11 mm. For a regular pupil smaller than 4 mm, one can choose a diameter equal to or less than 9 mm because the lens centers. The central thickness of the lenses varies from 0.12 to 0.15 mm in minus corrections and in phakic eyes. In aphakic eyes (in the range of + 15.00 D), the central thickness should be approximately 0.25 mm. The material most commonly used is polyfluorosiliconemethacrylate, and the preferred Dk is 96, with thinner lenses providing better oxygen exchange. However, contact lenses with Dks in the 40 to 70 range are less flexible and may be used to correct more significant corneal irregularities. Lenses with a Dk of 100 or more are used in eyes with less regular or irregular astigmatism.[6,8,12]

The contact lens should have good centration and movement; the tear film between the lens and cornea, when examined with fluorescein at the biomicroscope, should be thin and uniform with a good exchange of fluorescein with each blink. The dioptric power of the final lens should be obtained using the trial lens power and overrefraction, corrected for vertex distance.[8]

16. What are the basic rules for fitting rigid gas permeable lenses after ocular trauma?

The lens should align with the area of the cornea least affected by the trauma (usually superior, although sometimes nasal or temporal).[8,10]

1. Fit the contact lens over the steepest area of the cornea.
2. Use a large diameter lens in order to position the lens well under the superior lid and to permit positioning of the lens over the irregular area.
3. Consider the use of posterior toric RGP lenses with a design not based on central keratometry.
4. Central toricity may be very great when the laceration approximates the optical center. The peripheral cornea and the mid-periphery may still maintain a shape close to spherical.[8,10]

17. When should one fit a hydrophilic lens post-trauma?

Use of a spherical or toric hydrophilic lens is only possible when the post-traumatic cornea has a minimum of irregular scarring. Keratometry and videokeratoscopy provide significant information about the degree of irregularity of the astigmatism in the central cornea. If the reflected images are regular and free of distortions, the most precise refraction can be obtained. If the refraction is stable after two or three measurements in subsequent weeks, fitting of the contact lens can be initiated.[6,8]

If central corneal astigmatism is present, a spherical hydrophilic contact lens can be fitted, and the residual astigmatism is corrected with glasses. A hydrophilic lens should have a stable position and adequate movement. The patient is instructed to use the hydrophilic lens in a daily-wear routine.[6,8]

A careful overrefraction should be performed after 1 or 2 weeks to determine if there is residual astigmatism. If the residual astigmatism is well tolerated, a new correction does not necessarily need to be provided. However, if poorly tolerated, glasses can be prescribed over the hydrophilic lens. In the case of a patient who does not wish to have spectacles, a toric hydrophilic lens may be prescribed.

Prior to fitting a toric hydrophilic lens, one should verify that the topography and refraction are stable by means of serial measurements.[6,8] One should perform a trial with the toric hydrophilic lens to determine the axis of the cylinder; the dioptric power should be calculated based on the spectacle correction and with spherocylindrical correction over the trial lens.[6,8] In selecting a hydrogel trial toric lens, a trial lens with the closest axis measurement value possible should be used. The second most important parameter is the cylinder power, and third is the spherical power.

In follow-up examinations, corneal neovascularization should be looked for, especially in translimbal lacerations. This does not necessarily prevent the patient from using a hydrophilic lens, but the presence of new vessels indicates that there is hypoxia or mechanical trauma. To minimize problems, flatten the contact lens, decrease wearing time, attempt to control dehydration by using preservative-free drops frequently, and/or change the contact lens to a higher-Dk material to augment oxygen permeability. If there is no improvement in the vascularization, an RGP lens is then indicated.[6,8]

18. What are the other alternatives for fitting contact lenses post–corneal trauma?

The alternatives to RGP and hydrophilic contact lenses for post-trauma fitting include piggyback lenses and hybrid lenses (Softperm™).[8,10,11] The piggyback system, in which an RGP lens is fitted over a hydrophilic lens, is indicated in patients with intermittent intolerance of a rigid lens who need the rigid lens for significant central irregular corneal astigmatism.[8,10,11] The fitting should be accomplished in the following manner:

1. Fit a hydrophilic contact lens with high Dk/L with plano power and wait 30 minutes.
2. Perform keratometry or videokeratoscopy over the anterior surface of the hydrophilic lens.
3. Fit a gas permeable contact lens over the hydrophilic lens as one would fit over a normal cornea.
4. Evaluate the lens–lens relationship using biomicroscopy and, if nec-

essary, use high-molecular-weight fluorescein to prevent staining of the hydrogel or silicone hydrogel lenses and to help assess the rigid lens to soft lens/corneal fitting relationship.

5. When the RGP lens is fitted, proceed with an overrefraction over the two lenses.
6. The dioptric power is calculated for the RGP and should be ordered in a lens with a high Dk/L.

Complications are relative to adverse physiologic circumstances that produce hypoxia and neovascularization in the area of the scar. These can be minimized by choosing a lens for the appropriate parameters, permitting both lenses mobility during the blink.[8,10,11] The movement of the two lenses should be independent of one another. The use of these lenses may be only occasional or with some limitation of the number of hours used during the day in order to avoid complications.[8,10,11]

Softperm are hybrid lenses manufactured by CIBAVision. They combine a hydrophilic contact lens in the periphery and a rigid lens of butyl-styrene and silicone acrylate in the center in order to correct unusual refractive errors.[8]

The overall diameter of the Softperm lens is 14.5 mm, with the rigid central portion 8 mm in diameter and with an optical zone of 7 mm. The water content of the hydrophilic skirt is approximately 25%, and the lens Dk is 14×10^{-11}.[8] The rigid butyl-styrene center permits correction of high degrees of regular and irregular astigmatism present in the post-traumatic cornea. The hydrogel skirt provides distribution of the contact lens over the cornea, limbus, and sclera in order to position the optical zone directly over the pupil.[8]

The problems that occur with the Softperm lens are peripheral tightening with a decrease in adequate lens movement, physiologic complications due to poor mobility of the contact lens, and difficulty removing and handling the contact lens.[8] In follow-up examinations after fitting with a Softperm lens, the contact lens should be examined at the biomicroscope to determine if there are deposits, tears in the lens, and imperfections. The transition zone should be inspected.[8]

19. How should one follow up contact lenses carefully fitted in the post-trauma patient?

Follow-up of the contact lens fit post-trauma should be performed initially 2 to 3 days after dispensing the lens, with the patient using the lenses for 4 to 6 hours daily. One should evaluate the relationship between the lens and the cornea and the integrity of the corneal epithelium, if one is utilizing an RGP lens. If a hydrophilic lens was fitted, one should examine the lens–cornea relationship and check the peripheral limbus, especially if the lens appears tight and there is a mechanism that would produce hypoxia. In such cases, a new lens should be fitted.[6,8] The follow-up should be monthly in the first 3 months and twice a year after that. At all the examinations, one should perform biomicroscopy to determine if there are chips, tears, or scratches in the lens.

If there is any doubt about the condition of a contact lens, it should be removed and examined in detail. If necessary, it should be exchanged.[5,6,8]

20. What are the most frequent complications of contact lens fitting post-trauma?

The most frequent complications are:

- Epithelial edema
- Epithelial infiltrates
- Superficial punctate keratopathy
- Stromal edema
- Corneal erosion
- Neovascularization
- Keratometric and refractive alterations.[5,6,8]

21. How does one evaluate the visual results of contact lenses after ocular trauma?

Studies demonstrate that visual acuity improves with both RGP and hydrophilic lenses, as compared with spectacles. However, the RGP contact lens generally provides the best visual acuity by correcting both regular and irregular astigmatism.[10]

Visual acuity should be evaluated using a Snellen chart at 20 feet without correction and subsequently with spectacles and contact lenses to determine how much visual gain has been achieved with contact lenses.[10] Contrast sensitivity testing may be performed to determine if there are deficits that are not detected by the estimate of visual acuity.[10] Stereopsis testing should be performed when visual acuity in the traumatized eye is equal to or greater than 20/40 (6/12).[10] These tests should be repeated in 3 months if there is improvement in visual acuity with the use of the contact lens.[10]

Conclusions

The RGP contact lenses are most commonly indicated for visual rehabilitation in eyes that have suffered trauma and have regular and irregular astigmatism as well as corneal scarring. The contact lens should be used on a daily basis only. For success in fitting, it is necessary to have a motivated patient who understands the benefits of contact lens use for the improvement of visual acuity. After surgical repair of corneal lacerations, the contact lens should be fitted as soon as possible, even before the sutures have been removed, principally in children, in whom amblyopia can become a major problem.

References

1. Kara Jose N, Alves MR, Bonanome MTBC, Sousa NA Jr. Ferimento perfurante de globo ocular na infancia. *Rev Bras Oftalmol.* 1981;40:243–254.

2. McMahon TT. Ocular trauma. *Clinical Contact Lens Practice/Advanced Contact Lens Application* 1993:1–10.
3. Bennet E, Weismann, eds. *Clinical Contact Lens Practice,* rev. ed. Philadelphia: Lippincott-Raven, 1996;47A:1–10.
4. Alves MR, Kara Jose N, Prado J Jr, Usuba FS, Onclinx TM, Marantes CR. Ferimento perfurante ocular: 400 casos admitidos na Clinica Oftalmologica da Faculdade de Medicina de Universidada de Sao Paulo. *Arq Bras Oftalmol.* 1995;58:342–345.
5. Navon SE. Topography after repair of full-thickness corneal laceration. *J Cataract Refract Surg.* 1997;23:495–501.
6. Moreira SBM, Moreira H. *Lentes de Contato,* 2nd ed. Rio de Janeiro: Cultura Medica, 1998:307–309.
7. Weissman BA, Barr JT, et al. *Optometric Clinical Practice Guideline: Care of the Contact Lens Patient.* American Optometric Association, 2000.
8. Stein HA, Freeman MF, Stein RM, Maund LD. *Residents Contact Lens Curriculum Manual,* 2nd ed. New Orleans: EUA CLAO, 1999:143–159.
9. Brennan NA. Is there a question of safety with continuous wear? *Clin Exp Optom.* 2002;85:127–140.
10. Titiyal J, Das A, et al. Visual performance of rigid gas permeable contact lenses in patients with corneal opacity. *CLAO J.* 2001;27:163–165.
11. Kampolat A, Ciftci OU. The use of rigid gas-permeable contact lenses in scarred corneas. *CLAO J.* 1995;27:64–66.
12. Jankov M, Reggi JRA, Lui Netto A, Naufal SC, Dantas PEC, Dantas MCN. Topografia da cornea apos perfuracao corneal. *Arq Bras Oftalmol.* 2002;65:183–191.

18

Keratoconus

Timothy B. Edrington and Ari de Souza Pena

1. What is keratoconus?

Keratoconus, or conical cornea, is a noninflammatory ectasia of undetermined etiology characterized by thinning and subsequent protrusion of the corneal apex.[1] Although usually bilateral, it is also commonly asymmetric.[2] Keratoconus causes a progressive decrease in vision secondary to irregular astigmatism or corneal scarring. Its onset is reported as early as puberty; it tends to progress until 35 or 40 years of age.[3,4] Keratoconus patients enrolled in the Collaborative Longitudinal Evaluation of Keratoconus (CLEK) Study had an average self-reported age of diagnosis of 27 ± 9 years.[5]

2. What is the clinical picture of keratoconus?

A 15- to 35-year-old patient presents with varying degrees of astigmatism, usually associated with myopia. Keratoconus is characterized by symptoms of decreasing vision at distance and near, distortion of visual images, monocular diplopia, and ghosting of images. Frequent spectacle prescription changes are common. On retinoscopy, one observes scissoring reflexes.[6] In more advanced stages of the disease, an "oil droplet" figure may appear in the center of the retinoscopic reflex.

Keratoconus may be signaled by the presence of deformed keratometric mires with irregular contours. The mires are often blurred and doubled. Keratometric values are generally steeper than 47 D (7.18 mm radius of curvature). However, 5% of CLEK study patients had steep keratometric values flatter than 45 D (7.50 mm).[5] It is often difficult to determine precisely the principal corneal meridians. The major meridians are not 90 degrees apart (irregular astigmatism) in more advanced presentations.

Computed topography (videokeratoscopy) enhances the evaluation of the corneal surface, detecting irregularities in contour and localized areas of corneal steepening. Topographic analysis aids in the early diagnosis of keratoconus. Based on computed topography, Rabinowitz and McDonnell[7] consider the following findings confirmatory of the early diagnosis of keratoconus.

- Keratometry greater than 47.00 D.
- A difference of 3.00 D or more between points situated 3 mm above and 3 mm below the center of the cornea (I-S value).
- A difference in central keratometry between the two eyes of more than 1.00 D.

3. What are the biomicroscopic signs of keratoconus?

- Thinning of the corneal apex (seen with direct focal illumination using a thin slit-beam).
- Teardrop reflex (seen with diffuse illumination and caused by the more accentuated central curvature of the cone, which acts as a convex mirror). This is easier to observe with the pupils dilated.
- Vogt's striae in the posterior stroma, observed as oblique or vertical lines that may disappear with digital pressure to the upper eyelid.[8]
- Fleischer's ring, a pigmented ring in the basal epithelium just anterior to Bowman's membrane, partially (arc) or completely (ring) encircling the base of the cone, is composed of hemosiderin deposits.
- Anterior reticular scarring corresponding to ruptures in Bowman's membrane with the deposition of fibrous tissue.
- Increased visibility of corneal nerves.
- Ruptures in Descemet's membrane (seen in more advanced phases of the disease in direct illumination, retroillumination, and specular reflection).

Slit-lamp signs of keratoconus tend to increase in prevalence and severity as the condition progresses.[9]

4. What is the classification of keratoconus?

Several classification systems based on keratometry values exist including the following:

- Grade I (incipient): defined as keratometric values under 47.00 D
- Grade II (moderate): defined as values between 47.00 and 52.00 D with deformed mires
- Grade III (advanced): keratometric values greater than 52.00 and up to 60.00 D
- Grade IV (severe): keratometric measurements greater than 60.00 D

Classification can also be based on topography (Figure 18.1A,B):

- Round cone (nipple cone) is the most frequently occurring type. The ectasia is more central and circumscribed, and its extent can be measured with computer topography.
- Oval cone (sagging cone) is a more eccentric deformation in the inferior portion of the cornea. The apex of the cone is farther from the visual center.[10]

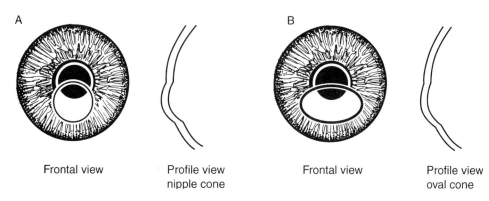

Figure 18.1. A: Round, nipple cone. B: Frontal view and profile of an oval (sagging) cone.

- Undefined (intermediate) cone is usually localized between a central and a sagging cone and corresponds to 15% to 20% of cases of keratoconus.

5. What are the clinical course and different phases of the evolution of keratoconus?

In the incipient and moderate phases, vision obtained with spectacle correction may be satisfactory, and the patient may be maintained in spectacles. In incipient, moderate, or advanced forms, if vision cannot be adequately corrected with spectacles, rigid gas permeable contact lenses are prescribed. Penetrating keratoplasty (PK) is indicated when the patient can no longer tolerate the comfort of rigid contact lenses or satisfactory vision is unattainable through the contact lenses. The literature indicates that 10% to 20% of keratoconus patients ultimately benefit from PK.[11] Up to 47% of post-PK eyes optically benefit from contact lens wear.[12]

6. What are the objectives of a good rigid gas permeable (RGP) contact lens fit in keratoconus?

One should attempt to achieve a lens-to-cornea fitting relationship with minimal apical touch or slight apical clearance. The lens should be designed with a peripheral curve system that permits good circulation of the tear film under the lens but without excessive edge lift.

Ideally, the lens fit should exhibit:

- Minimal apical touch or apical clearance
- No excessive areas of tear or debris pooling beneath the optic zone
- Good circulation of the tear film under the lens
- Good stability and comfort

With these conditions, the lens will cause the least amount of insult to the cornea.

7. What is the routine for choosing the Dk of a gas permeable contact lens in keratoconus?

Optimizing the fitting relationship is essential to rigid contact lens success. Even though keratoconus is not an oxygen-driven condition, patients should be prescribed mid- or high-Dk lenses to obtain adequate oxygen permeability as well as good in-eye wettability. For this reason, fluorinated silicone acrylate rigid contact lens materials may be preferable.

8. What is the technique for fitting rigid contact lenses in the early stages of keratoconus?

There are many different fitting philosophies described in the literature. Most may be classified as either apical touch (flat-fitting), divided support (alignment or three-point touch), or apical clearance (steep-fitting). In early or mild keratoconus, regular RGP fitting philosophies may be appropriate.

9. What is the method of lens fitting in more advanced phases of keratoconus?

In moderate and advanced cases, the practitioner should seek to attain minimal central touch (or apical clearance), as well as minimal intermediate compression. This is a three-point touch fitting relationship with minimal central touch and two zones of peripheral support. However, it is not always possible to attain a lens with a three-point touch fitting relationship.

Fitting Philosophies

Soper

One contact lens option is to fit a bicurve posterior surface (Soper type) when there is already significant protrusion of the cone occupying a large area of the cornea.

The characteristics of a Soper-type lens design include:

- Central posterior curve occupying a central optical zone between 6.0 and 7.5 mm
- A broad zone of intermediate curvature standardized at 45.00 D (7.50 mm)
- Peripheral curves of 40.00, 37.00, and 26.00 D
- The final diameter of the lens, which is based on the measurement of the optic zone increasing from 2 to 6.5 mm.[13,14]

The Soper lens design simulates a hat on the cornea. The goal is to achieve a slight apical clearance fitting relationship. In practice, the overall lens diameter is approximately 9.0 mm.

McGuire

The McGuire lens design is often prescribed for oval and more advanced cones. The goal is to achieve a feather or minimal touch apical fitting relationship. The McGuire design is made with four peripheral curves and a wide blend in the following manner:[10]

Example

Primary curve:	3.00 to 4.00 D flatter than the base curve
Secondary curve:	6.00 D flatter than the primary curve
Tertiary curve:	6.00 D flatter than the secondary curve
Quaternary curve:	6.00 D flatter than the tertiary curve

Final overall lens diameter is 9.0 to 9.4 mm

Edrington (CLEK Study)

A blended tricurve lens design is prescribed to achieve a minimal apical touch fitting relationship. A small overall lens diameter of 8.6 mm is generally prescribed. Select the initial trial lens base curve to equal the steep keratometric value or steep topography-simulated keratometric reading. Evaluate the fluorescein pattern. If the initial trial lens is flat (apical touch), select the next steeper base curve from the trial lens set and repeat fluorescein pattern analysis. If the initial trial lens is judged to be steep (apical clearance), apply the next flatter trial lens and repeat fluorescein pattern analysis. The goal is to determine, by bracketing, the steepest base curve in the trial lens set that provides minimal apical touch. Overrefract the trial lens with the best-fit base curve lens, and add the equivalent sphere of the overrefraction to the power of the trial lens. If there is excessive tear pooling around the base of the cone, consider decreasing the optic zone diameter. It is imperative that the peripheral curve system allow adequate tear exchange. If the diagnostic lens exhibits only minimal peripheral clearance, order a flatter peripheral curve system.[15]

Rose K

The Rose K lens is fitted with a 2.0 to 4.0 mm area of light apical touch with attention paid to achieving optimal peripheral clearance. A proprietary diagnostic lens set is available in base curves ranging from 5.10 to 7.60 mm in 0.10-mm increments. The fitting guide recommends selecting the initial base curve 0.2 mm steeper than the average keratometry values.[16] The standard overall diameter is 8.7 mm, and the optic zone decreases in diameter with steeper base curves.[17]

10. How does one manage the keratoconus patient fitted with contact lenses?

Every RGP lens wearer with keratoconus should be evaluated periodically, ideally at least every 6 months. The patient needs to be educated regarding symptoms and signs that would necessitate an un-scheduled visit.

At each examination, the lenses should be evaluated for the quality of their surfaces. Polishing the front surface and edge of the lens is very important in maintaining optimal lens wettability and patient comfort. The lens-to-cornea fitting relationship should be carefully evaluated with the aid of sodium fluorescein. A thorough slit-lamp biomicro-scopic examination of the cornea with the lens removed is critical to determine if the cornea is adversely affected by lens wear. Instill so-dium fluorescein to observe areas of corneal staining. If coalesced stain-ing is present at the apex of the cone, consider prescribing a steeper base curve to minimize physical trauma to the area of the staining. The presence of stipple staining or dimple-veil staining around the base of the cone is often due to excessive tear debris pooling beneath the optic zone. To decrease the pooling of tear debris, consider reducing the optic zone diameter by lens modification or reordering.

The development of new lens materials and fitting techniques has resulted in increased contact lens success. When the surface of a lens is diminished in quality because of warpage, deposits, or scratches, the lens should be replaced, generally after 1 to 2 years of use. When sig-nificant changes are noted in keratometry or corneal topography, the lenses should be refitted.

11. What are the problems of fitting and maintenance with progression of keratoconus?

As keratoconus progresses and the corneal apex steepens, fitting a con-tact lens becomes more challenging. Corneal scarring is often present with more advanced cases,[18] potentially causing decreased vision and photophobia.

12. Are there other treatment options for keratoconus patients?

Hydrophilic (Soft) Contact Lenses

Soft sphere or toric contact lenses may be prescribed in mild cases of keratoconus. Spectacles may be prescribed to wear over the soft contact lenses to correct residual astigmatism or to provide a reading add. As the condition becomes more advanced, soft lenses generally do not provide adequate vision because of corneal distortion and irregular astigmatism.

Piggyback Systems

In this technique, a soft lens is used as a carrier, and an RGP contact lens is fitted on top of the soft lens.[19] Some patients who are intolerant of rigid lens wear alone find that the addition of the soft carrier lens enhances comfort while still maintaining the superior vision afforded by the rigid lens. A piggyback system may also be prescribed as a bandage contact lens on a part-time wear basis to treat excessive 3 and 9 o'clock position peripheral corneal staining. When prescribing piggyback systems, instruct the patient how to insert, remove, clean, and disinfect the two lenses. It is advisable to prescribe a soft contact lens care system that will be suitable for both the soft and rigid lenses. Rigid lens care systems should not be used to care for soft contact lenses. Disposable soft or silicone hydrogel lenses should be prescribed on a daily-wear basis for the "carrier."

Hybrid Lenses (SoftPerm™)

Hybrid lenses have a rigid optical center made of gas permeable material and a hydrophilic (soft) skirt. Theoretically, these lenses provide the optics of a rigid lens and the comfort of a soft lens. Practically, however, they can be associated with difficulties related to tightening of the fit, reduced oxygenation of the cornea, and frequent breakage.

Large-Diameter Rigid Lenses

Rigid lenses with diameters of 10.5 to 15 mm have recently been marketed for the vision management of keratoconus and other irregular corneal conditions. Although large rigid lenses generally improve lens centration and patient-reported comfort, it is often challenging to obtain an optimal fitting relationship. When fitted to lightly touch the apex of the cone, there tends to be excessive clearance, sometimes with bubbles present, around the base of the cone. If fitted flatter to minimize clearance around the base of the cone, harsh bearing of the corneal apex may result.

Scleral Lenses

Scleral lenses are generally manufactured from gas permeable materials with a high Dk. They can be utilized with relative success for patients who do not tolerate corneal lenses.[20,21]

Refractive Surgery Procedures

LASIK and other currently available refractive surgery procedures are generally contraindicated in keratoconus patients. Keratoconus is a corneal thinning disorder, and LASIK further thins the cornea. Intracornial rings, crescent-shaped corneal inserts, have been utilized to reduce corneal surface distortion in keratoconus, thereby avoiding or delaying the need for a corneal transplant.[22,23]

13. What is the treatment of acute hydrops in keratoconus associated with contact lenses?

In acute hydrops, there is the sudden onset of corneal edema due to the rupture of Descemet's membrane, permitting the influx of aqueous into the corneal stroma. This causes decreased vision, photophobia, and frequently discomfort. Although rare, hydrops generally occurs in advanced forms of the disease.[24] Most of the time, hydrops is treated conservatively with hypertonic agents. It commonly resolves gradually, leaving central scarring, and may often flatten the apex of the cone. It is generally necessary to suspend contact lens wear. One study reported that 4 of 22 eyes eventually obtained a corneal transplant.[25]

14. What are the indications for corneal transplant in keratoconus?

The vast majority of patients with keratoconus can be managed with contact lenses. Indications for keratoplasty in keratoconus are:

- Unsatisfactory vision with contact lens use
- Intolerance of contact lens use, including limited wearing time
- The presence of dense central corneal opacities resulting in decreased vision and/or extreme photophobia
- Central corneal scarring with decreased acuity after the resolution of acute hydrops

15. What is the appropriate basic trial lens set for fitting keratoconus patients?

There are many excellent keratoconus fitting philosophies and recommended keratoconus trial lens fitting sets. A 13-lens trial set recommended by Edrington is shown in Table 18.1.[26]

Table 18.1. Recommended trial set

Base curve (D/mm)	Power (D)	Overall/optic zone diameters (mm)	Secondary curve radius (mm)	Third curve radius/width (mm)	Center thickness (mm)
47.00 (7.18)	−5.00	8.6/7.0	8.25	11.00/0.2	0.13
48.00 (7.03)	−5.00	8.6/7.0	8.25	11.00/0.2	0.13
49.00 (6.89)	−5.00	8.6/7.0	8.25	11.00/0.2	0.13
50.00 (6.75)	−7.00	8.6/6.5	8.25	11.00/0.2	0.13
51.00 (6.62)	−7.00	8.6/6.5	8.25	11.00/0.2	0.13
52.00 (6.49)	−7.00	8.6/6.5	8.25	11.00/0.2	0.13
53.00 (6.37)	−7.00	8.6/6.5	8.25	11.00/0.2	0.13
54.00 (6.25)	−7.00	8.6/6.5	8.25	11.00/0.2	0.13
56.00 (6.03)	−9.00	8.6/6.0	8.00	11.00/0.2	0.14
58.00 (5.82)	−9.00	8.6/6.0	8.00	11.00/0.2	0.14
61.00 (5.53)	−10.00	8.6/6.0	8.00	11.00/0.2	0.14
65.00 (5.19)	−12.00	8.6/6.0	8.00	11.00/0.2	0.14
70.00 (4.82)	−15.00	8.6/6.0	8.00	11.00/0.2	0.14

References

1. Krachmer JH, Feder RS, Belin MW. Keratoconus and related noninflammatory corneal thinning disorders. *Surv Ophthalmol.* 1984;28:293–322.
2. Zadnik K, Steger-May K, Jink BA, et al. Between-eye asymmetry in keratoconus. *Cornea.* 2002;21:671–679.
3. Amsler M. Le keratocone fruste au javal. *Ophthalmologica.* 1938;96:77–83.
4. Tuft SJ, Moodaley LC, Gregory WM, Davison CR, Buckley RJ. Prognostic factors for the progression of keratoconus. *Ophthalmology.* 1994;101:439–447.
5. Zadnik K, Barr JT, Edrington TB, et al., and the CLEK Study Group. Baseline findings in the Collaborative Longitudinal Evaluation of Keratoconus (CLEK) Study. *Invest Ophthalmol Vis Sci.* 1998;39:2537–2546.
6. Swann PG, Waldron HE. Keratoconus: the clinical spectrum. *J Am Optom Assoc.* 1986;57:204–209.
7. Rabinowitz YS., McDonnell PJ. Computer-assisted corneal topography in keratoconus. *Refract Corneal Surg.* 1989;5:400–408.
8. Vogt A. Reflexlinien durch faltung spiegelnder grenzflachen im bereiche von corneo, linsenkapsel und netzhaut. *Albrecht von Graefes Arch Ophthalmol.* 1919;99:296.
9. Zadnik K, Barr JT, Gordon MO, Edrington TB, the CLEK Study Group. Biomicroscopic signs and disease severity in keratoconus. *Cornea.* 1996; 15:139–146.
10. Caroline PJ, McGuire JR, Doughman DJ. Preliminary report on a new contact lens design for keratoconus. *Contact Intraocular Lens Med J.* 1978; 4:69–73.
11. Kennedy RH, Bourne WM, Dyer JA. A 48-year clinical and epidemiologic study of keratoconus. *Am J Ophthalmol.* 1986;101:267–273.
12. Brierly SC, Izquierdo L Jr, Mannis MJ. Penetrating keratoplasty for keratoconus. *Cornea.* 2000;19:329–332.

13. Soper JW, Jarrett A. Results of a systematic approach to fitting keratoconus and corneal transplants. *Contact Lens Med Bull.* 1972;5:50–59.
14. Raber IM. Use of CAB Soper cone contact lenses in keratoconus. *CLAO J.* 1983;9:237–240.
15. Edrington TB, Barr JT, Zadnik K, et al. Standardized rigid contact lens fitting protocol for keratoconus. *Optom Vis Sci.* 1996;73:369–375.
16. Caroline PJ, Norman CW, Andre MP. The latest lens design for keratoconus. *Contact Lens Spectrum.* 1997;12:36–41.
17. Betts AM, Mitchell GL, Zadnik K. Visual performance and comfort with the Rose K lens for keratoconus *Optom Vis Sci.* 2002;79:493–501.
18. Barr JT, Edrington TB, Fink BA, Weissman BA, Gordon MO. Factors associated with corneal scarring in the Collaborative Longitudinal Evaluation of Keratoconus (CLEK) Study. *Cornea.* 2000;19:501–507.
19. Soper JW. Fitting keratoconus with piggy-back and Saturn II lenses. *Contact Lens Forum.* 1986;11:25–30.
20. Tan DTH, Pullum KW, Buckley RJ. Medical applications of scleral contact lenses: gas-permeable scleral contact lenses. *Cornea.* 1995;14:130–137.
21. Pullum KW, Buckley RJ. A study of 530 patients referred for rigid gas permeable scleral contact lens assessment. *Cornea.* 1997;16:612–622.
22. Colin J, Cochener B, Savary G, Malet F. Correcting keratoconus with intracorneal rings *J Cataract Refractive Surg.* 2000;26:1117–1122.
23. Colin J, Cochener B, Savary G, Malet F, Holmes-Higgin DH. INTACS inserts for treating keratoconus. *Ophthalmology.* 2001;108:1409–1414.
24. Tuft SJ, Gregory WM, Buckley RJ. Acute corneal hydrops in keratoconus. *Ophthalmology.* 1994;101:1738–1743.
25. Grewal S, Laibson PR, Cohen EJ, Rapuano CJ. Acute hydrops in the corneal ectasias: associated factors and outcomes. *Trans Am Ophthalmol Soc.* 1999;97:187–198.
26. Edrington TB, et al., a standardized rigid contact lens fitting protocol for keratoconus. *Optom Vis Sci.* 1996;73:369–375.

19

Cosmetic and Prosthetic Contact Lenses

Paulo Ricardo de Oliveira and Jeffrey J. Walline

1. What is the difference between a cosmetic contact lens and a prosthetic contact lens?

A cosmetic contact lens is a tinted or painted contact lens used to enhance or alter the appearance of a normal eye. A prosthetic contact lens is a tinted or painted contact lens used to improve the appearance of a disfigured eye or to help correct the vision of a poorly functioning eye.[1-3] The term *tinted contact lenses* can be used to refer to both cosmetic and prosthetic contact lenses.

2. Do all tinted contact lenses improve vision?

Tinted contact lenses may or may not have refractive power. Contact lenses used to improve visual acuity have a clear pupil or a pupil with a translucent tint. Contact lenses used to improve the appearance of a nonseeing eye may have a black, opaque pupil. Tinted contact lenses may be used to reduce glare or photophobia in order to improve vision. Cosmetic contact lenses may occasionally induce irregular astigmatism.[4]

3. What are the types of cosmetic contact lenses?

Cosmetic contact lenses are nearly always soft contact lenses because rigid gas permeable contact lenses may be too small and may move too much to cover the entire iris. Cosmetic contact lenses may have a translucent tint or an opaque tint.

4. What are the indications for cosmetic contact lenses?

Cosmetic contact lenses are typically fitted because the patient wants to alter the color of the iris. Translucent, cosmetic contact lenses typically serve to enhance the natural color of the eye. They may make blue eyes a deeper blue, or they may make green eyes more obvious. Opaque cosmetic contact lenses may make brown eyes blue (Figure 19.1), blue eyes lavender, or may change the color of the eyes to aquamarine, amber, hazel, or any number of other colors. Opaque cosmetic contact lenses may also be used in theatrical settings to make the eyes appear more dramatic, "zombie-like," or animal-like. Contact lenses are also available with professional team logos or with simple designs.

5. What are the types of prosthetic contact lenses?

Prosthetic contact lenses may be polymethylmethacrylate (PMMA) contact lenses, rigid gas permeable (RGP) contact lenses, scleral contact lenses, or soft contact lenses.

6. What are the general indications for prosthetic contact lenses?

Prosthetic contact lenses may be used to improve the appearance of a disfigured cornea, sclera, iris, or crystalline lens. Any part of the eye may become disfigured due to trauma, ocular disease, systemic health problems, or congenital defects. Prosthetic contact lenses may also be used to disguise an enucleated eye, to patch an eye during vision therapy, to reduce glare or photophobia (Figures 19.2 and 19.3), or to treat intractable binocular diplopia.

7. What are the indications and contraindications for PMMA or RGP prosthetic contact lenses?

Both PMMA and RGP prosthetic contact lenses can be painted with exquisite detail to match a healthy contralateral eye, whereas soft con-

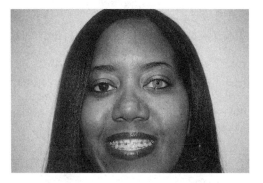

Figure 19.1. A brown-eyed patient wearing a blue, opaque cosmetic contact lens on her left eye.

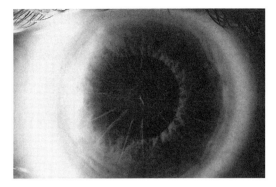

Figure 19.2. This patient complained of glare and halos, especially in dim lighting, after radial keratotomy.

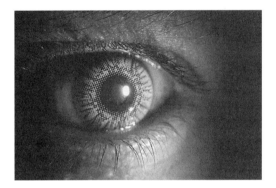

Figure 19.3. A prosthetic contact lens painted on the back surface with a 4-mm clear pupil to decrease glare and halos for the patient in Fig. 19.2.

tact lenses cannot be as individualized. Disfigured corneas often exhibit irregular astigmatism, and PMMA or RGP prosthetic lenses can correct poor vision due to irregular astigmatism while improving the appearance of the disfigured eye. Disfigured eyes with moderate to severe neovascularization should be fitted with highly oxygen-permeable, RGP prosthetic contact lenses because they allow maximal amounts of oxygen to reach the cornea. Because PMMA and RGP contact lenses are smaller, and because they move on the cornea more than soft contact lenses, they should not be used to mask anomalies that affect peripheral parts of the cornea or large portions of the anterior segment.

8. What are the indications and contraindications for fitting a scleral contact lens?

A scleral contact lens is indicated when a corneal contact lens will not center properly on the cornea or when one wishes to improve the appearance of the sclera. Scleral contact lenses require a greater level of expertise to fit them properly; fitting them requires substantial chair time, and they are available from only a limited number of sources, so they are relatively expensive. They should be used only after all other types of contact lenses have failed to correct the problem.

9. What are the indications and contraindications for fitting a soft prosthetic contact lens?

Soft, prosthetic contact lenses should be used when a significant proportion of the anterior eye is disfigured, when the patient is a previous soft contact lens wearer, or when the patient only wants to wear the contact lens occasionally. Soft contact lenses are contraindicated in eyes with moderate to advanced neovascularization, moderate to extreme dry eye, and irregular astigmatism. Soft contact lenses may also be difficult to handle for people with motor coordination problems.

10. How does one fit a PMMA or an RGP prosthetic contact lens?

A trial lens fitting will almost always be necessary on disfigured corneas. If possible, PMMA and RGP contact lenses should be fitted using keratometry readings and manifest refraction data. Keratometry readings are often not possible to obtain on disfigured eyes that require prosthetic contact lenses due to irregularities of the corneal surface. If only one cornea is severely affected, measuring the corneal curvature of the contralateral eye may yield a reasonable estimate for the initial contact lens parameters. Generally, PMMA or RGP prosthetic contact lenses should be fitted with a large diameter to cover the defect, and they should be fitted relatively tight to decrease the movement of the contact lens. Assessing the fluorescein pattern is often difficult or impossible on an opaque prosthetic contact lens. Particular attention should be paid to the centration and movement of the contact lens as well as to the corneal slit-lamp findings to determine whether the fit of the contact lens is appropriate.

11. How does one fit a scleral prosthetic contact lens?

Scleral prosthetic contact lenses can be fitted by taking an impression of the eye or by performing a trial fitting, but ocular impressions are rarely performed. Fitting a scleral contact lens is a two-step process. The first step is to approximate the radius of curvature of the sclera. Once an optimal scleral radius is achieved, the size and curvature of the optic zone should be determined. A refraction over the final trial lens should always be performed to determine the power of the contact lens.

12. How does one fit a soft cosmetic or prosthetic contact lens?

Soft cosmetic or prosthetic lenses are fitted using trial lenses with vary-ing base curves, diameters, thicknesses, and colors. The color of the contact lens should be determined compared to the contralateral eye in natural sunlight and under artificial lighting. If a contact lens is to be painted after the initial fitting, the flattest contact lens possible should be chosen because the painting process may cause the contact lens to tighten.

13. How does one disinfect soft cosmetic contact lenses?

There are specific criteria for each brand, and one should follow the recommendations of the manufacturer before choosing a method of disinfection. The tint may fade if hydrogen peroxide disinfecting so-lutions or alcohol-based daily cleaning solutions are used, but the rec-ommended method of cleaning or disinfecting the contact lens varies for each brand of contact lens.

14. Does an opaque cosmetic contact lens with a clear pupil reduce the patient's visual field?

In general, an opaque cosmetic contact lens with a clear pupil reduces the patient's visual field minimally, if at all. A smaller pupil size will limit the amount of light that reaches the back of the eye. A patient may complain that the vision is too dim, especially in poorly lit situations.

15. How and when should topical medication be used in the presence of a cosmetic contact lens?

Topical medication in the form of drops can be used routinely, but a soft contact lens can be damaged by certain topical medications. If the patient is wearing a cosmetic contact lens, it is best to apply the med-ication at least 10 minutes before inserting the contact lens or after removing the contact lens. If medication instillation is necessary more often, the patient should be told to remove the contact lenses prior to drop instillation and to insert them after waiting for 10 minutes.

Prosthetic Contact Lens Case Report

M.S., a 40-year-old Caucasian male police officer, reported for an eye examination with complaints of glare and halos around lights, especially in dim conditions, since undergoing bilateral radial keratotomy nearly 1 year earlier. He had been treated for glare and halos with varying concentrations of pilocarpine to constrict his pupils, which caused transient poor vision for 30 to 60 minutes. He reported a bout of iritis in the right eye 10 years ago, but he had no other significant personal or family ocular or systemic problems. He did not report any allergies or previous surgeries.

His uncorrected visual acuity was $20/30^{-1}$ in the right eye and $20/20^{-1}$ in the left eye. Manifest refraction was $+0.25 -1.75 \times 035(20/15)$ in the right eye and $+0.25 -2.25 \times 170 (20/20)$ in the left eye. His pupils were 7 mm in diameter in room light and 4 mm in diameter in bright light. He had 15 radial incision scars with a 2.5-mm clear zone in the right eye and eight radial keratotomy incision scars with a 3-mm clear zone in the left eye (Figure 19.2).

The patient was fitted with Durasoft 3 Colors™ contact lenses in both eyes to cover most of the radial incisions and to reduce the glare and halos. After 1 week of contact lens wear, the patient said that the contact lenses slightly reduced the glare but not enough to alleviate the discomfort. The contact lenses were mailed to Adventures in Colors (Denver, CO) to paint the back surface black with 2.0-mm clear pupil in each eye.

After the patient wore the contact lenses with the 2.0-mm clear pupil for 2 weeks, he reported significant reduction of the glare and halos, but he reported that his vision was too dim, especially when he worked at night. New contact lenses were ordered with a 3.0-mm clear pupil in the right eye and a 4.0-mm clear pupil in the left eye (Figure 19.3).

After wearing the contact lenses with larger pupils, the patient reported much better vision in dim situations without glare and halos. Visual fields were performed on the patient, and no reduction in peripheral vision was noted with the contact lenses.

References

1. Massare J, Freeman M. Cosmetic soft contact lenses. In: Kastl PR, ed. *Contact Lenses—The CLAO Guide to Basic Science and Clinical Practice.* Dubuque, IA: Kindall/Hunt Publishing, 1995:253–261.
2. Moreira S, Moreira H. Lentes de contato cosmeticas e proteticas. In: Moreira S, Moreira H, eds. *Lentes de Contato.* Rio de Janeiro: Cultura Medica, 1993:262–264.
3. Efron N. Tinted lenses. In: Efron N, ed. *Contact Lens Practice,* 1st ed. Boston: Butterworth-Heinemann, 2002.
4. Schanzer MC, Mehta RS, Arnold TP, Zuckerbrod SL, Koch DD. Irregular astigmatism induced by annular tinted contact lenses. *CLAO J.* 1989;15:207–211.

20

Therapeutic Contact Lenses

Paulo Ricardo de Oliveira and Melissa D. Bailey

1. What are the indications for the use of a therapeutic contact lens?

- Pain reduction caused by defects or lesions of the corneal epithelium
- More rapid restoration and preservation of corneal epithelial integrity
- Protection of the cornea in cases of corneal drying
- Protection of the cornea in cases of mechanical injury secondary to entropion and trichiasis
- Restoration of the anterior chamber after shallowing caused by small corneal perforations
- Delivery of medications to the ocular surface

2. What are the primary indications for the use of a therapeutic contact lens?

- Abrasions, erosions, and corneal ulcers
- Filamentary keratitis
- Neurotrophic keratitis
- Neuroparalytic keratitis
- Herpes simplex keratitis
- Dry eye syndrome
- Ectatic dystrophies
- Corneal dystrophies with epithelial compromise
- Bullous keratopathy
- Entropion, trichiasis, and lid defects
- Corneal lacerations with small perforations
- Postoperative discomfort
- After suturing the cornea or surgical correction of lid injuries

3. How should one choose a therapeutic contact lens?

The choice of a therapeutic contact lens depends basically on the objective. The water content, thickness, oxygen transmissibility, diameter, base curve, and power must be consistent with the problem that needs to be resolved. Collagen contact lenses are used when the eye care practitioner wants to soak the lens in a medication prior to applying the contact lens. Low-water-content contact lenses are used to prevent drying of the cornea. If the lens needs to be worn for an extended period of time, consider a silicone hydrogel lens that is designed to be worn on an extended basis.

4. What are the principal benefits of using a therapeutic contact lens?

- Alleviation of pain
- Treatment of corneal disease
- Improvement of visual acuity

5. What are the basic principles that must be observed when fitting a therapeutic contact lens?

To choose the base curve for the therapeutic contact lens, take readings of the patient's central corneal curvature with a keratometer or corneal topographer. In the event that central corneal curvature readings are not available or that it is not possible to obtain this measurement due to the condition of the cornea, choose a lens with an average base curve. In general, a therapeutic contact lens should be fit tighter than usual, providing adherence and stabilization. The contact lens diameter should be fairly large, covering the entire cornea, with less mobility than normal. Nonetheless, try to conserve some tear exchange. A therapeutic contact lens should either be thin with low water content or thicker with high water content, depending on the indication and the need for oxygen transmissibility. The cornea should not be further traumatized by the contact lens, and the patient should report good comfort with the lens in place.

6. How should the therapeutic contact lens be maintained?

The frequency of examination visits to reassess the condition of a therapeutic contact lens depends on the ocular disorder under treatment. When the threat of corneal perforation is present or there is a loss of corneal sensation, the cornea should be observed daily. In cases of superficial keratitis, bullous keratopathy, or recurrent erosion, the patient can be seen weekly. The eye care practitioner must evaluate the condition of the contact lens and determine if replacement is necessary. Many manufacturers make recommendations about the frequency of lens replacement, and those recommendations should be considered. Practitioners often use ordinary disposable contact lenses as therapeutic contact lenses, and these lenses may be changed daily, weekly, every 2 weeks, or at the discretion of the doctor.[1]

7. How does one proceed when it is necessary to measure intraocular pressure during the use of a therapeutic contact lens?

The lens should be removed from the eye very carefully. If fluorescein is used for tonometry, the eye should be irrigated thoroughly afterward. Another possibility is to use non-contact tonometry, measuring the pressure with the lens on the eye. The intraocular pressure measurement obtained will be a few millimeters higher than without the lens. Intraocular pressure measurements can also be obtained with a hand-held contact tonometer, such as the Tonopen™, through the lens, without difficulty.

8. How and when should one use topical medications with a therapeutic contact lens?

Topical medication can be used as necessary. The use of topical antibiotic is recommended in the majority of cases. When possible, preparations without preservatives should be used to avoid toxic and sensitivity reactions. Artificial tears should be preservative-free when they are used several times a day and/or for a long period of time. Hypertonic solutions may cause dehydration of the therapeutic contact lens and lead to tight-lens syndrome in these patients.

9. When is a therapeutic contact lens indicated for bullous keratopathy?

A therapeutic lens is indicated for relief of pain. The use is of short duration, generally while the patient is awaiting corneal transplantation or a surface stabilization procedure. In such cases, the lens should be used for as short a time as possible to avoid secondary infection or neovascularization.

A therapeutic contact lens can be used for longer periods in eyes with no hope of visual recuperation. In such cases, one may observe the development of neovascularization and formation of fibrosis under Bowman's membrane, which diminishes bullous formation, permitting discontinuation of the therapeutic lens.

10. How long are therapeutic contact lenses used for recurrent corneal erosion?

It generally takes a period of several months for the epithelial cells of the cornea to form a firm adhesion to the epithelial basement membrane. An extended wear contact lens may be used as therapeutic contact lenses to protect the fragile epithelium while the new adhesions form.[2]

11. When are therapeutic contact lens used to treat dry eye?

Therapeutic contact lenses can be used to provide comfort to patients with severe dry eye. The use of therapeutic contact lenses should be reserved for cases in which artificial tears, moisture chamber glasses, punctal occlusion, and other techniques have not provided the patient a minimum of comfort. It is important to remember that dry eye patients tend to form deposits more readily on contact lenses. If there are significant breaks in the corneal epithelium, there is also the possibility of ocular infection. Thus, when therapeutic contact lenses are prescribed to treat severe dry eye, the patient should be closely monitored.

The most appropriate type of contact lens for this situation is a low-water-content contact lens that tends to conserve the precorneal tear film and reduce tear evaporation. Conversely, high-water-content contact lenses significantly increase evaporation. When the aqueous layer of the precorneal tear film is evaporated, the eye still remains dry, and the lens may become tight as a consequence of dehydration. A low-water-content contact lens may prevent this situation.

12. Can therapeutic contact lenses be used to treat descemetocele formation or corneal perforation?

A therapeutic contact lens is used when a descemetocele or corneal perforation is very small, generally smaller than 2 mm, and when there is no incarceration of uveal tissue and no traction of the uveal tissue toward the wound. The contact lens should be fitted slightly tighter than normal, producing edema of the cornea. The edema leads to apposition of the borders of the lesion and impedes the flow of aqueous humor. It also facilitates reformation of the anterior chamber and scarring of the cornea at the site of the wound. A therapeutic contact lens can be used over cyanoacrylate adhesive to decrease patient discomfort and to protect the glue from the action of the lids, which can dislodge it. This may also prevent the cyanoacrylate from irritating the lids and causing giant papillary conjunctivitis.[3]

13. What are the goals of using a therapeutic contact lens following corneal transplantation?

A therapeutic contact lens may be used to aid reepithelialization of the transplanted corneal tissue and to make the patient more comfortable in the early postoperative period.[4] When patients are more comfortable, postoperative examinations are easier, especially in children. The contact lens protects exposed sutures and suture-related surface irregularities and also controls the symptoms of filamentary keratitis. The therapeutic lens reduces the postoperative inflammatory reaction in all patients. The risk of infection in these patients is significant; therefore, therapeutic contact lenses should be used for the minimum amount of time.

14. When should a therapeutic contact lens be used to treat corneal dystrophies?

Patients with certain corneal dystrophies often also have epithelial erosion. These erosions often cause pain, foreign-body sensation, photophobia, and tearing. When patients have recurrent episodes of these symptoms, a therapeutic contact lens may be helpful in treating the erosions and the associated symptoms.

15. When should a therapeutic contact lens be used to treat a chemical burn?

During the first and second weeks after a chemical injury, the inflammatory reaction may be so intense that it is impossible to fit a contact lens. When this inflammatory reaction decreases, however, a contact lens can be used to facilitate reepithelialization, to prevent and treat the frequent breakdown of epithelial adhesions, and to protect the cornea from eyelids that have abnormal surfaces due to scar tissue formation. Artificial tears and prophylactic antibiotics should be used frequently in these patients.

16. When should a therapeutic contact lens be used to treat neurotrophic keratitis?

Neurotrophic keratitis is characterized by slow-healing epithelial defects and loss of corneal sensation. Therapeutic contact lenses may assist with the process of reepithelialization and provide the patient with more comfort. Nonetheless, these patients should be followed very rigorously. Serious complications can occur. Due to the loss of corneal sensation, the patient may not notice pain from these complications.

17. What are the advantages of using a disposable contact lens as a therapeutic lens?

The major advantage is decreased cost and the option of frequent replacement. Thus, the patient can receive a new lens at each visit, eliminating the need to clean and disinfect the contact lens. In the United States, only a small number of contact lenses are approved by the Food and Drug Administration (FDA) for therapeusis, although many contact lenses are prescribed for therapeutic purposes as an off-label use. Although not specifically approved by the FDA for this use, silicone hydrogel contact lenses have been used on a continuous wear basis for a number of conditions including bullous keratopathy, chemical burns, recurrent corneal erosions, corneal perforations, neurotrophic ulcers, and corneal lacerations.[5] The silicone hydrogel lens may be a good choice when high oxygen permeability is needed and when the lens needs to be worn for an extended period of time.

18. What are the contraindications to the use of therapeutic contact lenses?

The most important contraindications are ocular infection of any kind, as well as the inability of the patient to return to the office for adequate follow-up. There are also relative contraindications such as seborrheic blepharitis, lacrimal system abnormalities, poor personal hygiene, and the presence of a filtering bleb.

19. What are the most common complications resulting from the use of a therapeutic contact lens?

- Corneal erosion
- Corneal ulcer
- Corneal neovascularization
- Central or peripheral corneal infiltrates
- Corneal edema
- Tight lens syndrome: edema of the cornea, perilimbal injection, iridocyclitis with hypopyon without infection

20. When and how should one use collagen lenses?

Collagen lenses are generally used to facilitate epithelialization and offer more comfort to the patient after a surgical procedure. Collagen lenses may also be used as a mode of administration of ophthalmic drugs. Generally, the collagen contact lens will dissolve over a period of 12 to 72 hours. Prior to insertion, the collagen contact lens may be soaked in a solution, such as a topical antibiotic, and this may provide the benefit of constant and time-released administration of the medication in which the lens was soaked.

References

1. Srur M, Dattas D. The use of disposable contact lenses as therapeutic lenses. *CLAO J.* 1997;23:40–42.
2. Rhee DJ, Pyfer MF, and Wills Eye Hospital (Philadelphia). *The Wills Eye Manual: Office and Emergency Room Diagnosis and Treatment of Eye Disease.* Philadelphia: Lippincott Williams & Wilkins, 1999.

3. Carlson AN, Wilhelmus KR. Giant papillary conjunctivitis associated with cyanoacrylate glue. *Am J Ophthalmol.* 1987;104:437–438.
4. Arora R, Gupta S, Taneja M, et al. Disposable contact lenses in penetrating keratoplasty. *CLAO J.* 2000;26:127–129.
5. Lim L, Tan DT, Chan WK. Therapeutic use of Bausch & Lomb PureVision contact lenses. *CLAO J.* 2001;27:179–185.

Selected Readings

Aquavella JV. Therapeutic contact lenses. In: Aquavella JV, Rao GN, eds. *Contact Lenses.* Philadelphia: JB Lippincott, 1987:140–163.

Aquavella JV. Therapeutic contact lenses. In: Kastl PR, ed. *Contact Lenses: The CLAO Guide to Basic Science and Clinical Practice;* vol 3. Dubuque, Ia: Kendall/ Hunt, 1995:67–77.

Donshik PC, Lembach RG. Therapeutic soft contact lenses. In: *CLAO Regional Basic Contact Lens Course.* New Orleans: Contact Lens Association of Ophthalmologists, 1995:66–69.

Mannis MJ. Therapeutic contact lenses. In: Smolin G, Thoft RA, eds. *The Cornea.* Boston: Little, Brown, 1994:723–737.

Mondino BJ, Weissman B, Mantley R. Therapeutic soft contact lenses. In: Stenson SM, ed. *Contact Lenses.* Norwalk/Los Altos: Appleton & Lan Lange, 1987:155–183.

Moreira SMB, Moreira H. Lentes de contato terapeuticas. In: Moreira SMB, Moreira H, eds. *Lentes de Contato.* Rio de Janeiro: Cultura Medica, 1993:259–261.

21

Maintenance and Handling of Contact Lenses

**Cleusa Coral-Ghanem
and Melissa D. Bailey**

1. What is the importance of contact lens maintenance?

The contact lens alters the natural defense mechanisms of the eye. As deposits form on the contact lens, an inflammatory reaction and/or infection may develop.

The use of the contact lens alters the ocular defense mechanism by:

- Limiting tear exchange
- Interrupting the tear film
- Reducing the efficiency of debris removal from the ocular surface
- Interfering with the normal protective function of a mucin layer
- inducing microtrauma due to both metabolic and mechanical effects
- Augmenting retention of microorganisms on the ocular surface
- Functioning as a vector, facilitating infection

The biofilm secreted by the eye coats the contact lens in a very short period of time. This attracts pathogens, particularly *Pseudomonas*. The bacteria adhere to the contact lens polymers; this adherence is stimulated by the presence of deposits on the contact lens surface.

The contact lens does the following:

- Maintains optical quality
- Prevents surface damage that facilitates the formation of deposits
- Removes environmental deposits
- Reduces the number of pathogenic microorganisms
- Increases the life of a lens.

2. What types of deposits form most frequently on contact lenses?

Three types of deposits form on contact lenses: organic, inorganic, and environmental.

Organic Deposits

The organic deposits are proteins, lipids, carbohydrates, pigments of organic origin, and deposits composed of microorganisms with other substances.

The tear proteins that frequently contribute to the formation of deposits are lysozyme, lactoferrin, and albumen. They are present in approximately equal amounts. Lysozyme and lactoferrin are positively charged proteins, and albumen is a negatively charged protein.

Contact lenses carry a negative charge, and thus proteins that are more positively charged are more prone to form deposits on contact lenses. For example, among the proteins, lysozyme, which carries a positive charge and a low molecular weight, is the substance most commonly deposited on ionic contact lenses and on high-water-content lenses (group IV, Food and Drug Administration, FDA). Lysozyme also adheres to ionic low-water-content contact lenses (group III, FDA). It does, however deposit on nonionic contact lenses of both low and high water content (materials and FDA groups II and III). The absorption of proteins by different contact lens materials depends principally on the electrical charge of the material and not on the water content.

Mucoprotein films consist of denatured proteins and appear as discrete, scattered deposits in fine layers. They are often semiopaque and whitish. These protein films can cover small parts or the entire surface of the contact lens. To observe them more easily, the patient should be asked to stop blinking, which allows drying of the surface of the contact lens.

Lipids are generally found in small amounts on hydrophilic lenses but may represent important deposits on rigid gas permeable lenses, especially on those that contain silicone, which makes the contact lens hydrophobic. Lipid deposits on the lens surface are seen as greasy areas or oily spots. Studies clearly indicate that protein accumulation primarily depends on the material, while lipid deposits depend on the individual characteristics and may be present in lens materials of FDA groups I, II, III, and IV.

Inorganic Deposits

The inorganic deposits are calcium salts, phosphates and carbonates of calcium, ferrous oxide, salts, and pigments derived from inorganic chemicals.

The most common types of inorganic deposits are "jelly bumps," which occur most frequently on extended-wear contact lenses. The jelly bumps are round, nodular deposits composed primarily of calcium, lipids, and cholesterol. These deposits are difficult to remove, and therefore the patient may be required to replace the contact lens. The formation of a jelly bump begins with the deposition of calcium, which forms the white base of the deposit. The calcium is then covered with an oily coat of lipid, and finally an external coat of mucoprotein. Removal of the jelly bumps often produces a defect in the surface of the contact lens. As jelly bumps grow in size and quantity, they may affect the patient's vision and cause discomfort.

Pigment deposits and lens discoloration may occur as the result of various factors such as nicotine, adrenaline, vasoconstricting solutions, and components of fluorescein. This type of deposit can be the result of both organic and inorganic elements. Yellow and brown granular particles deposited on the surface of the lens have been identified as similar structurally to melanin. The production of melanin is stimulated by substances present in certain medications, while nicotine and other aromatic substances are found in tobacco smoke. Epinephrine and other compounds used in eye medications may discolor the contact lens as they are absorbed. In certain circumstances, some preservatives, principally those derived from chlorhexidine and ascorbic acids, increase discoloration of the contact lens. There is a biochemical mechanism in which a hydrogel acts as an inert matrix for these reactions that rarely involve the polymer of the contact lens.

Environmental Deposits

The most common environmental deposits are rust spots and particles from cosmetics. Rust spots are caused generally by the use of tap water or by foreign matter in the environment. They are generally orange and circular. Deposits from cosmetics have an iridescent, greasy appearance and may be caused by mascara, hair spray, creams, etc.

Microorganisms normally inhabit the lens surface. Many species of fungi and yeast have been identified on hydrophilic lenses. Fungi have enzymatic activity that degrades the polymer of the contact lens. The most common bacteria found on contact lenses that can lead to infection are *Pseudomonas aeruginosa, Staphylococcus aureus,* and *Staphylococcus epidermidis.* Another microorganism, *Acanthamoeba,* is found on contact lenses much less frequently, but it can lead to a much more serious infection. *Acanthamoeba* may have the ability to adhere to and invade the cornea, even without any epithelial defect or dysfunction.

Contact lenses and contact lens maintenance products provide many plastic surfaces that facilitate adherence of bacterial and other microorganisms. Contact lens solutions may develop a biofilm; however, contact lens cases are particularly disposed to this type of contamination.[1]

3. Why is it important to remove deposits?

Aside from the fact that deposits can cause discomfort and visual disturbance, they may also produce mechanical abrasions and immunoallergic reactions and facilitate adherence of microorganisms and, subsequently, infections. The nature and quantity of the deposits vary considerably with the biochemistry of the individual's tear film, the length of time the contact lens has been used, the type of contact lens, and the environment.[2,3]

4. How are contact lens solutions formulated?

Contact lens solutions are formulated to accomplish three objectives: cleansing, rinsing, and disinfection. The solution must be compatible with the lens material, the tear film, and the ocular tissue. There must be equilibrium among the following properties: tonicity, the degree of acidity and alkalinity (concentrations of hydrogen ions—pH) in water, buffering agents, viscosity, cleaning agents, and antimicrobial agents.

5. What is tonicity?

Tonicity is the quantity of salt contained in a solution. The standard for tonicity of a contact lens solution is the intracellular salt content of the body, 0.9% sodium chloride, or 300 milliosmoles (mOsm). An isotonic solution is one in which the tonicity is equal to 0.9% sodium chloride. When the solution contains other salts used for other functions, the amount of sodium chloride must be reduced, so that the solution remains isotonic. Contact lens solutions are formulated to be isotonic, with the goal of maintaining the equilibrium of the ocular tissues and the water contained in the contact lens. An example of isotonic solution is natural tears. Tears do not provoke any swelling or dehydration in the corneal cells.

Hypertonic solutions are those that have tonicity greater than 0.9% sodium chloride. An example of a hypertonic solution is seawater. A hydrophilic contact lens in a hypertonic solution dehydrates and shrinks. Water shifts from areas of lower tonicity to higher tonicity to equalize the salt concentration between the two areas. Hypotonic solutions provoke the opposite effect of hypertonic solutions. A hydrophilic contact lens in the presence of hypotonic solution (tap water or distilled water) absorbs water and increases in thickness. If the cornea is placed in a hypotonic solution, it becomes edematous. The contact lens and cornea regain normal equilibrium in the presence of an isotonic tear film.

6. What are the degrees of acidity and alkalinity (pH), and how can they interfere with the comfortable use of contact lenses?

Tear film pH normally varies between 7.0 and 8.5.[4] This varies from person to person and throughout the day in each individual. Thus a contact lens solution can vary from 6.0 to 8.5 and still provide reasonable comfort.[5]

An ophthalmic solution with a pH between 6.6 and 7.4 is considered neutral and provides good ocular comfort. Changes in the pH may affect the stability, sterility, and viscosity of the contact lens solution. When solutions are outside the acceptable range of pH, they may provoke discomfort, burning, punctate keratopathy, and tearing.

7. What is the purpose of buffering agents, and which are most commonly used?

Buffering agents, either acid or alkaline, are used in contact lens solutions to stabilize the pH in the range of 7.0 to 7.4, i.e., within limits that do not adversely affect ocular comfort or the efficacy of the solution. The most common buffering agents used in contact lens solutions include borates, phosphates, citrates, and trimethamines.

8. How do viscosity agents work, and which are the most commonly used?

Viscosity agents establish the relative density of a solution; the concentration is dependent on the purpose for which the product is intended.

In contact lens care solutions, the cleaners are more viscous than the lubricants, and the lubricants are more viscous than the soaking agents. Lubricants and wetting agents contain viscous ingredients to prolong contact of the solution with the contact lens, to reduce friction, and thereby to improve comfort.

Viscosity agents most commonly used in contact lens solutions include methylcellulose hydroxyethylcellulose, hydroxypropyl methylcellulose (HPMC), polyvinyl alcohol, glycolhexaline, carbomide, and dextran.

9. What are surfactant cleaners, and which are most commonly used?

Surfactants are detergent substances that affect surface tension and are effective for removing oils, fat, mucus, and cosmetics. They are most effective at a slightly alkaline pH of 7.4.

Surfactants may be either ionic or nonionic. The surfactants are classified as anionic (negative charge), cationic (positive charge), and amphoteric (positive or negative charge, or both, depending on the pH of the solution). The most commonly employed surfactants are the amphoteric ionic and the nonionic surfactants because they offer stability, compatibility, and low toxicity. Many surfactant solutions contain viscosity agents, chelating agents, buffers, and preservatives. Some also contain polymeric microspheres, which act as abrasive cleaners. The surfactant cleaning agents may be used separately or in association with multiuse solutions. The surfactant agents most commonly used for contact lenses include miranol, sodium salts, tiloxopol, propaline glycol, and polyvinyl alcohol.

10. What is the function of antimicrobial agents, and which are most commonly used?

Antimicrobial agents have two basic functions: first, to prevent microbial proliferation as bacteriostatic agents, and second, to destroy microorganisms when used as bactericidal agents. To eliminate potentially harmful microorganisms in contact lenses, we use disinfecting agents. In many cases, preservative agents are used as disinfectants, as preservatives may have antibactericidal properties when used in higher concentrations.

The bacteriostatic agents are generally less irritating to the eyes than bactericidal agents, which frequently cause sensitivity and toxic reactions. The antimicrobial agents most commonly used in contact lens solutions include quaternary ammonia and biguanides, oxidative agents, systems that produce chlorine and chlorine bases, alcohol, organic mercurial compounds, weak acids, and EDTA (ethylenediamine-tetraacetic acid, disodium edatate).

11. What are the most common hypersensitivity reactions caused by contact lens solutions?

Contact lens solutions contain chemical preservatives that may induce toxic or allergic reactions. A toxic reaction may occur within minutes or hours of contact lens wear, producing conjunctival hyperemia, superficial punctate keratitis, and symptoms of burning and pain. An allergic reaction may occur weeks or months later and is associated with different symptoms and signs: burning, itching, photophobia, conjunctival hyperemia, superficial punctate keratitis, corneal infiltrates, superior limbic keratoconjunctivitis, nummular keratitis, dendriform lesions, and corneal vascularization. The toxic reactions most commonly encountered are caused by benzalkonium chloride chlorhexidine, incomplete neutralization of hydrogen peroxide (H_2O_2), inadequate rinsing of cleaning solution, residues of enzymatic cleaners, and contamination of the contact lens with substances such as hand creams or perfumes. The most frequent allergic reaction is the result of thimerosal exposure.

12. What are the characteristics of quaternary ammonia and biguanide as antimicrobial agents?

These agents are effective against bacteria, have only slight activity against fungus, and do not adhere to contact lens materials. Because they are large molecules, they are not absorbed by the contact lens. This group includes benzalkonium chloride, alkyl, triethanol, ammonium chloride, chlorhexidine, gluconate, and polymers, including polyhexamethyl biguanide (PHMB), polyaminopropyl biguanide, and polyquad (polyquarternium-1).

Benzalkonium chloride can be used with solutions for polymethylmethacrylate (PMMA) in concentrations up to 0.01% without problems. This preservative, however, may adversely affect silicone acrylate contact lenses as well as fluorosilicone acrylate lenses. These materials are gas permeable, and when they are in contact with benzalkonium chloride, they may absorb the chemical each time the lens is exposed, eventually reaching toxic concentrations. Benzalkonium chloride is toxic to human and animal tissues and can cause cellular injury at concentrations even as low as 0.001%.[6] Also, benzalkonium chloride intensifies the hydrophobicity of the contact lens surface, aiding deposit formation.

Alkyl-triethanol-ammonium chloride and chlorhexidine gluconate are effective against bacteria, but they are not very effective against fungi. Both are generally used in solutions with thimerasol as a preservative and disinfectant. Thimerosal, however, is active against fungi. Chlorhexidine can bind to contact lens materials and to protein deposits, augmenting its concentration in the eye and causing hypersensitivity reactions. The breakdown products of chlorhexidine can change the color of the contact lens to yellow or yellowish green.

PHMB is a high-molecular-weight substance used in a 0.001% concentration and has a broad spectrum of action as well as low toxicity. Dymed is a high-molecular-weight preservative that does not penetrate contact lens polymers, and it is effective for disinfection in concentrations as low as 0.00005%. It is a polymer made of repeating units of biguanide, separated by one chain of six carbons. Dymed contains a positive charge in the biguanide group that selectively activates and disintegrates microorganisms that have negative charges in their membrane. It is the preservative used in Renu™ and Renu Plus™ (Bausch & Lomb).

Polyquad (polyquarternium-1) is a cationic polymer effective against bacteria with low activity against fungus. Its molecular structure is large, not permitting it to be absorbed by the contact lens materials, nor does it adhere to the lens surface. When it is used in concentrations of 0.001%, to 0.005%, it acts as a preservative and disinfectant. It is used in Opti-Free™ and Opti-Free Express™ (Alcon), where it is combined with Aldox, an antifungal agent.

13. What is the oxidative agent used for contact lens solutions?

Hydrogen peroxide (H_2O_2) in a concentration of 3% is the oxidative agent utilized for both hydrophilic and rigid gas permeable contact lenses. It has excellent antimicrobial activity against bacteria and fungi. However, neutralization of hydrogen peroxide is an indispensable step before utilizing contact lenses disinfected with this agent.

14. What are products of chlorine and chlorine bases that act as antimicrobial agents?

These systems, utilized primarily in Europe, use tablets such as halezone and hypochlorite. In this system, the patient places a tablet in sterile solution to begin the process of disinfection. The bactericidal activity of chlorine depends on the pH of the solution and is greater at an acidic pH.

15. What are the alcohols used in lens maintenance systems?

Chlorbutanol has a broad spectrum of action, but because it acts slowly and requires a low pH to remain stable, it is rarely used as a base preservative in contact lens solutions except for solutions used with PMMA lenses. It is used in a concentration of 0.5%, at which it is soluble in water. Benzyl and isopropyl alcohol are more stable in solution than chlorbutanol; however, benzyl and isopropyl alcohol share other problems. They interact with the hydrophilic contact lens, and when liberated in the tear film, produce various degrees of toxicity and irritation. Because they convert to aldehydes, they can irritate the eye and discolor and harden the hydrophilic contact lens. Benzyl alcohol serves as a preservative and disinfectant in solutions for rigid contact lenses. Solutions that contain alcohol should not be used with an ocular prosthesis because they may cause the color in the prosthesis to fade.

16. What is the action of thimerosal in contact lens solutions?

Thimerosal, a mercurial agent with bactericidal activity against a broad spectrum of bacteria and fungi, is used in concentrations of 0.001%. It functions as a preservative, and at concentrations of 0.0005% it also functions as a disinfectant. Thimerosal is relatively nontoxic. Nonetheless, it may cause sensitivity reactions when it adheres to protein deposits on the surface of the contact lens. Sensitivity to thimerosal is more common in patients who wear hydrophilic contact lenses than in patients who wear rigid contact lenses. This is due to differences in the tear exchange under the lens. With a hydrophilic lens, there is a relative stagnation of the tear film under the contact lens, so the lens has a more prolonged contact with the eye, facilitating allergic reactions.

17. What are the weak acids that can be used as preservatives?

When saturated, boric acid is isotonic. It is not commonly used as a preservative due to its low antimicrobial activity. Sorbic acid works best as a preservative at lower pH values in the range of 6.6. Solutions formulated with sorbic acid may cause punctate keratopathy or burning in certain patients due to its acidity. Alone, sorbic acid is gentle to the ocular tissues and probably does not cause toxic or sensitivity reactions.

18. What is EDTA?

EDTA is a chelating agent that ligates metallic ions necessary for microbial growth. It is not bactericidal but improves the activity of other preservatives against gram-negative bacteria such as *Pseudomonas.*

19. What is the importance of cleaning the contact lens, and what types of cleaners are used?

Contact lenses should be cleaned and disinfected after each use. Therefore, we use solutions that are designed to work well and still remain compatible with the eye and the contact lens materials. Contact lenses are cleaned by rubbing and rinsing; therefore, the solutions used should be of low viscosity. More viscous solutions require more intense rinsing. Cleaning is the most important step in maintenance. Cleaning removes residues and reduces the number of microorganisms. Contamination of the contact lens is reduced from a million colonies to 3000 when the contact lens is simply cleaned. It is further reduced to less than 300 colonies when the cleaning is accompanied by complete rinsing. Cleaning and rinsing eliminate 99.9% of microbial contaminants.[7] From the microbiologic standpoint, a clean contact lens is much easier to disinfect than a dirty contact lens because contact lens contaminants may inactivate the preservative. Thus, when a contact lens reaches the disinfection stage, the microbial contamination should already be substantially reduced. Two types of cleaners are used:

Surfactant Cleaners

Surfactants are solutions for daily use that contain detergent substances that remove mucus, lipids, cosmetics, and environmental contaminants, including microorganisms, but that are not efficient in removing proteins.

Enzymatic Cleaners

An enzyme is a substance that accelerates chemical reactions to break down proteins. These cleaners contain enzymes that break down proteins (proteolytic enzymes), removing them from the surface of the contact lens. The use of enzymatic cleaners is optional, and the frequency of use depends on the individual characteristics of the patient as well as the length of lens wear. Disposable contact lenses and frequent replacement contact lenses often do not require enzymatic cleaners. Some enzymatic cleaners are sequential (utilized prior to disinfection), and others are used simultaneously (during the disinfection step).

20. What are the characteristics of enzyme systems?

Some enzyme systems contain the active agent, papaine. It is derived from papaya and has the following characteristics: it is inactivated by thermal disinfection and by 3% hydrogen peroxide; it is supplied in the form of a pill for weekly use; it may adhere to the hydrophilic contact lens polymer, causing hypersensitivity reaction; and it is available commercially as Hydrocare™ (Allergan).

Another multienzymatic system contains pancreatine. It is derived from porcine pancreas and has the following characteristics: it acts to remove proteins, lipids, and mucin; it should be avoided in patients with allergies to pork; and it is provided as tablets for weekly use or in liquid form for daily use. Commercially available systems that use pancreatine are Polyzyme™ (Alcon), Opti-Free Enzymatic Cleaner™ (Alcon), and Opti-Free Supraclens™ (Alcon).

Subtilisine A is an enzyme that is derived from the fermentation of bacillus licheniformis and has the following characteristics: it breaks down a large variety of proteins; it does not require activation; it is available for simultaneous or sequential enzymatic cleaning; it may be used with all systems of cleaning and disinfection; and it is used weekly in the form of a tablet. Commercially available products using this enzyme include Ultrazyme™ (Allergan), FizziClean™ (Bausch & Lomb), and Remove™ (Allergan).

21. What solutions can be used to rinse contact lenses?

After cleaning, the contact lens should be rinsed to remove the residual cleaner, remaining loose deposits, and microorganisms. Rinsing should be performed with multiuse solutions or saline solutions that are either preserved or nonpreserved. Some of these solutions are available in multiple unit packages of 10 to 15 mL.

Multiuse solutions are recommended for rinsing. Although commercially available saline solutions have a similar rinsing effect, the formulation of these solutions may vary, for example, in pH and thus may cause burning and punctate keratopathy.

Preserved saline solutions are available in plastic containers. Although the preservative functions to limit the microbial growth in solution, contamination can occur. The user should be instructed not to touch the tip of the dropper and to keep it closed when not being used.

Nonpreserved saline solutions are available in plastic containers of 10 to 15 mL or in aerosol cans with a unidirectional valve to prevent the entrance of microorganisms. These should be disposed of as frequently as the manufacturer's recommendation.

22. Why is contact lens disinfection important, and what methods are utilized?

Different microorganisms, including bacteria, fungi, and viruses, can be found as normal flora on the eye. The healthy eye is capable of resisting infection due to the presence of natural barriers, including an intact corneal epithelium, the act of blinking, and naturally occurring antibacterial agents in the tear film. Nonetheless, under appropriate ambient conditions, bacteria can multiply rapidly, increasing by tens of millions overnight. The association between infectious keratitis and contamination of contact lens care systems has been well documented.[8–10] Among the microorganisms, *Pseudomonas aeruginosa* is most commonly associated with infectious ulceration. *Pseudomonas* easily adheres to the contact lens polymer, and this adherence is encouraged by the presence of deposits on the surface.

Fewer than five species of *Acanthamoeba* have been associated with corneal ulceration, but *Acanthamoeba* infection is often associated with contact lenses. The most common sources of contamination by *Acanthamoeba* are homemade saline, water from public pools, and infrequent disinfection. Because *Acanthamoeba* infections are painful and difficult to treat clinically, the contact lens user needs to be instructed in their prevention.

Effective cleaning of the contact lens begins with effective digital massage of the contact lens, using surfactant or a multiuse solution. Digital cleaning and rinsing removes 99% of *Acanthamoeba* on a contact lens prior to chemical disinfection.[11] The care regimen (chemical or oxidative) is most effective when all the steps of the system are undertaken (i.e., cleaning, rinsing, and disinfection). The effect of chemical disinfection alone has minimal effect against *Acanthamoeba* and HIV.[12]

Thermal disinfection refers to a process through which living or vegetative microorganisms are killed or inactivated. This normally involves the destruction of the cell wall or membrane and/or the inhibition of protein synthesis in the microbe. Certain microbes are capable of producing spores that are not killed by the process of disinfection and theoretically are capable of germinating and producing ocular infection. For this reason, ideal contact lens sterilization (15 minutes at 121°C at 15 pounds per square inch (PSI) in the autoclave) would inactivate or kill all microorganisms and their spores. Nonetheless, this is an impractical approach, and repeated cleaning cycles may damage the lens polymer.

23. How is thermal disinfection achieved?

It is important to perform rigorous cleaning of the contact lens prior to thermal disinfection because the heat denatures proteins that then become fixed to the contact lens surface. The temperature should be 80°C for a minimum of 10 minutes. Heat disinfection units require a total of 45 minutes, including heating, disinfection, and cooling. This was the first method for disinfection of hydrophilic lenses. Despite its efficacy, it fell into disuse after the development of less sensitizing chemical disinfection systems and higher-water-content lenses.

Thermal disinfection is the most efficient method for the elimination of microorganisms, including *Acanthamoeba*. It is simple and inexpensive. It provokes no sensitivity reactions. It is rapid. It neutralizes residual enzymatic cleaners. This method, however, is contraindicated in high-water-content hydrophilic lenses, cosmetic contact lenses, and rigid gas permeable lenses. It shortens the useful life of the contact lens. It does not always reach the temperature required for disinfection (80°C for 10 minutes) in the interior of the contact lens case, and it does not protect the contact lens against contamination. It is often mistaken by the patient to be a method of cleaning.

24. How does nonoxidative chemical disinfection work?

Nonoxidative chemical disinfection is accomplished by immersing the contact lens for 4 to 6 hours in solutions that contain antimicrobial agents (chlorhexidine, thimerosal, dymed, polyquad, polyhexamide, and TrisChen). Advantages include broad-spectrum antimicrobial activity, utilization with a broad variety of contact lens materials, and convenience and practicality of use. Disadvantages include the need for a 4-hour exposure time, a more limited spectrum of antimicrobial activity, especially against fungi, and a higher incidence of hypersensitivity reactions to the preservatives.

25. What is the purpose of multiuse solutions?

Multiuse solutions are designed to clean, rinse, and disinfect contact lenses, providing all of these functions in a single solution. A balance must be achieved among the properties of the contact lens solution (tonicity, pH, viscosity, cleaning agents, antimicrobial agents, and buffering agents), but this may diminish the effectiveness of any one of these functions, making it necessary for the patient to use additional agents. Multiaction solutions designed for cleaning, rinsing, disinfecting, and removing protein deposits are preferred by patients who demand less time and effort. Nonetheless, for those situations in which there is excessive formation of deposits or oiliness on the contact lenses, more specific solutions are recommended for cleaning.

Many users of hydrophilic contact lenses who use multipurpose solutions do not demonstrate biomicroscopic changes but complain of a dry sensation. Placing the patient on a care regimen with 3% hydrogen peroxide without preservatives may alleviate the symptoms of dry eye. One study of adolescents demonstrated that patients using 3% hydrogen peroxide had fewer epithelial changes and inflammatory reactions than those who used ReNu™ and OptiFree™ multipurpose solutions.[13]

The multipurpose solutions do not require the use of a separate cleaner and disinfectant. An important part of cleaning and treatment with a surfactant is the use of mechanical friction for 10 to 20 seconds on each side of the contact lens. The surfactant adheres to lipids and debris on the surface of the contact lens and is subsequently removed with rinsing. Multipurpose solutions do not contain enzymes and do not remove proteins chemically. Protein deposits may carry positive or negative charges. Calcium, which has two positive charges, acts to form a bond between proteins on the surface of the contact lens. Multipurpose solutions avoid this bond, which serves as a base for the formation of deposits.

26. What multipurpose solutions are most commonly used for hydrophilic lenses?

Commonly available multipurpose solutions include Complete Comfort Plus™ (Allergan), OptiFree Express™ (Alcon), ReNu Plus™ (Bausch

& Lomb), and SOLOcare™ (CIBAVision). These solutions contain a substance that works like a surfactant cleaner.

Complete Comfort Plus™ uses a surfactant cleaner (poloxamere 237) to remove protein and debris during manual cleaning of the contact lens. More proteins are removed through the action of electrolytes incorporated in the solution, whose strong ionic forces attract molecules of protein with the opposite charge while the contact lens is immersed in the solution. They also contain the lubricant HPMC, which restores the surface of the contact lens during the period of immersion, making it more comfortable for the user.

OptiFree Express, in addition to the surfactant poloxamine, contains sodium citrate, which interacts with cationic organic molecules, dislocating the lysozyme that is bound to the lens polymer. Sodium citrate is also able to chelate calcium and other metals. Optifree Express now has Aldox, an antifungal, antimicrobial agent, which was not included in previous versions of the solution.

ReNu Plus contains poloxamine and hydranate, a multifunctional molecule with four negative charges that forms a complex with calcium, breaking the bonds of this deposit. In addition, hydranate promotes dispersion, as it adheres to proteins with positive charges and makes them repellant to the surface of the contact lens.

SOLOcare contains the surfactant poloxamere 407, a copolymer of polyoxyethylene polypropylene, as a cleaning agent to remove proteins and debris on the contact lens.

These four solutions contain preservatives, including quaternary ammonium and biguanides: polyhexamethylene biguanide (Tris Chem™) is present in Complete; polyquad is present in OptiFree Express, which also contains the antifungal Aldox; dymed is present in ReNu; and polyhexamide is in SOLOcare. The four multiuse solutions contain EDTA, which, as was discussed above, is nonbactericidal but augments the activity of the preservatives. For appropriate disinfection, the contact lens should be soaked in solution for at least 4 hours.

27. What multiuse solutions are most commonly used to clean rigid gas permeable contact lenses?

These include Boston Simplicity™ (Bausch & Lomb) and Unique pH™ (Alcon). The multipurpose solution Boston Simplicity uses surfactants. In addition, to maintain the ideal viscosity and promote comfort, the makers of Boston Simplicity incorporate a combination of polymers and the agent neutraclens. Neutraclens surrounds the surfactants and prevents irritation while still removing deposits. Neutraclens also distributes a lubricant on the lens surface, helping to prevent formation of deposits. The Boston Simplicity formulation contains polyaminopropyl biguanide, chlorhexidine gluconate, and EDTA as preservatives.

The multipurpose solution Unique pH™ (Alcon), for PMMA and rigid gas permeable contact lenses, contains the surfactant tetronic 1304. Tetronic 1304 facilitates removal of deposits after rubbing the contact lens. Unique pH also contains boric acid, which functions as a buffer; propylene glycol, which provides tonicity; sodium hydroxide and chlorhydric acid, which are utilized to adjust the pH to 7; polyquad (polyquarternium-1) as a disinfectant and preservative; EDTA as a chelating agent; and hydroxypropyl-guar (HP-guar), a polysaccharide extracted from the guar plant. HP-guar is a neutral polymer that is compatible with the other ingredients. The contact lens is coated with HP-guar when it is immersed. When the contact lens is placed on the eye and comes in contact with the tear film, HP-guar becomes as viscous as mucin. In the presence of borate, HP-guar forms a double-bond with the tear film. The product is a liquid of low viscosity, a desirable condition for manipulation of the lens (cleaning and rinsing with the contact lens outside the eye). The solution Unique pH does not need to be removed from the contact lens prior to insertion, and it is compatible with the enzymatic cleaner OptiFree SupraClens™.

28. What are the advantages and disadvantages of multipurpose solutions?

The advantages include:

- Broad-spectrum antimicrobial activity
- Utilization with a variety of contact lens materials
- Simplicity of use
- Reduced time spent training the user
- Ease of transport
- Good cost-benefit relationship

The disadvantages include:

- Possibility of hypersensitivity reactions
- The need for 4 hours for disinfection
- Antimicrobial activity limited to a few microorganisms
- Decreased efficacy compared with specific solutions

29. How does oxidative chemical disinfection work, and what are its advantages and disadvantages?

Oxidative chemical disinfection is accomplished using 3% hydrogen peroxide, which is a disinfectant with excellent antimicrobial activity against a broad variety of microorganisms. An oxidative reaction transforms the molecule of hydrogen peroxide into water and oxygen. Stabilizers such as sodium stanate, nitrate, and phosphonic acid may be added to promote continuation of the reaction in the recipient.

In its generic form, hydrogen peroxide can be found commercially at a lower cost than formulations especially prepared for contact lenses. Generic forms of hydrogen peroxide, however, cannot be used for contact lens care and maintenance because they have variable concentrations of heavy metals and undesirable residues that may discolor the lens.

Three percent hydrogen peroxide has a pH of 4.0 (acid), a tonicity equal to zero (hypotonic), and high osmolarity (900 mOsm). To make this cleaning system compatible with the eye, it is necessary to neutralize the solution by lowering the concentration of H_2O_2 to less than 50 to 60 parts per million (PPM), adjust the pH to approximately neutral (7.0 to 7.4), and to approximate isotonic conditions (equal to 0.9% sodium chloride). To achieve ocular compatibility, two methods of neutralization are used: catalase (Oxisept™ system, Allergan) or a platinum disk (AOSept™ system). The time necessary to neutralize with catalase or the platinum disk is 6 hours. The efficacy of the neutralization disk depends on its age and how well it is preserved. Older disks can become covered with residue. This leads to incomplete neutralization of the hydrogen peroxide, which can raise the levels of hydrogen peroxide to toxic levels; therefore, the neutralization disks require periodical replacement.

Excessive exposure of the contact lens to hydrogen peroxide may cause an increase in the base curve of a hydrophilic contact lens, depending on pH and tonicity. These changes may last for 30 to 60 minutes after neutralization of the peroxide. High-water-content ionic polymers, especially those that contain methacrylate, are more affected than low-water-content neutral polymers. This problem is eliminated when one uses a catalytic disk for neutralization.

30. What chemical oxydizing solutions are available and can be used?

The oxidizing solutions most commonly available in oxidizing systems include OXYSEPT Comfort Plus™ (Allergan) and AoSept™ (CIBA Vision).

OXYSEPT Comfort Plus™ (Allergan)

This system accomplishes disinfection and neutralization of 3% hydrogen peroxide in one procedure. It includes a disinfecting solution in a catalase pill, which transforms the 3% hydrogen peroxide into water and oxygen. To neutralize the 3% hydrogen peroxide in the Oxysept Comfort Plus™ system, the manufacturer has added a pill with the polymer HPMC. The body of the pill contains a catalase and neutralization indicator. When the pill is added to 3% hydrogen peroxide, the HPMC polymer absorbs water and retains humidity. After 20 minutes, during which the contact lens remains in direct contact with 3% hydrogen peroxide, the pill begins to dissolve, and catalase is gradually released. When neutralization is achieved, the solution turns pink. After 6 hours of disinfection and neutralization, all of the lubricant is released, and the viscosity of the solution is similar to that of human tears.

AO Sept™ (CIBAVision)

In the AO Sept™ system, neutralization is achieved by means of a disk. The disk is inserted into the small cylindrical container with a basket that holds the contact lenses. Old disks covered with residues may not completely neutralize the peroxide, and the remaining solution that fails to neutralize may cause significant ocular irritation.

31. What are the advantages and disadvantages of oxidative chemical disinfection with 3% hydrogen peroxide?

Advantages

- It penetrates the surface of the contact lens to remove small molecules in the hydrogel pores.
- It promotes cleaning action of the surface by oxidizing peptide chains, breaking down proteins and lipids.
- It promotes disinfection. In 10 minutes, it can kill both bacteria and viruses. Forty minutes are required to eradicate fungi, and 2 hours are required to eliminate *Acanthamoeba*.
- It can be utilized with all contact lens materials, both rigid and hydrophilic.

Disadvantages

- It is toxic to the eye and may fail to neutralize.
- Exposure of hydrogen peroxide that is not neutralized may produce ocular irritation, intense hyperemia, keratitis, tearing, chemosis, burning, and punctate keratopathy.
- The solution loses its disinfecting capacity after neutralization.

32. What is the purpose of wetting solutions?

Wetting solutions serve to wet contact lenses and reequilibrate the water content of contact lenses, making them more comfortable during initial placement and also during wear. They enhance the distribution of tears on the contact lens surface, improving optical function. Wetting solutions may contain a low concentration of nonionic surfactant that helps in cleaning the contact lens surface; a viscosity agent to reduce friction; buffering agents; and preservatives. Formulations designed for use with hydrophilic contact lenses may be used with rigid contact lenses, although the inverse is not true.

Wetting agents are especially indicated for patients with relative tear deficiency and decreased blinking. In addition, they are used for people who sleep in their contact lenses, work in very dry conditions, or use computers for lengthy periods of time. Nonetheless, any contact lens wearer may benefit from wetting agents, especially if the wetting agents are instilled several minutes prior to contact lens removal. While wetting is not an absolutely necessary step in contact lens care, it may contribute substantially to the success of contact lens use.

33. What are the steps for contact lens maintenance?

Step 1: Cleaning the Contact Lens Case

The case must be cleaned at least once a week with hot water and soap. The case should then be air dried, and after drying, kept closed. In general, disposable cases are recommended, and cases should be replaced at least every 6 months. Materials that foster the growth of microorganisms can accumulate in contact lens cases, and contamination may occur from the user's fingers or from a dirty contact lens. It has been demonstrated that in cases of ocular infection the pathogens identical to those that caused the infection are frequently found in the contact lens case or under the fingernails of the user. Such contaminated contact lens cases may be the vector for ocular infection.

Step 2: Hygiene of Hands, Eyes, and Ocular Adnexa

Prior to inserting a contact lens, wearers should wash their hands with soap to remove foreign material, grease, nicotine, and contaminants that may damage the contact lens or infect the eye. Soaps with antiseptic cream, chemical deodorants, or strong fragrances should be avoided because these substances can be inadvertently instilled in the eye during transfer of the lens. The hands should be dried on lint-free towels, and nails should be kept clean. It is also important to remove contact lenses prior to using creams/cleansers to clean eyelid margins and eyelashes.

Step 3: Cleaning

Wearers should use a cleaning solution that contains detergent substances that are indicated for their type of contact lens. These solutions are not effective for the removal of proteins. The excessive friction that is required to remove proteins from contact lenses may produce scratches or grooves in the hydrophilic lens or may deform the rigid gas permeable lens. For this reason, wearers should use enzymatic cleaners, which specifically remove proteins, in addition to the cleaning solution.

Step 4: Rinsing

Rinsing is indicated to remove loose deposits and cleaning solution from the surface of the contact lens. With the contact lens in the palm of the hand, the user should direct a stream of solution at the lens, either multiuse solution or saline, lightly rubbing the lens surface back and forth. A second rinse without rubbing is then performed. Some solutions permit placement of the lens in the eye without rinsing.

Step 5: Disinfection

After cleaning and rinsing, the contact lens should be placed in a disinfectant to eliminate pathogenic microorganisms. Some systems use a separate solution for this step. In multipurpose solution systems, the same solution is used for both steps. Wearers usually place their lenses in the disinfecting solution overnight.

Step 6: Neutralization

Neutralization is necessary for strong disinfectants that may irritate the eye. For example, hydrogen peroxide solutions are neutralized during the disinfection step.

Step 7: Wetting

Wetting drops are used before insertion of the contact lens, during contact lens wear to alleviate symptoms of dryness, and to aid in removing a contact lens.

34. What should guide the professional in indicating to the user the correct method of cleaning and disinfection?

The following factors should be taken into consideration:

Contact Lens Material

All forms of disinfection can be used with low-water-content contact lenses.
   With high-water-content lenses, one can use all forms of disinfection except thermal disinfection.

Contact Lens Type

Hydrophilic contact lenses that are not frequently changed require the use of specific solutions such as daily surfactant and weekly enzymatic cleaning. Contact lenses that are exchanged every 3 months or more frequently can be managed with multiuse solutions, especially in wearers who do not have a tendency to form deposits.

Tear Film Deficiency/Blepharitis

Patients with tear film deficiency have a greater propensity to have preservative reactions and may be more susceptible to deposit formation. Patients with dry eyes and/or blepharitis frequently have a higher lipid level in the tear film. For this reason, they should use an enzymatic cleaner that contains lipase.

Use of Systemic or Ocular Medication

Antihistamines

The antihistamines have various degrees of effects, similar to atropine, including the tendency to alter tear film integrity.[14,15] Their use can unmask clinically significant dry eye that would otherwise remain subclinical.

Isotretinoin

The use of isotretinoin shortens tear breakup time as the result of a decrease in the secretion of lipid from the meibomian glands.[16,17] This drug may cause dry eye symptoms, and 20% of isotretinoin and 8% of contact lens wearers present with symptoms of contact lens intolerance.[16]

Beta Blockers

A reduction in lacrimal secretion can be related to the collateral effects of beta blockers, administered either systemically or topically. Propranolol, practolol, timolol, and various others may be related to dry-eye symptoms.[18–20]

Birth Control Pills

The use of birth control pills has been anecdotally associated with contact lens wear problems. There are no studies that prove the effect of contraceptive agents on contact lens intolerance. The possible etiologic mechanisms include alteration of tear production and an induced change in the corneal curvature.[21,22]

Aspirin

Aspirin that is taken orally may be excreted in the tear film and absorbed by a hydrophilic contact lens, producing epithelial defects.[23,24]

Anticholinergic Drugs

Atropine and related drugs may cause drying of the mucous membranes. Scopolamine and certain other antinausea medications may produce dry eye symptoms and difficulty using contact lenses. Other drugs with possible anticholinergic activities, such as phenothiazines, anxiolitic agents, and tricyclic antidepressants, have been associated with dry eye and contact lens intolerance.[25]

Work Environment

Wearers who work in a polluted work environment may require specific solutions to maintain contact lens hygiene. The practitioner may also suggest daily disposable lenses.

History of Allergy

In patients with allergies, 3% hydrogen peroxide or thermal disinfection may be the best answer, as these patients may be more likely to develop sensitivity to chemical cleaners and preservatives.

Practicality and Cost

The best maintenance and care plan for wearers is the one that has the greatest probability of being followed. If they feel the cleaning procedures are impractical or if the system is too costly, they may be less likely to adhere to proper cleaning and maintenance.

35. How should rigid gas permeable lenses be maintained?

Maintenance of the rigid gas permeable (RGP) lens should include either specific solutions or multiuse solutions. Specific solutions include products such as Duracare™ and Totalens™ (Allergan), Opti-Soak™ (Alcon), and Optimum (Lobob). Multiuse solutions include products such as Boston Simplicity™ (Bausch & Lomb) and Unique-pH™ (Alcon). The RGP lens may form the same types of deposits as hydrophilic lenses but usually to a lesser extent. Microorganisms easily adhere to a contact lens with deposits. A clean lens makes it difficult for these organisms to adhere as easily.

Steps to follow include:

1. Hand washing, avoiding soaps with perfume or creams.
2. Handling the contact lenses right to left, in the same order always, to avoid switching the contact lenses.
3. Placing of two or three drops of cleaning solution on the surface of the contact lens, wetting the lens completely.
4. Gently rubbing each side of the contact lens in the palm of the hand, back and forth for approximately 20 seconds, with the concave surface up.
5. Complete rinsing with multiuse solution or saline, avoiding tap water.
6. Disinfecting with specific or multiuse solutions, and placing the con-

tact lens in a storage solution and disinfectant for 4 hours or for the entire night. The wearer should use new solution each night and should make sure that the contact lens is completely submerged.

7. Rinsing with multiuse or saline solution prior to inserting the contact lens.
8. Placing wetting drops on the contact lens prior to inserting it in the eye.
9. Emptying the storage case, rinsing it, and drying it while open.

The following steps are recommended in addition:

1. Always clean the contact lens immediately after removal from the eye.
2. Use very light rubbing action during the cleaning. Significant pressure on a RGP lens can cause damage and modify the parameters of the lens. This is particularly important for wearers who have switched to RGP lenses from PMMA lenses, as the RGP lens is more fragile.
3. The RGP contact lenses should not be rubbed between fingers, because they may be broken or deformed in this manner.
4. Thermal disinfection should not be used.
5. When an RGP contact lens is being used on an extended wear basis, it should be removed at least once a week for cleaning and disinfection.
6. To remove proteins, the wearer should use an enzymatic cleaner daily or enzyme cleaner in the pill form once per week.
7. Contact lens solutions should not be used after the expiration date. Extra rigid contact lenses should be stored dry and clean, in a container that is also dry and clean. Prior to using an RGP lens that has been in dry storage, it is recommended that the RGP contact lens be placed in conditioning/disinfecting solution for at least 4 hours to increase comfort.

36. How should rigid contact lenses be inserted and removed?

The wearer should be given the following instructions:

1. Close the drain in the sink or place a clean paper towel over the drain prior to handling a contact lens to avoid loss of the lens.
2. Wash the hands to remove dirt and microorganisms that may accumulate on the contact lens and cause ocular irritation or infection. Dry with a lint-free towel.
3. Rinse the lens with multiuse solution or sterile saline to remove traces of dirt, lint, and other particulate material. If foreign bodies adhere to the contact lens at the time of insertion, it may cause ocular discomfort.
4. Place the contact lens on the index finger of the dominant hand. With the middle finger of the other hand, lift the upper lid at the lashes. The middle finger of the dominant hand is then used to pull the inferior lid down (Figure 21.1).

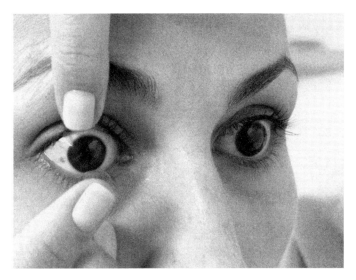

Figure 21.1. Correct technique for bimanual insertion of a rigid contact lens.

5. Using a mirror on a table and looking directly at the contact lens, the wearer can then place the contact lens on the cornea. After placement of the lens, the wearer may then release the eydids, first the inferior and then the superior lid.

Removal Method 1

1. Open a towel and place it on the table in order to avoid losing the contact lens.
2. Use the index finger of the right hand to remove the contact lens from the right eye and of the left hand to remove the contact lens from the left eye. The finger is placed at the junction of the lateral border of the lid (Figure 21.2).
3. Open the eyes wide and pull the lids to the side. At the same time, blink, looking straight ahead, to eject the contact lens. This procedure can be performed with either the index finger or the thumb of the same hand. The other hand can be positioned below the eye to catch the contact lens.

Removal Method 2

This method uses both hands for removal. The most important factor is grasping the contact lens between the lid margins to push the lens out with a blink.

1. Grasp the inferior lid with the dominant hand and the superior lid with the other.
2. Apply pressure with two fingers in the direction of the center of the eye at the edge of the contact lens (Figure 21.3).

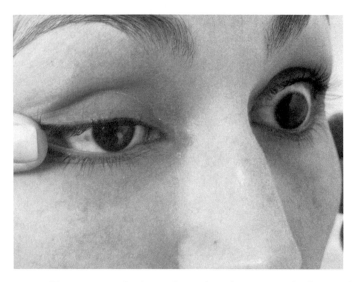

Figure 21.2. Traction on the lateral canthus for removal of a rigid contact lens.

3. The lid margin may evert, making it difficult to remove the contact lens if the lid is pressed incorrectly (Figure 21.4).

Removal Method 3

1. Grasp the suction cup with thumb and forefinger of the dominant hand.
2. Grasp the upper lid with the index finger of the other hand.
3. Look straight ahead, using a mirror.
4. Touch the suction cup to the surface of the contact lens. The suction cup will cling to the contact lens, facilitating removal (Figure 21.5A and B).

Wearers with poor palpebral tone, problems with lid margin position, and/or contact lenses of large diameter may have more success with methods 2 and 3.

37. How should gas permeable lenses be stored?

Steps in storage are as follows:

1. Wash hands with a neutral soap and dry on a lint-free towel.
2. Clean the contact lens case.
3. Remove the contact lens from the eye and place it in the palm of the hand.
4. Use the right hand to manage the right lens and the left hand to manage the left lens, to avoid switching the lenses.
5. Place two or three drops of cleaning solution on each surface of the contact lens, covering it completely.

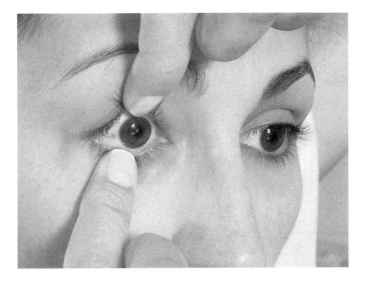

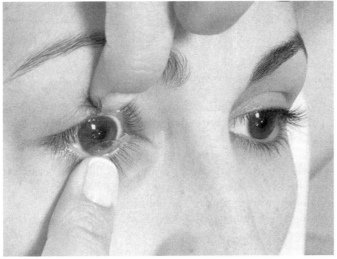

Figure 21.3. Alternate method for rigid contact lens removal using both hands to grasp the contact lens between the lid margins. Slight pressure on the lower lid will tilt the lens forward and away from the cornea.

6. Gently rub each side of the contact lens with the index finger for 20 seconds.
7. Rinse with multiuse solution or saline for 10 to 20 seconds.
8. Place the contact lens in a clean case, and before closing it, check to be sure that the edge of the lens is not caught in the top of the case.
9. Disinfect the contact lens.
10. Check to be sure that the contact lens is not everted before placing it on the eye.

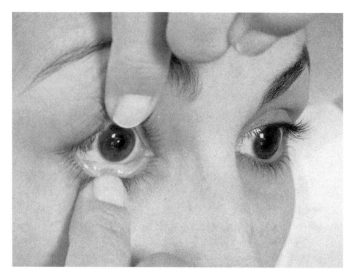

Figure 21.4. Incorrect method of manipulating the lower lid causing eversion of the lid.

The following practices are strongly recommended:

1. Always clean and disinfect the contact lens after removal from the eye. This applies to all types of contact lenses, including disposable contact lenses.
2. Avoid rubbing a dry contact lens, because at the time of removal there may be particulate matter on the lens that can scratch the surface during the cleaning process.
3. Check the expiration date of the solution.
4. If cleaning the contact lens becomes difficult, consider the use of ultrasonic cleaning.

38. How should a hydrophilic contact lens be inserted and removed?[26]

Step 1

Follow steps 1 through 3 described above for insertion and removal of an RGP lens.

Step 2

Examine the lens to be sure that it is clean and moistened without cracks or particulate matter. Then place the lens on the tip of the index finger and look at it against a bright light. If the lens appears damaged or dry, it should not be placed in the eye (Figure 21.6).

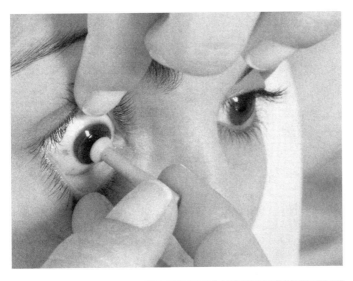

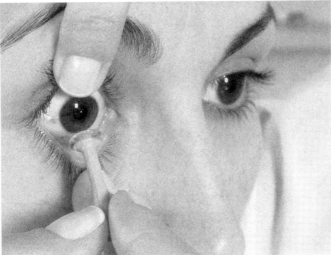

Figure 21.5. A: Correct placement of the suction cup. B: Removal of the rigid contact lens with the suction cup.

Step 3

Check to make sure that the contact lens is right side up. When placed in the eye inside out, it is uncomfortable, moves excessively, and may not provide good vision. To determine if the contact lens is inside out, place it on the tip of the index finger against a light, and look at the shape of its borders. If it is correctly oriented, the shape should be similar to that shown in Figure 21.7A. If inverted, it will appear as in Figure 21.7B.

As demonstrated in Figure 21.8A, if the edge of the lens forms a round arc when positioned on the tip of index finger, it is correctly

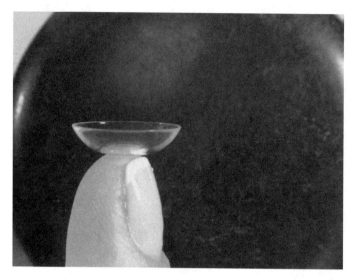

Figure 21.6. Examination of lens integrity by viewing the lens in profile placed on the fingertip.

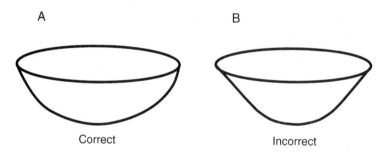

Figure 21.7. A: Correct configuration of the lens. B: Incorrect appearance of the an "inside-out" lens.

positioned. If the border splays outward, however, the lens is inside out (Figure 21.8B).

Step 4

Place the contact lens in the eye (Figure 21.9A and B)

1. Always handle the lens, right or left, with the corresponding hand to avoid switching the lens.
2. Position the lens on the tip of the right index finger, for example, and be sure that it is dry, to facilitate transfer of the contact lens to the eye.

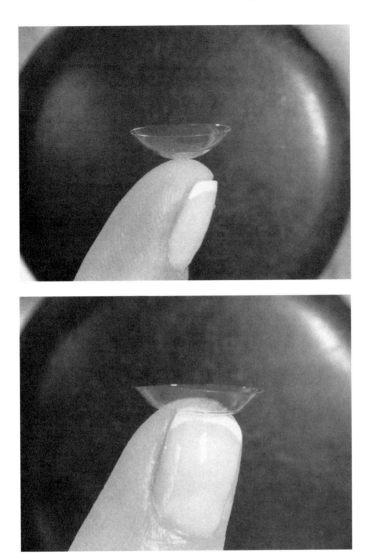

Figure 21.8. A: Correct configuration. B: Incorrect configuration with outward splaying of the border.

3. Place the middle finger of the same hand near the inferior palpebral margin, pulling the lid down inferiorly.
4. Use the fingers of the other hand to lift the superior lid.
5. Place the contact lens directly on the eye, using the index finger.
6. Look down and slowly remove the right hand, freeing the lower lid.
7. Look straight ahead and remove the left hand, freeing the upper lid.
8. Blink gently.

The same steps should be repeated for the contact lens in the left eye.

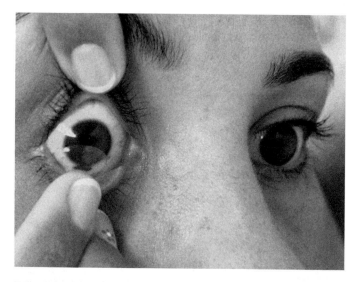

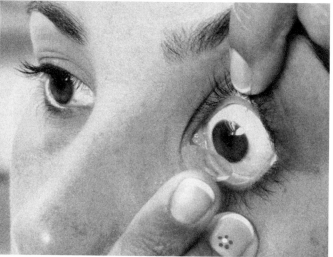

Figure 21.9. Placement of a hydrophilic contact lens in the A: Right eye. B: Left eye.

Step 5

Check vision alternately in each eye to be sure that the contact lens is in place. If vision is blurred or discomfort is felt, check to see if the contact lens is off-center, dirty, in the wrong eye, torn, or damaged. If, after placement in the eye, vision is still blurred or the eye is uncomfortable, a new lens should be tried, or the old lens should be set aside and the wearer should contact his/her eye care practitioner.

Removal Method

1. Wash, rinse, and dry hands.
2. Use wetting drops 5 to 10 minutes prior to removal to ensure that neither the eye nor the contact lens is dry. A moistened contact lens remains loose and is more easily removed from the eye. This avoids ocular irritation and tearing of the contact lens during removal from the eye.
3. Begin removing the first lens by looking at a distant target.
4. Be sure that the lens is in the eye.
5. Look up without lifting the head. Pull the inferior lid down with the middle finger. Place the tip of the index finger on the inferior border of the contact lens, and slide it off of the cornea and over to the white of the eye.
6. Gently grasp the contact lens between the index finger and thumb and remove it (Figure 21.10).

39. What is the basic care routine for daily wear hydrophilic lenses?

1. Daily cleaning with surfactant.
2. Daily enzymatic cleaning (solution) or weekly (tablet).
3. Daily disinfecting with chemical solutions or 3% hydrogen peroxide.
4. Individuals with a good tear film may substitute multiuse solution for specific solutions. It may be necessary to augment regular maintenance with surfactant and enzymatic cleaners.

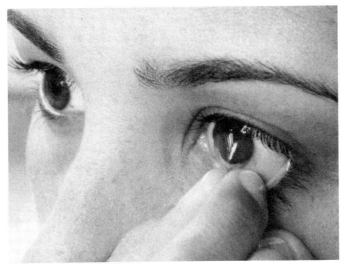

Figure 21.10. Removal technique of a soft contact lens.

40. What is the basic care routine for cosmetic hydrophilic lenses?

1. Daily cleaning with surfactant solution.
2. Daily enzymatic cleaning (solution) or weekly cleaning (tablet).
3. Daily chemical disinfecting.
4. Cleaning with abrasive solutions is *not* recommended.
5. Thermal disinfection is *not* recommended.

41. What is the basic care routine for extended wear hydrophilic lenses?

1. The lens should be removed at least once a week and, if possible, more frequently as the lens gets older.
2. Use surfactant solution and enzymatic cleaner.
3. Disinfect with specific solutions or 3% hydrogen peroxide.
4. High water-content lenses should not undergo thermal disinfection.

42. What is the basic care routine for hydrophilic lenses used only occasionally?

1. Cleaning with surfactant or multiuse solutions.
2. Chemical solution for disinfection and storage.
3. Change of the storage solution every time the contact lens is used.

Lenses should not be stored in saline.

43. What is the basic routine for care of disposable lenses?

1. Cleaning and disinfection with multiuse solution or 3% hydrogen peroxide.
2. Enzymatic cleaning can be dispensed with in lenses that are discarded at least every 3 months in wearers who do not have giant papillary conjunctivitis.

44. What is the basic care routine for hybrid contact lenses?

1. Instill lubricant in the contact lens prior to removing it from the eye.
2. Clean the lens with surfactant solution, rubbing gently for 20 seconds.
3. Avoid everting the contact lens.
4. Disinfect with 3% hydrogen peroxide or chemical solution, avoiding chlorhexidine.

Enzyme cleaner is recommended for wearers who have a tendency to deposit formation. Hybrid contact lenses should not be disinfected thermally.

45. How does one proceed when a contact lens is dislocated in the eye?

A contact lens may dislocate over the conjunctiva during insertion or wear. To re-center it, the following method should be used:

1. Look in the direction of the dislocated contact lens. Blink gently. The contact lens should move automatically in the direction of the center of the eye, returning to the correct position.
2. Close the lids and massage the contact lens gently through the closed lid.
3. Push the dislocated lens over the cornea with the eye closed, placing slight pressure with the finger on the border of the superior or inferior lid.

46. What are the recommended intervals for use and exchange of different types of conventional contact lenses?

Contact lens type	Wearing time	Period of exchange
PMMA	10 hours	Years
Daily wear RGP	15 hours or all waking hours	18 to 24 months
Extended wear RGP	Continuously up to 7 days	12 months
Daily wear hydrophilic	12 hours or all waking hours	12–18 months
Extended wear hydrophilic	Continuously up to 7 days	Up to 12 months

47. What is the recommended period for the use and exchange of disposable and planned replacement contact lenses?

1. Daily disposable: One day of use followed by disposal.
2. Weekly disposable: Up to 7 days of continuous wear with disposal, or removal each night with disposal after 2 weeks. Examples include Acuvue 1 and 2 (Vistakon J&J); Focus Week (CIBA Vision); Hydron Biomedics 55 (Ocular Sciences); Precision UV (Wesley Jessen); SofLens 66 (Bausch & Lomb); etc.
3. Monthly disposable: Silicone hydrogel contact lenses generally can be used during sleep for up to 30 days. These lenses must be discarded after 30 days. It is recommended that they be removed once

weekly for cleaning and disinfection. Examples include Night & Day (CIBA Vision); Purevision (Bausch & Lomb).
4. Programmed exchange: Daily wear lenses are discarded monthly. Examples include Surevue and Vistavue (Vistakon J&J); FreshLook tinted lenses (Wesley Jessen); Focus Toric and Focus Progressives (CIBA Vision).

Some wearers may require more frequent exchange of contact lenses if deposits form, if the lens breaks or tears, or if other problems with lens maintenance occur.

48. What is the appropriate wearing time immediately after fitting of a contact lens?

Daily Wear Contact Lenses

1. One should initiate wear beginning with 6 hours a day, increasing by 2 hours a day.
2. An alternative approach is to initiate wear at 4 hours a day, adding 2 hours every 2 days until one reaches 10 hours a day. If, during the gradual adaptation to a rigid contact lens, the process is interrupted, it should be reinitiated until a maximum of 10 to 12 hours is reached.

Occasional Use Contact Lenses

Individuals who use a contact lens for weekend events or for sports should not wear the lens for more than 8 hours at a time.

Extended Wear Contact Lenses

There are two possible approaches:

1. In the first week, the lens can be worn all day, with removal at bedtime. If there is no irritation or blurring of vision, the patient can begin wearing the lenses continuously. However the eye care practitioner should reevaluate the patient after the first week.
2. The lenses can be left in for the first 24 hours with a follow-up examination with the eye care practitioner the next day. The period of extended wear can then be determined by the ophthalmologist or optometrist.

The general rule is that all extended wear lenses should be removed at least once a week for cleaning and disinfection.

49. What are the most frequent symptoms during the fitting and adaptation to a rigid gas permeable lens?

Normal Symptoms

- Sensation of a wet eye and the intermittent blurring of vision with increased tearing.
- Lid irritation that can cause excessive or incomplete blinking. The incomplete blink (an unconscious reaction to diminish the discomfort caused by the edge of the lens on the lid) should be corrected with the fitting.
- Difficulty with upgaze.
- Light sensitivity.

Abnormal Symptoms

- Sudden burning or pain. Acute pain may be caused by particulate matter under the contact lens.
- Constant halo around lights.
- Ocular irritation and progressive redness.
- Difficulty with contact lens removal with adherence of the contact lens to the eye.
- Blurred vision with glasses for more than 1 hour after removal of the contact lens.

50. How can practitioners avoid contamination of contact lenses in the office?

1. Wash hands before every manipulation of the contact lens.
2. Wash hands after contact with the patient's eyes.
3. Disinfect trial lenses. The quickest way is to use 3% hydrogen peroxide when one wants to test a contact lens in another patient. The most practical is to change the chemical solution every time a lens is manipulated.
4. Rinse with multiuse solutions or saline.
5. Discard preserved saline solutions after 2 weeks.
6. Discard saline solutions without preservatives at the end of each day.
7. Avoid tap water, filter water, or mineral water for rinsing of lenses.
8. Vigorously clean and follow programmed exchange of the contact lens cases.
9. Monitor the expiration date on the contact lens solution labels.
10. Impress upon all staff the need for the prevention of contamination.

51. How should hydrophilic contact lenses be stored in the office?

1. Change the disinfectant solution every time the contact lens is used as a trial lens.
2. Change the solution in all open containers every 15 days.
3. Perform periodic laboratory culture of the contact lens stock.
4. Monitor the expiration date on the contact lens labels.

52. How should rigid gas permeable lenses be stored in the office?

Rigid gas permeable contact lenses should be maintained clean and dry, in a clean, dry case. Alternatively, RGP contact lenses can be maintained in solution. However, there does not appear to be any significant difference with regard to the rate of contamination in these two forms of storage. Dehydration of the contact lens may have a slight effect on the contact lens parameters and the wettability of the lens surface.

53. How can incompatibility reactions among solutions be avoided?

The manufacturers have tested the compatibility of their products with ocular tissues and the most commonly employed materials in contact lenses, but it is not possible to test cross-compatibility among all of the solutions and existing materials. For this reason, it is important to closely follow the instructions of each manufacturer. Systemic medications excreted into the tear film and, more commonly, any medication that is placed on the eye topically may interact with the contact lens. Examples of incompatibilities between contact lens materials and solutions are as follows:

- Thimerosal, when heated, may cloud the contact lens or the case.
- Hydrocare™ solution may cause mild keratitis when used with contact lenses made of silicone elastomeres.
- Rigid gas permeable lenses undergo a polymeric alteration when in contact with alcohol, acetone, perfumes, or gasoline.
- Hydrophilic contact lenses stored in surfactant solution may turn opaque or discolored.
- Chemical disinfection, when used in combination with thermal treatment of contact lenses, may discolor or alter the polymer.
- High-water-content hydrophilic lenses may become opaque, discolored, or wrinkled when submitted to thermal disinfection.
- Thermal disinfection with saline solution that has been previously used may turn the lens gray.

In addition to issues of compatibility between contact lens solutions and materials, there are examples of incompatibility between solutions; e.g., solutions such as chlorhexidine should not be used with enzymatic cleaners that contain papaine. To avoid incompatibilities, it is best not to mix solutions manufactured by different companies; to give instructions to patients about contact lens care in writing; to ask at every visit which methods and what products the patient is using; and to let the patient know about the possibility of incompatibilities of the contact lens with specific solutions.

54. Can one swim while wearing contact lenses?

The primary reason to avoid swimming while wearing contact lenses is the risk of bacterial infection, as the water is generally contaminated. Aside from this risk, one should consider that swimmers, divers, skiers, and surfers require good distance vision to avoid accidents and to maximize performance.

In lakes and oceans, there may be contamination from chemical products and sewage, particularly after heavy rains. Nonetheless, studies have demonstrated that the presence of chemical products and microbes in contact lenses used by swimmers is not significant. In pool water, *Staphylococcus, Streptococcus, Pseudomonas aeruginosa,* and *Acanthamoeba* may proliferate. The latter two cause severe corneal ulceration when associated with contact lens use. To minimize contamination, large quantities of chlorine are added to pools periodically. The chlorine, besides altering the color of the contact lens, may adhere to the polymer and produce significant ocular irritation. The risks of ocular infection must be explained in detail to the patient. Nonetheless, it is the responsibility of the contact lens wearer to weigh the risks of using contact lenses under these conditions.

55. What are the recommendations for the individual who wants to swim with contact lenses?

In the pool:

1. Use protective goggles.
2. Clean and disinfect the contact lens carefully after swimming, or consider wearing daily disposable lenses during swimming that can just be discarded after swimming.
3. Wait 20 minutes after swimming before removing the contact lens. This permits reequilibration of the contact lens with the tears, making the lens looser and preventing any damage to the corneal epithelium during removal.
4. Use wetting drops prior to removing the contact lens to loosen the contact lens and to help eliminate any chemical or microbial contaminants.
5. Have two pairs of contact lenses, with one pair for use during swimming, that can be set aside, cleaned, and disinfected while the other pair is worn.

6. Discard contact lenses after swimming when the risk of infection is the greatest.
7. Have a pair of glasses in case the contact lenses are lost.

In the ocean:

1. Close the eyes underwater. After surfacing, blink rapidly to remove water from the eye. When contact lenses are in contact with salt water, they do not fit as tightly.
2. Have glasses available in case the contact lenses are lost.

56. How does one avoid contamination of the contact lenses with cosmetics or hair care products?

Cosmetics can deposit on the contact lenses and may cause allergic reactions; they can form a greasy film on the contact lens, obscuring vision and thereby reducing wearing time and comfort. We recommend the following practices:

1. Use unscented and hypoallergenic cosmetics.
2. Use cosmetics made by established companies with a record of quality control.
3. Wash hands thoroughly to remove any residue prior to handling of the contact lenses. Oily cosmetics are difficult to remove from the fingers and from the contact lens.
4. Apply cosmetics when the contact lens is already in place to reduce the risk of contaminating the lens. Presbyopic patients, however, may find it easier to apply makeup without a contact lens. They may wish to place the lens in position after cosmetic application.
5. Avoid iridescent eye shadow, because the particles may get into the eye and remain under the contact lens. Compact eye shadows are preferred over liquid, oils, or creams, which are more difficult to remove from the contact lens. Use eye shadow in moderate quantities only. Facial powder in a compact is preferred over loose powder and should be applied with care. Remove any excess powder from around the eyes.
6. Apply eyeliner with an attempt to avoid any obstruction of the meibomian glands. Otherwise, this may cause blepharitis, hordeola, or chalazia. For the contact lens wearer, pencil liners are better than liquids or pastes. Avoid using saliva to moisten the brush or cosmetic.
7. Wash mascara brushes frequently and change them every 3 months. Mascara brushes should not be shared. Mascara is a combination of greasy pigment, wax, and chemical preservatives, generally in a liquid base, which is an optimal medium for the growth of microorganisms.
8. Apply mascara lightly and distant from the base of the lashes. Never use a sharp object to separate the lashes. Avoid waterproof mascara and mascara designed to elongate the lashes. These con-

tain nylon and rayon fibers that are dry and may loosen, entering the eye. The tears carry these fibers under the contact lens, where they can irritate or cause injury to the cornea. Water-resistant mascara (not waterproof) is recommended for the contact lens user because it is soluble in water and may be removed easily with emulsifying agents. The waterproof mascara, however, requires using oily products to remove it. If these oily products remain on the lid margin, they may contaminate the contact lens, even after thorough rinsing.

9. Close and tightly cap the cosmetics immediately after use to avoid contamination. Do not expose cosmetics to heat.

10. Remove the contact lens before removing makeup.

11. When applying cream to the lids at night, take care not to touch the lashes, and preferably, after 20 minutes, remove the excess cream with a tissue. Cream can penetrate the eye during the night, entering the tear film and causing decreased vision in addition to burning and pain the next day.

12. Aerosol solutions and their sprays should be used prior to the insertion of the contact lens. If it is necessary to apply hair spray while wearing a contact lens, the eyes should be closed, and the place where the spray was applied should be left quickly, because the aerosol remains in the air for a period of time.

13. Avoid wearing contact lenses during hair coloring or chemical treatments to the hair.

14. Avoid the use of cosmetics and contact lenses in eyes that are red, inflamed, or infected.

References

1. Driebe WT Jr. Contact lens cleaning and disinfection. In: Kastl PR, ed. *Contact Lenses. The CLAO Guide to Basic Science and Clinical Practice*, vol 2. Dubuque, IA: Kendall/Hant Publishing, 1995:237–262.

2. Caroline PJ, Obin JB, Gindi JJ, et al. Microscopic and elemental analysis of deposits on extended wear soft contact lenses. *CLAO J.* 1985;311–316.

3. Kleist FD. Appearance and nature of hydrophilic contact lens deposits. II. Inorganic deposits. *Int Contact Lens Clin.* 1979;6:177–186.

4. Carney LG, Hill RM. pH profiles: part 1—one pH, or many? *J Am Optom Assoc.* 1975;46:1143–1145.

5. Brawner L, Essop DG. A review of contact lens solutions. *Contacto.* 1962;6:49–51.

6. Burstein NL. Preservative cytotoxic threshold for benzalkonium chloride and chlorhexidine digluconate in cat and rabbit corneas. *Invest Ophthalmol Vis Sci.* 1980;19:308–313.

7. Shih K, Sibley MJ. The microbiological benefit of cleaning and rinsing contact lenses. *Int Contact Lens Clin.* 1985;12:234–242.

8. Patrinely JR, Wilhelmus KR, Rubin JM, Key JE. Bacterial keratitis associated with extended wear soft contact lenses. *CLAO J.* 1985;11:234–236.

9. Mayo MS, Schiltzer RL, Ward MA, Wilson LA, Ahearn DG. Association of *Pseudomonas* and *Serratia* corneal ulcers with use of contaminated solutions. *J Clin Microbiol.* 1987;25:1398–1400.

10. Donzis PB, Mondino BJ, Weismann BA. *Bacillus* keratitis associated with contaminated contact lens care systems. *Am J Ophthamol.* 1988;105:195–197.

11. Penley CA, Willis SW, Sickler SG. Comparative antimicrobial efficacy of soft and rigid gas-permeable contact lens solutions against *Acanthamoeba*. *CLAO J*. 1989;15:257–260.
12. Liedel KK, Begley CG. The effectiveness of soft contact lens disinfection systems against *Acanthamoeba* on the lens surface. *J Am Optom Assoc*. 1996; 67:135–142.
13. Soni OS, Horner DG, Ross J. Ocular response to lens care systems in adolescent soft contact lens wearers. *Optom Vis Sci*. 1996;73:70–85.
14. Erickson OF. Drug influences on lacrimal lysozyme production. *Stanford Med Bull*. 1960;18:34.
15. Crandall DC, Leopold IH. The influence of systemic drugs on tear constituents. *Ophthalmology*. 1979;86:115.
16. Fraunfelder FT, Baico JM, Meyer SM. Adverse ocular reactions possibly associated with isotretinoin. *Am J Ophthalmol*. 1985;100:534.
17. Ensink BW, Van Voorst Vader PC. Ophthalmological side effects of 13-cis-retinoic therapy. *Br J Dermatol*. 1983;108:637.
18. Scott D. Another beta blocker causing eye problems. *Br Med J*. 1977;2:1221.
19. Mackie IA, Seal DV, Pescod JM. Beta-adrenergic receptor blocking drugs: tear lysozyme and immunological screening for adverse reactions. *Br J Ophthalmol*. 1977;61:354.
20. Almog Y, Monselise M, Almog CH, et al. The effect of oral treatment with beta blockers on tear secretion. *Metab Pediatr Syst Ophthalmol*. 1983;6:343.
21. Chizek DJ, Franceschetti AT. Oral contraceptives: their side effects and ophthalmological manifestations. *Surv Ophthalmol*. 1969;14:90.
22. Frankel SH, Ellis PP. Effect of oral contraceptives on tear production. *Ann Ophthalmol*. 1978;10:1585.
23. Valenic JP, Leopold IH, Dea FJ. Excretion of salicylic acid into tears following oral administration of aspirin. *Ophthalmology*. 1980;87:815.
24. Miller D. Systemic medications. *Int Ophthalmol Clin*. 1981;21:177.
25. Berman MT, Newman BL, Johnson NC. The effect of a diuretic (hydrochlorothiazide) on tear production in humans. *Am J Ophthalmol*. 1985; 99:473.
26. Coral-Ghanem C. *Lentes de Vontato: Manual do Usuario*. Joinville: Oftalmologia e Clinica de Lentes de Contato: Solucoes, 2002:41–44.

22

Complications Associated with Contact Lens Use

Newton Kara-José, Cleusa Coral-Ghanem, and Charlotte E. Joslin

1. How do complications occur with contact lenses?

The contact lens wearer can have complications that either are directly induced by or are the result of existing problems that are aggravated by the presence of a contact lens. The contact lens is in direct contact with the eye and induces alterations through (1) trauma, (2) reduced corneal and conjunctival wetting, (3) decreased corneal oxygenation, (4) stimulation of allergic and inflammatory responses, and (5) infection.

The principal causes of complications are:

- Inadequate lens-to-cornea fitting relationship
- Insufficient contact lens oxygen transmissibility
- The presence of preexisting ocular pathology
- Interference by environmental factors
- Intolerance of contact lens material
- Poorly maintained contact lenses
- Contaminated contact lenses and lens cases
- Use of incorrect contact lenses

2. What are the principal symptoms of complications?

Two principal symptoms alert one to ocular changes that can be attenuated by the use of contact lenses, delaying diagnosis of ocular lesions. They are:

1. Pain. All chronic contact lens wear contact lenses may cause corneal hypesthesia. Hydrophilic contact lenses are used to alleviate dis-

comfort in cases of epithelial lesions or to reduce contact of exposed nerve ends with the lid and air.

2. Decreased visual acuity. One of the principal mechanisms of defense of the eye is diminished visual acuity in the presence of some irregularity of the anterior surface of the cornea. The contact lens replaces the surface and serves as the new refracting surface for the eye and can mask the irregularities that would ordinarily signal ocular problems. This is particularly true in rigid gas permeable contact lenses, and to a lesser extent, in soft contact lenses.

Other symptoms frequently encountered include:

- Conjunctival hyperemia
- Contact lens intolerance

3. How can the incidence of contact lens–related complications be reduced?

Reducing the incidence of complications depends on:

- Correct selection of the contact lens candidate
- Accurate selection of the contact lens to provide an adequate fit
- Appropriate patient education regarding the care, handling, and limitations of contact lens use
- Patient compliance with duration of use and follow-up examinations, as well as early recognition of the signs and symptoms of abnormalities

Contact lenses alter the corneal physiology, and the relationship between the lens and cornea is a dynamic process. Ill-fitting lenses or noncompliant patients risk exacerbating, or even inducing, disease. Conversely, contact lenses can also alleviate disease and provide therapeutic effects. As a result of this dynamic relationship and the possible complications, follow-up should be ongoing. The examination should be meticulous and complete, both in the selection of the contact lens candidate and in the evaluation of effects on the eye induced by the contact lens. It is the responsibility of the contact lens practitioner to instruct and educate the patient regarding adequate fit, care and maintenance, duration of use, and risks of complications.

Despite a long history of successful contact lens use without complications, the dynamic relationship among the eye, the contact lens, and ambient factors can result in unforeseen complications at any time.

4. What are the principal complications of contact lenses?

Lids

- Blepharitis
- Meibomianitis

Conjunctiva

- Giant papillary conjunctivitis
- Superior limbic keratoconjunctivitis
- Infectious conjunctivitis
- Conjunctivitis secondary to mucoprotein deposits
- Conjunctival hyperemia
- Acute red eye

Cornea

- Superficial punctate keratitis
- Corneal de-epithelialization
- Corneal edema
- Corneal distortion
- Hypesthesia
- Desiccation: 3 and 9 o'clock position staining
- Sterile infiltrates
- NeovascularizationS
- uperior arcuate epithelial lesions
- Opacities
- Microbial keratitis
- Pseudodendritic keratitis

5. How does the cornea receive oxygen during contact lens wear?

The cornea is predominantly supplied with oxygen through the atmosphere, but small amounts of oxygen are also supplied through the aqueous and limbal vasculature.[1,2] The amount of atmospheric oxygen pressure available to the eye through the tears in open eye conditions at sea level (155 mm Hg) is much greater than that available through the aqueous (55 mm Hg) or under closed eye conditions (55 mm Hg).[3,4] Under closed eye conditions, the majority of oxygen to the cornea is supplied through the palpebral conjunctiva.[5] Numerous factors beyond individual variability affect corneal oxygen demand, including corneal temperature and pH levels, previous ocular surgical history, previous contact use, and contact lens material and design.[6–8]

The use of contact lenses reduces the amount of oxygen available to the cornea, and this reduction is based on both lens design and lens material. Multiple measures exist for assessing the oxygen supply to cornea through a contact lens, but the most commonly used are oxygen permeability (Dk) and oxygen transmissibility (Dk/L). Oxygen permeability is a property of the lens material itself and is independent of lens design or thickness. Oxygen transmissibility is dependent on lens center thickness (L) and accounts for the difference in the oxygen availability to the cornea between lenses manufactured of the same material but with different center thickness (i.e., an aphakic lens versus a -3.00-

D lens). Higher permeability and transmissibility values indicate more oxygen is available to the cornea.

Holden and Mertz[9] determined the critical oxygen levels to avoid corneal edema in daily and extended wear contact lens use. These oxygen transmissibility levels, known as the Holden-Mertz criteria, suggest that $Dk/L = 24.1 \times 10^{-9}$ is necessary for daily wear use and that $Dk/L = 87 \times 10^{-9}$ is necessary for extended wear use.

Contact lenses can be divided into three main types based on the mechanism through which the cornea is oxygenated during lens wear:

1. Polymethylmethacrylate (PMMA) lenses, also known as hard contact lenses, are infrequently used today because they are impermeable to oxygen ($Dk = 0$). In eyes fitted with PMMA lenses, corneal oxygenation is dependent entirely on oxygen dissolved in the tear film and on lacrimal exchange with the blink.
2. As the name implies, rigid gas permeable lenses are a technical advancement beyond PMMA lenses. Oxygen is supplied to the cornea through the lens material in addition to lacrimal exchange with the blink. Up to 20% of the tear volume is exchanged per blink.[10] Rigid gas permeable (RGP) lenses currently are available with an oxygen permeability up to $Dk = 250$.
3. Hydrogel, or soft contact lenses, are nearly entirely dependent on oxygen diffusing across the lens material. Only 1% of the tear volume is exchanged with each blink.[10] The highest oxygen permeability currently available in hydrogel lenses is $Dk = 140$.

6. What causes corneal edema in contact lens use? What is the clinical presentation of patients with corneal edema, and how is it managed?

Causes and Mechanism of Action

Corneal edema in contact lens use may result from either acute or chronic hypoxic corneal conditions. Most commonly, the hypoxia is caused by a continuum of two factors: (1) Contact lens materials are inappropriately selected given the individual corneal physiologic demands and the patient's contact lens wearing schedule. (2) Contact lenses are inadequately fitted.

Types of Corneal Edema

Epithelial Edema

Epithelial edema resulting from contact lenses is rare in healthy corneas, but it can result from hypoxia. Lens type alters the amount of corneal hypoxia.

PMMA lenses
The PMMA lenses are most likely to cause epithelial edema because they are oxygen impermeable.[11]

Soft and Rigid Gas Permeable Contact Lenses
In soft contact lens wear, historical data are rather inconclusive about the corneal epithelial edema response to hypoxia based on measurements conducted using instruments with limited reproducibility. Optical coherence tomography (OCT), a new method of optical imaging with very high instrument reproducibility for corneal thickness measurements, demonstrates that corneal epithelial thickness does not increase in response to transient hypoxia resulting from eye closure (3 hours) with soft contact lens wear.[12]

Similar studies examining transient epithelial thickness changes during rigid gas permeable contact lens wear have not been performed with OCT. However, studies have been conducted that examine different measures of epithelial stress under hypoxic conditions. The effects of epithelial hypoxia can also be examined by measuring the changes in the permeability of the corneal epithelium, such as that which occurs following overnight wear of RGP lenses.[13] In RGP lenses, the increase in epithelial permeability in overnight wear is dependent on the dose of hypoxia, with medium Dk lenses increasing permeability more than high Dk lenses.[14] This suggests that transient epithelial edema resulting from hypoxic stress could occur if hypoxic levels were sufficient, such as that reported with PMMA lenses.[11]

Hypotonic Tear Film
Epithelial edema in healthy corneas can be created by a hypotonic tear film (from excessive epiphora or reflex lacrimation).[15]

Stromal Edema

Stromal edema occurs frequently from all types of contact lens wear. Corneal stromal swelling develops following both acute and chronic hypoxic conditions. Following transient, overnight wear of contact lenses, stromal swelling increases, with lower Dk/L lenses producing greater stromal swelling than higher Dk/L lenses. Similar outcomes resulted in chronic conditions after 1 month of continuous wear.[12,16]

Corneal Edema and Lens Material

In 1984, Holden and Mertz determined the critical oxygen levels necessary to avoid corneal edema in daily and extended wear contact lens use. Subsequent research has supported these findings and demonstrated that materials of increasing oxygen permeability produce decreasing amounts of corneal edema.[17] Significant advances in polymer technology have allowed the recent development of contact lens materials with excellent oxygen permeability that produce no increase in corneal thickness when lenses are worn overnight compared to baseline, pre–contact lens thickness. With the advent of this new technology, the Food and Drug Administration (FDA), in the fall of 2001, approved two new silicone hydrogel contact lenses for up to 30 nights of continuous wear. The oxygen permeability of these new lenses (at a Dk = 110 and = 140, balafilcon and lotrafilcon, respectively) offers a better safety profile to prevent corneal edema in both continuous and daily wear.

Corneal Edema and Lens Fit

Because the cornea receives nearly all the oxygen through the atmosphere or the precorneal tear film, all contact lenses can reduce the amount of oxygen to the eye to the point of clinical significance. As described earlier, lenses that require lacrimal exchange to oxygenate the cornea may be more likely to cause corneal edema if they are inadequately fitted. Other factors that alter the oxygen supply to the cornea include:

1. Effects of refractive power on lens thickness (i.e., an aphakic lens versus a -3.00-D lens)
2. Effects of lens design on lens thickness, including:
   • Prism ballasting for astigmatism correction
   • Eccentric lenticularization
   • Bifocal segments
3. Status of lens surface, i.e., presence of lens deposits

The "overwear syndrome" develops as a result of prolonged lens wear in hypoxic conditions. It is classically seen with PMMA lenses and hence is infrequently seen today compared with the past. Patients may develop large abrasions from excessive contact lens wear and remain initially asymptomatic because the hypoxic conditions create corneal hypesthesia. After removal of the contact lens and following gradual return of corneal sensation, severe pain develops from the corneal abrasion. Treatment should initially focus on the corneal abrasion, including prophylactic antibiotics and cycloplegic agents to alleviate pain, and should later focus on refitting the patient into a more oxygen permeable lens material.

Symptoms and Signs of Epithelial Edema

Sclerotic scatter illumination at the slit-lamp biomicroscope can be used to detect corneal epithelial edema, also known as central corneal clouding. Epithelial edema is usually central and reduces the transparency of the cornea, so a cloudy area is obvious when viewed against the dark background of the pupil. Epithelial edema may create symptoms of light sensitivity, glare, and halos. PMMA wearers were also found to have an increase in myopia and steepening of the cornea associated with epithelial edema.

Symptoms and Signs of Stromal Edema and Associated Findings

Microcysts

Microcysts likely represent pockets of cellular breakdown products. They are likely to be extracellular as the epithelial turnover rate is only 7 days, but resolution of microcysts requires a few months following discontinuation of lens wear. Microcysts are visible in the epithelium and migrate from the deep epithelium anteriorly until they reach the surface of the cornea, at which time they stain with sodium fluorescein dye. There is a link between microcysts and corneal hypoxia, and they are traditionally seen in three conditions: (1) upon initiation of contact lens wear; (2) under hypoxic contact lens–wearing conditions, such as extended wear; and (3) when the cornea again receives adequate oxygenation, such as with discontinuation of contact lenses or when the lens material is changed to allow a significantly higher oxygen amount of oxygen to the cornea.[18–20]

Stromal Striae and Folds

Striae develop if the level of stromal edema exceeds 5% and may represent refractile changes resulting from collagen fibril separation with increasing stromal hydration. If the level of stromal edema exceeds 10%, posterior stromal folds develop that represent a buckling of the cornea relative to Descemet's membrane.[21]

Stromal Vascularization

Both superificial and deep stromal vascularization can develop in the presence of persistent corneal edema. Further detail is provided later.

Treatment of Corneal Edema

1. Select a lens material with a higher oxygen permeability.
2. Decrease contact lens wearing time.
3. Provide an optimal contact lens fit.

7. How do contact lenses influence epithelial integrity, and what changes are visible clinically?

Causes and Mechanism of Action

Contact lenses alter the physiology and morphology of the epithelium and can influence corneal integrity. The intact corneal epithelium serves as the first line of defense against microorganisms, and only a few organisms, including *Neisseria gonorrhoeae*, *Corynebacterium diphtheriae*, and *Listeria* species, have penetrated an intact epithelium.[22] Physiologic changes in the epithelium that result from contact lens wear can include edema, decrease in mitosis, delay in epithelial cell turnover, epithelial thinning, and compromised junctional integrity.[1-6] By altering the epithelium, contact lenses can challenge corneal health and increase the likelihood for infection, as is demonstrated by the increased incidence of *Pseudomonas aeruginosa* infections in contact lens wearers compared to non–contact lens wearers.[23-25] While most of these changes are subclinical occurrences that occur in normal lens wear, it is critical to monitor for more pronounced changes that further endanger the epithelial integrity.

Conditions of contact lens wear that can further endanger the epithelial integrity include:

1. Inadequate lens oxygen transmissibility
2. Inappropriately fitted contact lens
   - Rigid lenses
     - Excessively flat base curve
     - Inadequate peripheral edge clearance
     - Inferiorly decentered
     - Poorly polished lens or lens edge
   - Soft lenses
     - Tight lens
3. Mechanical trauma secondary to lens insertion or removal
4. Damaged contact lenses
   - Deposits on anterior and posterior lens surfaces
   - Torn or cracked lenses
5. Debris between lens and cornea
6. Tear film instability

Symptoms and Signs of Epithelial Disruption

Signs include the following:

- Punctate epithelial keratopathy (Color Plate 22)
- Superficial epithelial arcuate line (Color Plate 23)
- Epithelial abrasions
- Foreign body track
- 3 and 9 o'clock position desiccation staining
- Dellen (Color Plate 24)
- Microcysts
- Vacuoles
- Mucin balls
- Dimple veiling

Symptoms that may vary based on severity:

- Foreign body sensation
  Photophobia

Treatment of Epithelial Defects

The presence of epithelial defects resulting from contact lens wear must be monitored closely, and treatment may be warranted, depending on the severity of the epithelial defect, to prevent against infection. The presence of other clinical signs of epithelial disruption should be followed and modifications to contact lenses should be made to provide the ideal lens fitting relationships. Mucin balls likely are not detrimental to contact lens wear.[26] If recurrent epithelial keratopathy persists, subepithelial corneal opacities and scarring may develop in the area of epitheliopathy.

Considerations should include:

• Temporary cessation of contact lens wear
• Prophylactic antibiotic therapy in the presence of epithelial defects
• Refitting of contact lenses
• Patient education

8. What are the causes of corneal hypoesthesia in contact lens wearers?

All contact lens use reduces corneal sensitivity. Some types of lenses are more likely to cause corneal hypesthesia, and historically PMMA lenses are the greatest culprits. Alterations in corneal sensitivity may be acute or chronic and may develop following both short-term and long-term contact lens wear. The consequences of corneal hypesthesia may include an inability to detect painful ocular conditions that signify a potentially threatening situation.

Acute Hypesthesia

• In adapted PMMA lens wearers, corneal sensitivity decreases on average 110% over a 12-hour period following lens insertion.[27]
• In adapted soft contact lens wearers, placement of a soft lens with a water content of 38% reduces sensitivity approximately half as much as a PMMA lens does.
• The majority of corneal sensation recovery occurs within the first hour for both PMMA and soft lens wearers, but complete recovery in PMMA lens wearers takes longer and is dependent on the cumulative years of lens wear.[28-30]

Chronic Hypesthesia

Long-term wearers of both soft and RGP contact lenses demonstrate a similar loss of corneal sensitivity.

• The amount of hypesthesia produced in both types of lens wear appears to stabilize after a few months of lens use.[31]
• Corneal hypesthesia in daily lens wearers does not appear to be dependent on the cumulative years of lens use.[31]
• In contrast, for PMMA wearers, the duration of lens wear is significantly related to loss of corneal sensitivity.[32]

Mechanism of Action

Although the exact mechanisms for corneal hypesthesia remain elusive, possible mechanisms include:

- Sensitization to the mechanical trauma produced by contact lenses. This is most likely the cause of hypesthesia in RGP lens wearers.[31]
- Corneal metabolic changes that affect corneal nerves. Soft contact lenses most likely produce hypesthesia through this mechanism.[31]
- Acidosis of the cornea, reducing corneal sensitivity.

Signs and Symptoms of Hypesthesia

- Most patients remain asymptomatic of the hypesthesia. Paradoxically, it may be corneal hypesthesia that allows contact lens wear to be comfortable:
- Lack of pain in contact lens wearers should not be used as a diagnostic factor to rule out complicating conditions when a patient should exhibit pain.

Treatment for Hypesthesia

Utilize high oxygen permeable lens materials when fitting contact lenses.

9. How does contact lens wear alter the endothelium?

Acute Changes: Endothelial Blebs

Edematous endothelial cells can be observed through confocal microscopy and specular reflection following acute hypoxia caused by contact lens use.[18]

Chronic Changes: Endothelial Polymegethism

Chronic use of contact lenses with low oxygen permeability reduces the uniformity of the endothelial cell size and shape and decreases the total number of endothelial cells.[33] While this is generally not visible at the slit lamp, significant changes to the endothelium can reduce the functioning of the endothelial pump and alter corneal hydration.

10. How should contact lens–induced corneal distortion be managed?

Mechanisms of Action

Corneal warpage is an alteration of the corneal curvature that results from a molding effect produced by contact lens wear. It can change the refractive error by altering the myopia (or hyperopia), by changing the magnitude or axis of the regular astigmatism, or by inducing irregular astigmatism. It is diagnosed by using corneal topography or keratometry, in which serial curvature changes or topographic (or keratometric mire) irregularity are present. Irregular astigmatism usually causes a decrease in best-corrected spectacle visual acuity that improves with an RGP overrefraction. Irregular astigmatism resulting from corneal disease, such as keratoconus, must be differentiated.

Corneal warpage can result from the wear of any contact lens, but it is more common in certain lens designs:

- Historically, wearers of PMMA lenses were most susceptible to corneal warpage, particularly if they were long-term PMMA wearers. Corneal warpage likely resulted from both a mechanical shape change due to ill-fitting lenses and from focal edematous changes resulting from inadequate corneal oxygenation. Fortunately, few patients still wear PMMA lenses.
- Most patients with normal corneas who wear well-fitted soft and RGP contact lenses do not exhibit corneal warpage, although there are a few exceptions.
- Types of contact lenses that are most likely to cause corneal molding inadvertently include posterior aspheric multifocal RGP lenses and thick, low-water-content soft contact lenses. Both lens types induce warpage due to their fitting characteristics. Posterior surface, aspheric multifocal lenses are traditionally fitted several diopters steep, while thick, low-water-content soft contact lenses frequently exhibit minimal lens movement.
- All types of ill-fitting contact lenses can easily induce corneal warpage.

Treatment of Corneal Distortion

1. In contact lens patients with corneal warpage, it is important to distinguish between the absence and presence of irregular astigmatism and a subsequent decrease in the best-corrected visual acuity.
2. Contact lens refitting should be considered in all patients with a decrease in best-corrected spectacle visual acuity resulting from corneal warpage with irregular astigmatism.
3. For contact lens patients who have corneal molding but do not have irregular astigmatism or a subsequent decrease in spectacle visual acuity, it may not be necessary to refit the contact lens. For example, a presbyopic patient may have superior distance, intermediate, and near contact lens visual acuity using a posterior surface, aspheric RGP design and would be dissatisfied if refitted into a design less likely to induce corneal molding.

Other Types of Corneal Distortion

Other types of corneal distortion that may result from contact lens wear include a corneal impression ring, bulbar conjunctival imprint, and myopia reduction.

Corneal Impression Ring

An RGP contact lens with an inappropriate peripheral edge lift can cause localized corneal distortion as evident by the presence of an impression ring, or edge imprint. Epithelial compromise may be present as indicated by sodium fluorescein staining. The presence of an impression sign indicates the need to alter the contact lens edge lift or refit the lens entirely. If the remainder of the lens fit is appropriate, the peripheral curvature can be flattened to modify the edge profile and prevent an impression ring.

Bulbar Conjunctival Imprint

Soft contact lenses and large-diameter RGP lenses may produce a conjunctival imprint. The presence of a conjunctival imprint suggests a lens that is excessively tight. If the lens is a soft lens, consider flattening the base curve. In large-diameter RGP lenses producing imprints, the peripheral curves must be flattened.

Myopia Reduction

The ease with which corneal warpage can be induced has led to further development of lens designs to change the shape of the cornea intentionally for temporary myopia reduction. In June 2002, the FDA approved the first (rigid) contact lens for overnight wear in for myopia reduction. The Corneal Refractive Therapy (CRT) Lens, by Paragon Vision Sciences, was approved for all ages for the correction of up to -6.00 D of myopia with up to -1.75 D of refractive astigmatism.

11. What are the best methods to prescribe spectacles for contact lens wearers?

Prescribing spectacles in contact lens wearers can be complicated if contact lens–induced corneal warpage is present. Corneal warpage is an alteration of the corneal curvature that results from a molding effect produced by contact lens wear. It can change the refractive error by altering the myopia (or hyperopia), by changing the magnitude or axis of the regular astigmatism, or by inducing irregular astigmatism.

1. If a contact lens wearer desires spectacles for supplemental use and there is neither a decrease in best-corrected spectacle acuity nor complaints of spectacle blur post–lens removal, then glasses should be prescribed based on habitual conditions. There is no reason to delay the manifest refraction after contact lens removal during the examination.

2. In cases where contact lens fitting may induce corneal warpage, such as when using a lens design known to induce corneal warpage or in keratoconus patients, it is advisable to delay writing a spectacle prescription for supplemental use until a few weeks after the contact lens fit has been stabilized.

3. If there is a decrease in best-corrected spectacle visual acuity asso-

ciated with contact lens–induced corneal warpage, contact lens re-fitting should be considered. Spectacle prescriptions should ideally be delayed in contact lens refitting until there is a stabilization of the refractive error and a return to the initial best-corrected spectacle visual acuity.

4. In contact lens wearers with stable corneal warpage and no irregular astigmatism or decrease in best-corrected spectacle acuity, it may be appropriate to maintain the same lens design. As discussed earlier, an example may be a presbyopic patient who is satisfied with posterior surface multifocal RGP lenses. Spectacles can be prescribed for supplemental use, and the patient should be informed that cessation of contact lens use may require a change in the spectacle prescription.

12. How and why does corneal vascularization occur, and how should it be managed?

Causes and Mechanism of Action

Corneal neovascularization develops in contact lens wearers in response to the same inciting factors that cause neovascularization in non–contact lens wearers. Some common causes are corneal hypoxia and inflammation. Hypoxia, which can lead to corneal edema, is one of the most common inciting factors in contact lens wearers. Corneal neovascularization most often develops as a result of chronic hypoxia in contact lens wearers (Color Plate 25).

Common Lens Types Associated with Hypoxia

- Tight soft lenses. In patients with borderline dry eyes, a decrease in tear flow can alter the fit of the lens as dehydration occurs. Evaluation of lens fit initially after insertion may demonstrate an appropriate fit, which may become inadequate following several hours of lens wear. Patients are usually symptomatic and describe ocular dryness, an increase in lens awareness, and occasionally a decrease in vision following increased wearing times.
- Thick, low-water content soft lenses.
- PMMA lenses.
- Extended wear of contact lenses that provide insufficient corneal oxygenation in closed-eye conditions.
- Hybrid lenses (hydrogel skirt, rigid center) with low oxygen permeability.

Lens-Related Causes of Inflammation

- Persistent corneal trauma due to an inappropriate lens fit, which can produce corneal changes ranging from mild superficial punctate keratopathy to contact lens–associated acute red eye (CLARE) to cor-

neal abrasions. Contact lens–induced keratopathies may be severe enough to induce intraocular inflammation, such as iritis.
- Sensitivity reaction to preservatives in lens care products and topical medications.

Symptoms and Signs of Corneal Vascularization

- Clinically, superficial corneal vascularization should be distinguished from deep stromal vascularization, and documentation should include measurement with the slit lamp. Contact lens–associated neovascularization is superficial and extends more than 1 mm beyond the limbus in only 10% of contact lens patients.[34] Vascular patterns in which a spike, branch, or sprout is present at the end of the vessel should be closely monitored for progression.[35] The formation of neovascularization is a static process consisting of remodeling changes, so recently formed vessels can regress if the inciting factor is removed early enough in the formation of the vessel. Established vessels do not regress, and treatment of the condition results in a patent vasculature without red blood cells. These vessels, called ghost vessels, can rapidly refill with red blood cells in the presence of hypoxic or inflammation stimuli.[36]
- Associated findings present with corneal neovascularization may include the presence of adjacent ghost vessels, early corneal opacification, corneal exudate, limbal hyperemia, and conjunctival injection.

Treatment of Corneal Vascularization

The goal in the management of corneal neovascularization is for the vessels to empty of red blood cells and become ghost vessels. If treated early enough in the neovascularization process, all clinical signs of vessels in the cornea should resolve.[36]

Treatment involves removing the inciting stimuli. This may include the following:

1. Change to a more highly oxygen permeable lens material.
2. Reduce contact lens wearing time.
3. Improve the lens-to-cornea fitting relationship to prevent corneal keratopathy.
4. Treat any preexisting conditions that may be adding to the corneal keratopathy, such as blepharitis.
5. Switch lens care products if a toxic reaction resulting from hypersensitivity is suspected.
6. In the presence of moderate-to-severe inflammation, consider a pulse of topical nonsteroidal antiinflammatory drugs (NSAIDs) or corticosteroids to aid in vessel regression.

13. What is the appearance of toxicity reactions in the cornea?

Causes and Mechanism of Action

Toxicity reactions from contact lens care products and topical ophthalmic medications may result if a hypersensitivity exists to the offending agent. Historically, many contact lens care products contained preservatives that produced toxic reactions. The use of most of these preservatives has been discontinued, and toxicity reactions are not nearly as common today. Thimerosal, a mercury-containing preservative, is regarded as a primary cause of toxic corneal reactions, and is rarely used anymore in ophthalmic products.[37] Benzalkonium chloride (BAK) is still used as a preservative in many topical ophthalmic medications and in some lens care products, but it does not cause hypersensitivity reactions as frequently as thimerosal.

Signs and Symptoms of Toxicity Reaction in the Cornea

Thimerosal toxicity reactions may produce a variable clinical picture, which may include:

1. Superificial punctate keratopathy.
2. Pseudodendrites (Color Plate 26): Appearance similar to dendrites produced by herpes simplex keratitis without the terminal bulbs. Lesions stain with sodium fluorescein dye.[38]
3. Subepithelial corneal opacities[39]: Similar in appearance to other causes of subepithelial opacities, including viral, bacterial, and chlamydial.
4. Contact lens–associated superior limbic keratoconjunctivitis (Color Plate 27)[40]: Similar entity to the superior limbic keratoconjunctivitis described by Theodore and Ferry,[41] but occurs in younger patients without history of thyroid disorder.

Treatment of Toxicity Reaction in the Cornea

1. Toxicity reactions require a discontinuation of the offending agent.
2. Consider therapeutic agents, such as anti-inflammatory medications, if sufficient inflammation exists, or prophylactic antibiotics, if significant epithelial involvement is present.

14. What types of keratitis can result from contact lens use?

While all types of keratitis can present in contact lens wearers, two main types of ulcerative keratitis are particularly associated with contact lens use. These are microbial keratitis, namely *Pseudomonas aeruginosa* and *Acanthamoeba* keratitis. Both can have significant visual morbidity. The following section discusses sterile marginal infiltrates, microbial keratitis including that caused by *P. aeruginosa* (Color Plate 28), and *Acanthamoeba* keratitis (Color Plate 29). These are the main types of keratitis resulting from contact lenses. Other types of keratitis (i.e., viral, herpetic fungal, parasitic, etc.) are not included in this discussion, as they are less commonly associated with contact lens use, but they should be considered in the list of differentials in any keratitis.

15. How is microbial keratitis differentiated from sterile marginal infiltrates, also known as contact lens peripheral ulcers (CLPUs)?

One of the most serious potential complications from contact lens wear is microbial keratitis, or a bacterial corneal ulcer. Although the incidence of microbial keratitis is low, contact lens wear is the primary risk factor for developing microbial keratitis, and the risk varies based on the type of lens and the wearing schedule. The estimated annualized incidence of microbial keratitis is 1.1 per 10,000 users of daily wear RGP lenses, 3.5 per 10,000 users of daily wear soft lenses, and 20.0 per 10,000 users of extended wear soft lenses ($p <.00001$ for comparison between all groups).[42] In traditional soft hydrogel lens materials, the relative risk for corneal ulcers is 10 to 15 times greater when lenses are worn for extended periods of time as compared to daily wear.[43] No studies have reported either the annualized incidence of microbial keratitis with silicone hydrogel ultrahigh Dk lenses or the relative risk for microbial keratitis in extended wear compared to daily wear silicone hydrogels.

While the incidence of microbial keratitis is very low, correctly differentiating microbial keratitis from sterile marginal infiltrates is critical to avoid potentially sight-threatening consequences. Sterile marginal infiltrates represent the greatest diagnostic dilemma to early microbial keratitis, and they are generally considered to be an immunologic response. Sterile marginal infiltrates may result from contact lens wear itself, from endotoxins created by bacteria present in conditions such as *Staphylococcus aureus*–associated blepharitis, or from a combination of the two.[44,45] Because virulent strains of microbial keratitis can perforate a cornea rapidly, accurate diagnosis and immediate management of microbial keratitis is crucial.

Clinical differentiating characteristics are as follows:

Sterile Marginal Infiltrates (Color Plate 30)

Stromal infiltrate characteristics include the following:

- Focal infiltrate, primarily anterior stromal.
- Diameter of infiltrate usually ranges from 0.1 to 1.2 mm.[45]
- Peripheral or mid-peripheral corneal involvement; infiltrates are

usually 2.5 mm or less from the limbus and involves a "clear zone" of cornea between the infiltrate and limbus.[45]

- Absence of overlying epithelial defects except in more severe cases.
- Absence of associated corneal thinning.
- Absence of cell, flare, or other inflammation in the anterior chamber.
- Minimal decrease in visual acuity.
- Minimal subjective pain.

Microbial Keratitis

Stromal infiltrate characteristics include the following:

- Stromal involvement may extend to deep stromal layers, with the exception of early ulcers.
- Presence of an epithelial defect. Although nearly all cases of microbial keratitis have an epithelial defect present, this is not an absolute rule. Culture-positive cases of microbial keratitis without epithelial ulceration have been reported, with the offending microorganisms representing both gram-positive and-negative organisms.[46]
- Central and paracentral involvement.
- Presence of corneal thinning, edema, necrosis, or neovascularization.

Other characteristics include:

- Presence of anterior chamber inflammation, including cell, flare, and hypopyon, which may result in miosis and posterior synechiae. Ability to assess the anterior chamber inflammation may be decreased due to the presence of a dense infiltrate.
- Significant decrease in visual acuity.
- Significant subjective pain.

16. What is the management of sterile infiltrates?

Sterile infiltrates represent an immunologic reaction (Color Plate 30).[44] Treatment usually consists of topical steroid drops along with prophylactic antibiotic coverage. For most cases, dosing four times daily is adequate, although dosing with increased frequency may be appropriate if multiple sterile infiltrates are present. Close follow-up care, especially early in treatment, should be provided to prevent inappropriate treatment of an early microbial keratitis and to monitor for improvement. Improvement usually occurs quickly following steroid initiation. While the diagnosis and treatment of the acute condition is of primary concern, it is critical to evaluate and treat thoroughly any chronic ocular surface disease, such as blepharitis or dry eye syndrome, which may increase the likelihood for future recurrence or additional complications.

17. What is the treatment of microbial keratitis?

Treatment of microbial keratitis requires immediate and frequent antibiotic coverage with agents susceptible to the offending microorganism. Classically, the treatment of microbial keratitis is based on the severity of the corneal ulcer and whether the ulcer appears to be sight-threatening or potentially sight-threatening.[47]

Rarely sight-threatening corneal ulcers include the presence of each of the following clinical findings:

- Anterior chamber response of grade 1+ or less (<10 cells per 1 mm field)
- Corneal infiltrate of 2 mm or less in size
- Corneal infiltrate of >3 mm from the visual axis

Sight-threatening corneal ulcers include the presence of any of the following characteristics:

- Anterior chamber response of grade 2+ or greater
- Corneal infiltrate of >2 mm in size
- Corneal infiltrate <3 mm from the visual axis
- Worsening of clinical course following 48 hours of treatment

Corneal ulcers that are rarely sight-threatening are commonly treated empirically with fluoroquinolone agents (ciprofloxacin, ofloxacin, and levofloxacin),[48] and most community acquired ulcers resolve with broad-spectrum therapy.[49] Empirical treatment always requires consideration of antibiotic resistance, which is increasing with fluoroquinolones.[50] Drug resistance to the fluoroquinolones has been reported with both gram-positive and -negative organisms, including *Pseudomonas aeruginosa*.[51]

Sight-threatening corneal ulcers are usually referred by optometrists and ophthalmologists to fellowship-trained, corneal subspecialists for treatment and management.[47] If electing to treat sight-threatening corneal ulcers, corneal cultures and Gram stains should be performed, and broad-spectrum antimicrobial treatment and cycloplegics should be initiated while culture and specificity results are pending. Therapeusis should be modified as appropriate based on laboratory results. Traditionally, Ancef (cefazolin) and fortified aminoglycosides (gentamicin or tobramycin) are each prescribed hourly, alternating every 30 minutes around the clock for the first 24 hours. Initial dosages are tapered with clinical improvement. The initial goal is closure of epithelial defects.[49] Hospitalization should be considered in any patient who the physician will not be able to use the drops as prescribed or if noncompliance is an issue.

Antimicrobial agents are tapered as wound healing improves, and steroid therapy may be added following epithelial defect closure to reduce corneal scarring and decrease the associated anterior chamber inflammation.

18. What are the risk factors for microbial keratitis?

Microbial keratitis usually results from trauma to the cornea, contact lens wear (and overwear, in particular), tear or eyelid dysfunction, corneal disease or damage, corneal innervation deficits, or conjunctivitis. Topical medications, such as corticosteroids or antivirals, or contaminated ocular medications, all increase the risk of a bacterial corneal ulcer. Systemic conditions associated with increased risk include diabetes, alcoholism or drug abuse, debilitating disease, immunosuppressive therapy, acquired immunodeficiency syndrome (AIDS), and burn.[52]

Sources of microbial contamination include the environment, the user's hands (beneath the nail), the eye and ocular adnexa, contaminated lenses or lens cases, and contaminated solutions.

19. What are the most common organisms for microbial keratitis in contact lens wearers, and what is the typical appearance?

Pseudomonas aeruginosa, a gram-negative organism, is one of the causes, if not the most common cause, of microbial keratitis in cosmetic contact lens wearers.[23–25] In patients wearing bandage soft contact lenses, the most common organisms were *Staphylococcus, Streptococcus,* and *Serratia*.[53] Virulent *P. aeruginosa* infections can rapidly progress, resulting in deep extension with necrosis and corneal perforation within 24 hours.

Many types of microbial keratitis have a nonspecific appearance, in which it may be difficult to determine the offending microorganism by appearance alone. However, several clinical signs are distinctive to *P. aeruginosa* and include the following[54]:

- Rapidly progressive course
- Ulcer characteristics:
  - Central or paracentral
  - Broad, and initially shallow
  - Necrotic extension, progressing to a stromal abscess that spreads concentrically, forming a ring ulcer
- Copious mucopurulent, yellowish-green exudate, which is adherent to the ulcer
- Epithelial edema resulting in a ground-glass appearance of the cornea

20. How is *Acanthamoeba* keratitis associated with contact lens use? How is it diagnosed and what is the treatment?

Acanthamoeba is a free-living ameba that resides in water, soil, and air. Two forms of the organism exist: a metabolically active trophozoite form and a more resistant, dormant cyst form. Both forms can adhere to contact lenses, which likely plays a significant role in *Acanthamoeba* keratitis, as contact lens wear allows for easy transfer of the organism to the cornea.[55] In vitro studies of unworn lenses provide conflicting data as to which form is most likely to adhere to various lens types, but most clinical cases of *Acanthamoeba* keratitis result from contaminated soft contact lenses.[55,56] A recent study from Moorfields Eye Hospital reported an annualized incidence in the United Kingdom of 1.13 to 1.26 per million non–contact lens wearing adults and between 17.53 to 21.14 per million adult contact lens wearers.[57]

Risk factors included contact lens wear (88% of patients with *Acanthamoeba* keratitis wore contact lenses), hard water as opposed to domestic soft water, irregular or inappropriate disinfection, and a recent history of swimming with contact lenses.[57] Historically, users of salt tablet–prepared saline as opposed to commercially available saline were also much more at risk for *Acanthamoeba* keratitis.[58] Patients frequently give a history of ocular and contact lens exposure to a lake or hot tub, and less frequently to tap water.

Unfortunately, many contact lens disinfection products available do not have appropriate amebicidal effects, particularly for the resistant cyst form.[59–61] Multipurpose solutions and two-step hydrogen peroxide systems, in which lenses are soaked in peroxide for 4 hours before neutralization, provided superior cysticidal effects, and rinsing appears to beneficial in trophozoite removal.[59,61,62]

The classic clinical presentation of advanced *Acanthamoeba* keratitis is a ring-shaped infiltrate with severe pain and photophobia disproportionate with the clinical appearance (Color Plate 31). Early disease may present as a nonspecific keratitis presentation and result in a delay in the correct diagnosis, as it is frequently misdiagnosed as other types of keratitis, ranging from viral to herpetic, fungal to microbial.[63] Linear infiltrates may develop along the corneal nerves, known as radial keratoneuritis, and their presence is considered a hallmark primarily of this disease.[64] *Acanthamoeba* keratitis must be considered in any patient refractory to treatment or in the face of negative cultures.

Acanthamoeba keratitis has traditionally been diagnosed through cultures, smears, and biopsy. More recently, confocal microscopy has been employed, as it provides a noninvasive method to diagnose the condition. Organisms can be seen in vivo in the epithelium and stroma, with the double-walled cystic form appearing as highly reflective, ovoid bodies approximately 10 to 25 μm in diameter.[65,66] Also visible through confocal microscopy are trophozoites and radial keratoneuritis.[66]

Immediate diagnosis of *Acanthamoeba* keratitis and initiation of appropriate therapeusis is critical for a good visual outcome. Patients in whom the diagnosis and treatment begins within 1 month of the onset of symptoms suffer less morbidity and end up with better visual acuity.[67] Medical treatment after correct diagnosis is challenging, primarily due to the resistant cystic form of the ameba, and a penetrating keratoplasty may be required. Medical therapy usually involves a multidrug regimen of antiamebic drugs, which usually include topical polyhexamethylene biguanide, propamidine isethionate, and neomycin.[68] All potential cases of *Acanthamoeba* keratitis should be referred to a corneal subspecialist for diagnosis and management.

References

1. Smelser G, Ozanics V. Importance of atmospheric oxygen for maintenance of the optical properties of the human cornea. *Science.* 1952;115:140.
2. Hill R, Fatt I. How dependent is the cornea on the atmosphere? *J Am Optom Assoc.* 1964;35:873.
3. Fatt I, Freeman RD, Lin D. Oxygen tension distributions in the cornea: a re-examination. *Exp Eye Res.* 1974;18:357–365.
4. Fatt I, Bieber MT. The steady-state distribution of oxygen and carbon dioxide in the in vivo cornea. I. The open eye in air and the closed eye. *Exp Eye Res.* 1968;7:103–112.
5. Efron N, Carney LG. Oxygen levels beneath the closed eyelid. *Invest Ophthalmol Vis Sci.* 1979;18:93–95.
6. Benjamin WJ, Hill RM. Human corneal oxygen demand: the closed-eye interval. *Graefes Arch Clin Exp Ophthalmol.* 1986;224:291–294.
7. Harvitt DM, Bonanno JA. pH dependence of corneal oxygen consumption. *Invest Ophthalmol Vis Sci.* 1998;39:2778–2781.
8. Vannas A, Holden BA, Sweeney DF, Polse KA. Surgical incision alters the swelling response of the human cornea. *Invest Ophthalmol Vis Sci.* 1985; 26:864–868.
9. Holden BA, Mertz GW. Critical oxygen levels to avoid corneal edema for daily and extended wear contact lenses. *Invest Ophthalmol Vis Sci.* 1984; 25:1161–1167.
10. Polse KA. Tear flow under hydrogel contact lenses. *Invest Ophthalmol Vis Sci.* 1979;18:409–413.
11. Bergmanson JP, Chu LW. Corneal response to rigid contact lens wear. *Br J Ophthalmol.* 1982;66:667–675.
12. Wang J, Fonn D, Simpson TL, Jones L. The measurement of corneal epithelial thickness in response to hypoxia using optical coherence tomography. *Am J Ophthalmol.* 2002;133:315–319.
13. McNamara NA, Fusaro RE, Brand RJ, Polse KA. Epithelial permeability reflects subclinical effects of contact lens wear. *Br J Ophthalmol.* 1998;82:376–381.
14. Lin MC, Graham AD, Fusaro RE, Polse KA. Impact of rigid gas-permeable contact lens extended wear on corneal epithelial barrier function. *Invest Ophthalmol Vis Sci.* 2002;43:1019–1024.
15. Schoessler JP, Lowther GE. Slit lamp observations of corneal edema. *Am J Optom Arch Am Acad Optom.* 1971;48:666–671.
16. Ichijima H, Imayasu M, Tanaka H, Ren DH, Cavanagh HD. Effects of RGP lens extended wear on glucose-lactate metabolism and stromal swelling in the rabbit cornea. *CLAO J.* 2000;26:30–36.
17. Lin MC, Graham AD, Fusaro RE, Polse KA. Impact of rigid gas-permeable contact lens extended wear on corneal epithelial barrier function. *Invest Ophthalmol Vis Sci.* 2002;43:1019–1024.
18. Holden BA, Sweeney DF, Vannas A, Nilsson KT, Efron N. Effects of long-term extended contact lens wear on the human cornea. *Invest Ophthalmol Vis Sci.* 1985;26:1489–1501.
19. Kenyon K, Polse KA, Seger RG. Influence of wearing schedule on extended-wear complications. *Ophthalmology.* 1986;93:231–236.

20. Zantos S. Cystic formations in the corneal epithelium during extended wear of contact lenses. *ICLC.* 1983;10:128.

21. Polse KA, Sarver MD, Harris MG. Corneal edema and vertical striae accompanying the wearing of hydrogel lenses. *Am J Optom Physiol Opt.* 1975;52:185–191.

22. Grayson M. *Diseases of the Cornea.* St. Louis: CV Mosby, 1979.

23. Alexandrakis G, Alfonso EC, Miller D. Shifting trends in bacterial keratitis in south Florida and emerging resistance to fluoroquinolones. *Ophthalmology.* 2000;107:1497–1502.

24. Dart JK. Predisposing factors in microbial keratitis: the significance of contact lens wear. *Br J Ophthalmol.* 1988;72:926–930.

25. Tan DT, Lee CP, Lim AS. Corneal ulcers in two institutions in Singapore: analysis of causative factors, organisms and antibiotic resistance. *Ann Acad Med Singapore.* 1995;24:823–829.

26. Dumbleton K, Jones L, Chalmers R, Williams-Lyn D, Fonn D. Clinical characterization of spherical post-lens debris associated with lotrafilcon high-Dk silicone lenses. *CLAO J.* 2000;26:186–192.

27. Millodot M. Effect of the length of wear of contact lenses on corneal sensitivity. *Acta Ophthalmol (Copenh).* 1976;54:721–730.

28. Tanelian DL, Beuerman RW. Recovery of corneal sensation following hard contact lens wear and the implication for adaptation. *Invest Ophthalmol Vis Sci.* 1980;19:1391–1394.

29. Millodot M. Effect of soft lenses on corneal sensitivity. *Acta Ophthalmol (Copenh).* 1974;52:603–608.

30. Velasco MJ, Bermudez FJ, Romero J, Hita E. Variations in corneal sensitivity with hydrogel contact lenses. *Acta Ophthalmol (Copenh).* 1994;72:53–56.

31. Murphy PJ, Patel S, Marshall J. The effect of long-term, daily contact lens wear on corneal sensitivity. *Cornea.* 2001;20:264–269.

32. Sanaty M, Temel A. Corneal sensitivity changes in long-term wearing of hard polymethylmethacrylate contact lenses. *Ophthalmologica.* 1998;212:328–330.

33. Yamauchi K, Hirst LW, Enger C, Rosenfeld J, Vogelpohl W. Specular microscopy of hard contact lens wearers II. *Ophthalmology.* 1989;96:1176–1179.

34. Cunha MC, Thomassen TS, Cohen EJ, Genvert GI, Arentsen JJ, Laibson PR. Complications associated with soft contact lens use. *CLAO J.* 1987;13:107–111.

35. Inomata H, Smelser GK, Polack FM. Corneal vascularization in experimental uveitis and graft rejection. An electron microscopic study. *Invest Ophthalmol.* 1971;10:840–850.

36. Zauberman H, Michaelson IC, Bergmann F, Maurice DM. Stimulation of neovascularization of the cornea by biogenic amines. *Exp Eye Res.* 1969;8(1):77–83.

37. Mondino BJ, Salamon SM, Zaidman GW. Allergic and toxic reactions of soft contact lens wearers. *Surv Ophthalmol.* 1982;26(6):337–344.

38. Udell IJ, Mannis MJ, Meisler DM, Langston RH. Pseudodendrites in soft contact lens wearers. *CLAO J.* 1985;11:51–53.

39. Mondino BJ, Groden LR. Conjunctival hyperemia and corneal infiltrates with chemically disinfected soft contact lenses. *Arch Ophthalmol.* 1980;98:1767–1770.

40. Sendele DD, Kenyon KR, Mobilia EF, Rosenthal P, Steinert R, Hanninen LA. Superior limbic keratoconjunctivitis in contact lens wearers. *Ophthalmology.* 1983;90:616–622.

41. Theodore FH, Ferry AP. Superior limbic keratoconjunctivitis. Clinical and pathological correlations. *Arch Ophthalmol.* 1970;84:481–484.

42. Cheng KH, Leung SL, Hoekman HW, et al. Incidence of contact-lens-associated microbial keratitis and its related morbidity. *Lancet.* 1999;354: 181–185.

43. Schein OD, Glynn RJ, Poggio EC, Seddon JM, Kenyon KR. The relative risk of ulcerative keratitis among users of daily-wear and extended-wear soft contact lenses. A case-control study. Microbial Keratitis Study Group. *N Engl J Med.* 1989;321:773–778.

44. Ficker L, Seal D, Wright P. Staphylococcal infection and the limbus: study of the cell-mediated immune response. *Eye.* 1989;3(pt 2):190–193.

45. Holden BA, Reddy MK, Sankaridurg PR, et al. Contact lens-induced peripheral ulcers with extended wear of disposable hydrogel lenses: histopathologic observations on the nature and type of corneal infiltrate. *Cornea.* 1999;18:538–543.

46. McLeod SD, Goei SL, Taglia DP, McMahon TT. Nonulcerating bacterial keratitis associated with soft and rigid contact lens wear. *Ophthalmology.* 1998;105:517–521.

47. McMahon TT. Diagnosis and treatment of corneal ulcers. *Contact Lens Spectrum.* 2001.

48. McLeod SD, DeBacker CM, Viana MA. Differential care of corneal ulcers in the community based on apparent severity. *Ophthalmology.* 1996;103:479–484.

49. McLeod SD, Kolahdouz-Isfahani A, Rostamian K, Flowers CW, Lee PP, McDonnell PJ. The role of smears, cultures, and antibiotic sensitivity testing in the management of suspected infectious keratitis. *Ophthalmology.* 1996;103:23–28.

50. Goldstein MH, Kowalski RP, Gordon YJ. Emerging fluoroquinolone resistance in bacterial keratitis: a 5-year review. *Ophthalmology.* 1999;106:1313–1318.

51. Chaudhry NA, Flynn HW Jr, Murray TG, Tabandeh H, Mello MO Jr, Miller D. Emerging ciprofloxacin-resistant *Pseudomonas aeruginosa. Am J Ophthalmol.* 1999;128:509–510.

52. Ormerod LD, Hertzmark E, Gomez DS, Stabiner RG, Schanzlin DJ, Smith RE. Epidemiology of microbial keratitis in southern California. A multivariate analysis. *Ophthalmology.* 1987;94:1322–1333.

53. Schein OD, Ormerod LD, Barraquer E, et al. Microbiology of contact lens-related keratitis. *Cornea.* 1989;8:281–285.

54. Liesegang TJ. Bacterial keratitits. In: Kaufman HE, Barron BA, McDonald MB, eds. *Cornea.* 2nd on CD-ROM ed. Woburn, MA: Butterworth-Heinemann, 1999.

55. Sharma S, Ramachandran L, Rao GN. Adherence of cysts and trophozoites of *Acanthamoeba* to unworn rigid gas permeable and soft contact lenses. *CLAO J.* 1995;21:247–251.

56. Seal DV, Bennett ES, McFadyen AK, Todd E, Tomlinson A. Differential adherence of *Acanthamoeba* to contact lenses: effects of material characteristics. *Optom Vis Sci.* 1995;72:23–28.

57. Radford CF, Minassian DC, Dart JK. *Acanthamoeba* keratitis in England and Wales: incidence, outcome, and risk factors. *Br J Ophthalmol.* 2002;86:536–542.

58. Schaumberg DA, Snow KK, Dana MR. The epidemic of *Acanthamoeba* keratitis: where do we stand? *Cornea.* 1998;17:3–10.

59. Cancrini G, Iori A, Mancino R. *Acanthamoeba* adherence to contact lenses, removal by rinsing procedures, and survival to some ophthalmic products. *Parassitologia.* 1998;40:275–278.

60. Hiti K, Walochnik J, Haller-Schober EM, Faschinger C, Aspock H. Viability of *Acanthamoeba* after exposure to a multipurpose disinfecting contact lens

solution and two hydrogen peroxide systems. *Br J Ophthalmol.* 2002;86:144–146.

61. Hughes R, Kilvington S. Comparison of hydrogen peroxide contact lens disinfection systems and solutions against *Acanthamoeba* polyphaga. *Antimicrob Agents Chemother.* 2001;45:2038–2043.

62. Kilvington S, Anger C. A comparison of cyst age and assay method of the efficacy of contact lens disinfectants against *Acanthamoeba. Br J Ophthalmol.* 2001;85:336–340.

63. Illingworth CD, Cook SD. *Acanthamoeba* keratitis. *Surv Ophthalmol.* 1998;42:493–508.

64. Moore MB, McCulley JP, Kaufman HE, Robin JB. Radial keratoneuritis as a presenting sign in *Acanthamoeba* keratitis. *Ophthalmology.* 1986;93:1310–1315.

65. Winchester K, Mathers WD, Sutphin JE, Daley TE. Diagnosis of *Acanthamoeba* keratitis in vivo with confocal microscopy. *Cornea.* 1995;14:10–17.

66. Pfister DR, Cameron JD, Krachmer JH, Holland EJ. Confocal microscopy findings of Acanthamoeba keratitis. *Am J Ophthalmol.* 1996;121:119–128.

67. Bacon AS, Dart JK, Ficker LA, Matheson MM, Wright P. *Acanthamoeba* keratitis. The value of early diagnosis. *Ophthalmology.* 1993;100:1238–1243.

68. Rutzen AR, Moore MB. Parasitic infections. In: Kaufman HE, Barron BA, McDonald MB, eds. *Cornea.* 2nd on CD-ROM ed. Woburn, MA: Butterworth-Heinemann, 1999.

23

Complications Associated with Material, Deposits, and Lens Design in Rigid Gas Permeable Lenses

Cleusa Coral-Ghanem and David A. Berntsen

1. What are the principal problems related to material and lens deposits in rigid gas permeable lenses?

The principal problems related to material and lens deposits in rigid gas permeable (RGP) lenses include flexure and warping of the lens, lacquer cracks, protein and material crazing, surface hazing, hydrophobic areas, surface deposits, and debris under the lens.

Contact Lens Flexure

Symptoms and Signs

1. Fluctuation of vision
2. Mild distortion of the keratometric mires when the patient blinks or distortion of the retinoscopic reflex, both with the contact lens on the eye.

Causes[1,2]

1. Tight/steep fitting lens
2. Thin lens
3. Large diameter optical zone
4. Flexibility of the material; increase in the flexibility is directly proportional to an increase in the oxygen permeability (Dk) value.

Management

1. Fit a contact lens with a flatter base curve, because a contact lens fitted steeper than K is generally more flexible than a lens on K.

2. Increase center thickness.
3. Decrease the Dk and counsel the patient against continuous wear.

Contact Lens Warpage

Contact lens deformation differs from flexure, because it represents a permanent alteration in contact lens shape and is acquired over time.

Symptoms and Signs

1. Reduction in visual acuity with an induced sphero-cylindrical over-refraction
2. Change in the contact lens parameters such that a formerly spherical base curve becomes Toric
3. Corneal warpage

Causes

1. Excessive digital pressure during the cleaning process
2. A high-Dk RGP lens (the higher the Dk of the material, the more prone it is to warping[3])
3. Highly toric cornea
4. A very tight lid
5. Extended wear
6. Excessive heat (e.g., a contact lens case left in the car in the sun)
7. Inadvertent exchange of the contact lenses between eyes; this situation occurs when there are small differences between the two eyes or the change in curvature is compensated for by the power.

Management

1. Decrease the Dk and advise against extended wear.
2. Use a mechanical cleaning system.
3. Clean the contact lens in the palm of the hand and not between the fingers. (On average, warping is three times more likely to occur when a RGP lens is cleaned between two fingers rather than properly cleaning the lens in the palm of the hand.[4])

Lacquer Cracks

This term, which refers to a surface with an appearance similar to cracked varnish, has been used generically to refer to two distinct problems: *crazing* of the surface and *cracking* of the surface.

Surface Crazing

This term is sometimes used to describe a protein-coated contact lens with a cracked protein film that can be mistaken for cracks in the lens itself. This form of *cracked protein crazing* is due to surface deposits and can be removed by polishing the lens surface. However, the term *crazing* is also used to describe fine cracks seen within the lens material itself due to excessive lens flexure or other factors resulting in surface material breakdown. In this case, there may be scratches deep within the material or layered deposits on the lens that are not removable by polishing because the problem is within the actual lens material.[5] In this case, the lens must be replaced as the crazing can lead to fine surface cracks.

Cracked Protein Crazing

Symptoms and Signs
1. Sharp plaques of deposits that look like superficial lines engraved in the material

Causes
1. Failure to care for the lens appropriately
2. Alterations in the tear film

Management
1. Polish the surface.
2. Repeat enzymatic cleaning.

Material Crazing

Symptoms and Signs
1. The appearance of layered deposits or scratches within the material that cannot be removed by polishing the lens surface

Causes
1. Excessive lens flexure or other excessive mechanical manipulation
2. Material breakdown caused by exposure to adverse conditions (i.e., repeated exposure to alcohol after repeated cleaning with Miraflow)

Management
1. Exchange of the contact lens

Surface Cracking

Symptoms and Signs
1. May be asymptomatic
2. Ocular irritation due to deposits within the cracks or corneal abrasion caused by posterior surface cracks
3. The appearance of "stained glass" on the transparent surface without deposits
4. Fissures that penetrate 10% into the matrix of the contact lens, seen at the electron microscopic level[5]

Causes
1. Physical factors
   - Heat
   - Polymer composition
   - Dehydration/evaporation
   - Abrupt changes in temperature
   - Alkaline pH
   - Ultraviolet radiation

2. Organic fluids
   - Undiluted alcohol
   - Various solvents
   - Various surfactants
3. Mechanical pressure
   - Manipulation/flexure
   - Polishing/modification of the contact lens
   - Manufacture process

Management: Exchange of the Contact Lens

The terms *cracking* and *crazing* are not synonymous. Cracked protein crazing creates deposits, both linear and plaquelike, on the surface of the material that resemble ceramic cracks or cracked varnish. Superficial cracking resembles a crystal with a cracked pattern in the clean surface. A combination of the two problems can also exist. After polishing and removal of the superficial crazing caused by a cracked protein coat, superficial cracking may be found in the lens surface. However, the term *crazing* is also used to describe a cracked varnish appearance within the lens material that is not due to surface deposits and can be found in the absence of surface cracks.

Surface Hazing

All RGP contact lenses are susceptible to evaporation of the tear film on the anterior surface. Surface hazing is first seen after the blink when the tear film on the surface of the contact lens begins to break up, thus causing dynamic blurring of the surface of the contact lens. It is believed that this problem occurs due to poor interactions of the mucin layer with the lens surface, resulting in reduced in vivo wettability. Hazing is most frequent and appears in a shorter period of time, in silicone acrylate contact lenses than in fluorosilicone lenses in which fluorine promotes a lens interaction with the tear film mucin.

Symptoms and Signs

1. Drying of the contact lens
2. Coating of the contact lens between blinks

Causes

1. Inadequate contact lens care
2. Environment
3. Lens polymer
4. Manufacturing methods
5. Low temperature and high humidity
6. Length of time between blinks

Management

1. The use of lubricating drops
2. Review of contact lens care methods
3. Exchange of contact lens material

Hydrophobic Areas (Figure 23.1)

Good surface wettability is one of the most important properties of the RGP contact lens.

Symptoms and Signs

1. Blurred vision with the contact lens
2. Hydrophobic areas on the contact lens surface

   A hydrophobic surface can be separated into two categories: initial and acquired.[6]

Initial Hydrophobic Areas

Early on, hydrophobic areas are seen in new RGP contact lenses. They are almost always the result of a problem with manufacture.

Causes

1. Persistence of products, such as contact lens laboratory pitch, used during the finishing phase of the contact lens
2. Lack of proper lens conditioning in solution prior to dispensing
3. Imperfect polishing
4. Excessive heating during lens polishing
5. An old or imperfect diamond used in the cutting

Management

1. After cleaning, leave the contact lens immersed in conditioning solution for 24 hours prior to dispensing it to the patient.
2. Remove adherent material with special solutions supplied by the appropriate laboratory.
3. Exchange the contact lens.

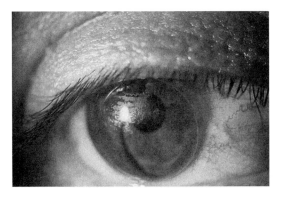

Figure 23.1. Hydrophobic areas on the surface of a rigid gas permeable lens.

Acquired Hydrophobic Areas

Acquired hydrophobic areas occur after weeks or months of use.

Causes

1. Tear film deficiency
2. Inadequate blinking
3. Oily film from some substance on the fingers or because of meibomian glands dysfunction
4. Contamination with cosmetics or soap that contains lanolin
5. Mucoprotein film
6. Use of solutions incompatible with the surface of the material
7. Alterations in the surface of the material (such as surface scratches)

Management

1. Use of surfactant plus enzymatic cleaner plus ultrasound.
2. Daily cleaning with an abrasive cleaner.
3. The patient should be instructed that cleaning of the contact lens should be done immediately after removal.
4. Review the type of soap the patient normally uses for hand washing and ensure that it does not contain lanolin.
5. Avoidance of contact between the patient's hands and creams prior to manipulating the contact lens.
6. Treatment of meibomianitis.
7. Change of contact lens material from a silicone acrylate to a fluorosilicone acrylate or from high-Dk to low-Dk material to diminish the formation of deposits.

Surface Deposits

The clinical appearance of deposits may vary significantly, depending on location.

1. On the anterior face, they are easily seen as a grayish translucent film via direct illumination.
2. On the posterior face, they can be detected in retroillumination. With time and the presence of multiple plaques, visualization becomes easier as hydrophobic alterations on the epithelium occur.
3. Peripheral plaques on the lens bevel are most commonly seen on the anterior surface of the lens and are detected as opaque residues deposited in the form of a ring around the optical zone.
4. Deposits on the posterior peripheral surface are rare and generally easy to remove.

Symptoms and Signs

1. Loss of sharp visual acuity to varying degrees
2. Ocular irritation
3. Contact lens deposits

Causes

1. Hydrophobic fragments in the tear film and other deposits
2. Improper cleaning technique or inadequate cleaning regimen

Management

1 Daily use of an abrasive cleaning solution
2. Weekly cleaning with enzymatic solution
3. Use of cleansing lubricant drops
4. Exchange of contact lens material (fluorosilicone acrylate materials in general are more deposit resistant)

Debris Under the Contact Lens

Debris and exfoliated cells trapped under the contact lens may be seen with direct or indirect illumination. They are most frequently encountered in users who sleep with contact lenses and may provoke adhesion and/or epithelial abrasions.

Symptoms and Signs

1. Specific visual complaints
2. Ocular irritation
3. Fragments trapped between the posterior surface of the contact lens and the anterior corneal surface, generally localized in the pupillary area

Causes

1. Tear film deficiency
2. Inadequate blink
3. Tight contact lens

Management

1. Start lubricant cleansing drops four times per day
2. Check the contact lens–cornea fitting relationship
3. Check contact lens maintenance

2. What are the problems associated with rigid contact lens design?

Problems in rigid contact lens design include persistent discomfort, peripheral corneal drying, adhesion and corneal molding, and tight or loose lens fit.

Persistent Discomfort

Causes

1. Inadequate peripheral curve design
2. Inadequate lens edge design

3. Poorly designed contact lens (tight, loose, small diameter)
4. Incorrect blinking
5. Deposits on the posterior surface of the contact lens
6. Lens care products that irritate the eye

Management

1. Design a new contact lens.
2. Recommend blinking exercises.
3. Check the lens care routine.
4. Inspect the lens edge design and roll the edges if necessary.

Peripheral Corneal Drying (3 and 9 O'Clock Position Staining)

This is the complication most frequently encountered in rigid contact lens users, occurring in approximately 50% of RGP patients.[7] This clinical picture is more common in continuous-wear patients than in patients who wear RGP lenses on a daily wear basis.[8] The drying may be localized or generalized. In severe cases, it can lead to peripheral corneal ulceration, neovascularization, and scarring.[2,9]

Symptoms and Signs

1. Redness of the eye or dryness sensation
2. Discomfort
3. Pain that increases with the number of hours of wear, principally when there is dellen formation (Figure 23.1).
4. Coalesced punctate keratitis that is frequently present in the nasal and temporal regions adjacent to the contact lens (Color Plate 32).
5. Localized conjunctival injection
6. Pingueculaum/pterygium formation and lipid deposit
7. Vascularized limbal keratitis[10,11]
8. Formation of scarring and hyperplasia (Figure 23.2), induced by extreme and chronic drying
9. Some patients have no symptoms

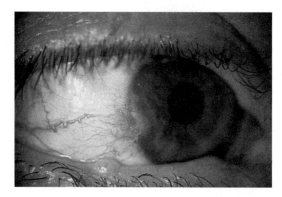

Figure 23.2. Peripheral corneal drying (3 and 9 o'clock position syndrome, 4+).

Causes

1. Tear film breakup near the lens edge associated with tear film deficiency or poorly wetting RGP material
2. Excessive friction of the contact lens at the limbus
3. Excessive edge lift resulting in adjacent corneal desiccation
4. Poor blinking
5. A thick contact lens edge
6. An interpalpebral fit in which the contact lens is decentered inferiorly will increase the interaction between the superior lid and the contact lens edge, resulting in irritation and alteration of the normal blinking reflex. Poor contact lens mobility results in poor lacrimal exchange and consequent drying of the corneal periphery.

Management

1. Select a better wetting lens material such as a low-Dk fluorosilicone acrylate material.
2. Alter the lens edge.
   - Round off the lens edge to increase patient comfort and facilitate blinking.
   - Use lenticular designs.
     - A plus lenticular design with a minus contact lens of -5.00 D or more minus.
     - A minus lenticular design with a highplus lens to facilitate lens movement and avoid inferior dislocation.
   - Decrease the elevation of the lens edge while carefully avoiding insufficient peripheral clearance that may also cause desiccation.[12] One way to determine the appropriate edge lift is to evaluate the fluorescein pattern that, ideally, demonstrates a band of peripheral fluorescein that is denser than the central fluorescein pooling.[13]
3. Make the contact lens thinner, with the edge slightly elevated.
   - Use a contact lens with low Dk to employ a contact lens that is thinner and lighter.
4. Check the contact lens material.
   - Use a low-Dk fluorosilicone acrylate.
   - Use a hyper-Dk fluoro-silicone acrylate with high wettability such as a Menicon Z™. (Note: these lenses may need more frequent replacement than lower-Dk fluorosilicone acrylate materials due to decreased stability.)
   - Move to a hydrophilic lens.
5. Position the contact lens superiorly if it tends to ride low.
   - Increase the diameter to improve lid attachment.
   - Use a base curve equal to the flatter meridian of the cornea (on K) or flatter.
   - Use lenticular designs with special edges.
   - Fit an aspheric or multispheric design.
   - Check the peripheral curves to improve the tear exchange.
6. Reduce the diameter and tighten the base curve if the patient is using a large contact lens.

7. Reevaluate the tear film in case of lacrimal deficiency.
   - Use lubricating drops.
   - Make the patient aware of limitations of use.
   - Counsel against the use of cosmetic lenses in dry eye.
8. Evaluate the blink. In cases of insufficient blinking, recommend exercises:
   - The eye is fixed on a distant object at the height of the eyes, and the patient blinks 20 times, performing a complete blink without altering facial expression (blink with normal intensity).
   - Repeat this exercise four times daily for at least 30 days.
9. Use topical corticosteroid and antibiotics judiciously as appropriate in cases of vascularized limbal keratitis or in other more severe pictures.
10. Avoid prolonged or continuous use.

Adhesion—Corneal Molding (Fixed Contact Lens Syndrome)

Adhesion, although it may occur in daily or RGP contact lens users, is much more frequent when the contact lenses are worn during sleep. The patient awakes in the morning with a contact lens stuck to the cornea and immobile. Many times the contact lens begins to move only 2 to 3 hours after awakening.

Symptoms and Signs

1. Discomfort or pain, principally after removal of the contact lens
2. Sensation of a tight contact lens
3. Contact lens difficult to remove
4. Blurred vision with glasses
5. Fixed contact lens, usually inferiorly positioned
6. Debris under the contact lens due to decreased tear flow (Color Plate 33)
7. Indentation in the cornea and conjunctiva after removal of the contact lens (Color Plate 34)

Causes

1. A tight contact lens fitted steeper than the flat keratometric reading may be subject to more adhesion.
2. A flat-fitting, large diameter lens with inadequate edge lift that impedes tear exchange and contact lens movement
3. Hydrophobic contact lens surface
4. Tense lids
5. Corneal topographic characteristics
6. A thin tear film under the contact lens with a decrease in the aqueous component (viscosity of the mucous layer greatly contributes to adherence of debris, which, under continual pressure from the lid, may contribute to adhesion of the contact lens)

Management

1. Observe the cornea to be sure that it returns to a normal physiologic condition so that the lens can be refitted
2. Review the parameters of the contact lens used.
   - Flatten the radius of curvature if the contact lens is fitted tight.
   - Fit a base curve on K or flatter, because a flatter lens is less likely to flex.
   - Increase the central thickness by 0.03 to 0.05 mm.
   - Consider an interpalpebral fit if the base curve of the contact lens is large and fitted flatter than the flat Keratometric reading.
   - Reduce the diameter and fit with apical clearance.
   - Smoother peripheral curves facilitate tear fluid exchange.
   - Change the RGP material.
3. Try aspheric and multispheric contact lenses.
4. Advise against prolonged/continuous use.

Prolonged adhesion can cause localized corneal distortion, superficial punctate keratitis, corneal erosion (Figure 23.3), and acute red eye.

Tight Contact Lens

Symptoms and Signs

1. Burning
2. Discomfort
3. Corneal edema
4. Absent or minimal contact lens mobility
5. The presence of an air bubble under the contact lens
6. Limbal hyperemia

Inadequate movement of the contact lens can cause epithelial irritation or toxic reactions from metabolic products trapped under the lens.

Management

1. Loosen/flatten the contact lens by reducing the optic zone diameter or flattening the base curve.

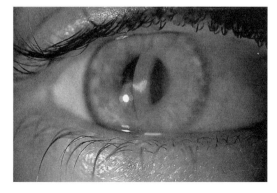

Figure 23.3. Corneal erosion caused by prolonged molding from a tight lens.

Loose Lens

Symptoms and Signs

1. Discomfort
2. Irritation of the superior lid
3. Visual complaints
4. Excessive contact lens movement with nasal or temporal decentration
5. Limbal injection

Management

1. Tighten/steepen the contact lens by increasing the optic zone diameter or steepening the base curve.

3. How does one manage contact lens decentration?

Contact lens decentration is classified as inferior, lateral, or superior.

Inferior Decentration

Symptoms and Signs

1. Visual disturbances
2. Drying[7] (3 and 9 o'clock position staining)
3. Sensation of the contact lens
4. Changes in blinking pattern
5. Corneal distortion[14]
6. Poor contact lens–cornea relationship[15]
7. Contact lens adhesion[16]

Causes

1. Excessively thick lens edge
2. Tight contact lens

Management

1. Fit on K or flatter than K, especially with negative powers.
2. Request a minus lenticular edge design in a low power minus contact lens (< -1.50 D) and in all plus power contact lenses to facilitate lid attachment and positioning of one quarter of the contact lens under the superior lid.
3. Request a plus lenticular design in contact lenses with high minus power to diminish trauma from the edge of the contact lens to the lid margin, facilitating a normal blink.
4. Verify that the design of the peripheral curve is large and flat enough, producing clearance of the lens edge.
5. Reduce the contact lens center thickness using a lower Dk material to avoid flexure. Increasing center thickness has a minimal effect on

the transmission of oxygen; however, it may cause the contact lens to be heavier, producing decentration.[17]
6. Consider a material with a lower specific gravity.

Lateral Decentration

Symptoms and Signs

1. Discomfort
2. Visual disturbance in some cases
3. Contact lens decentration nasal or temporal with blinking

Causes

1. Against-the-rule corneal astigmatism
2. Decentered corneal apex
3. Flat contact lens

Management

1. Steepen the base curve
2. Increase diameter
3. Use an aspheric back surface contact lens

Superior Decentration

Symptoms and Signs

1. Asymptomatic
2. A superiorly decentered contact lens: Superior decentration, when small, may be beneficial to vision as well as comfort. If it is excessive, the contact lens will put pressure on the superior limbus and may become adhered and may also result in corneal distortion[14,18–20].

Causes

1. Flat contact lens
2. Flat superior cornea
3. Thick edge

Management

1. Steepen the base curve.
2. Increase the thickness 0.03 to 0.04 mm.
3. Use a plus lenticular edge or anterior bevel.
4. Use a material with a higher specific gravity.

References

1. Bennett ES. Silicone/acrylate lens design. *Int Contact Lens Clin.* 1985;12:45.
2. Bennett ES, Egan DJ. Rigid gas-permeable lens problem-solving. *J Am Optom Assoc.* 1986;57:504–512.

3. Ghormley NR. Rigid EW lenses: complications. *Int Contact Lens Clin.* 1987; 14:219.

4. Carrell BA, Bennett ES, Henry VA, Grohe RM. The effect of rigid gas-permeable lens cleaners on lens parameter stability. *J Am Optom Assoc.* 1992; 63:193–198.

5. Grohe RM, Caroline PJ, Norman CW. Rigid gas-permeable surface cracking. Part I: clinical syndrome. *Contact Lens Spectrum.* 1987;2:37–45.

6. Grohe RM, Caroline PJ. RGP non-wetting syndrome. *Contact Lens Spectrum.* 1989;4:32–44.

7. Henry VA, Bennett ES, Forrest JF. Clinical investigation of the Paraperm EW rigid gas-permeable contact lenses. *Am J Optom.* 1987;64:313–320.

8. Schnider CM. Rigid gas-permeable extended wear. *Contact Lens Spectrum.* 1990;5:101–106.

9. Bennett ES. How to manage the rigid lens wearer. *Rev Optom.* 1986;123: 102–110.

10. Grohe RM, Lebow KA. Vascularized limbal keratitis. *Int Contact Lens Clin.* 1989;16:197–209.

11. Miller WL. Rigid gas-permeable surface defects associated with an isolated case of vascularized limbal keratitis. *Int Contact Lens Clin.* 1995;22:201–212.

12. Schnider CM, Terry RB, Holden BA. Effects of lens design on peripheral corneal desiccation. *J Am Optom Assoc.* 1997;68:163–170.

13. Bennett ES. Rigid gas-permeable lens problem solving. In: Bennett ES, Henry VA, eds. *Clinical Manual of Contact Lenses.* Philadelphia: Lippincott Williams & Wilkins, 2000:181–210.

14. Wilson SE, Lin DTC, Klyce SD, et al. Rigid contact lens decentration: a risk factor for corneal warpage. *CLAO J.* 1990;16:177–182.

15. Kikkawa Y, Salmon TO. Rigid lens tear exchange and the tear mucous layer. *Contact Lens Forum.* 1990;15:17–24.

16. Schnider CM, Bennett ES, Grohe RM. Rigid extended wear. In: Bennett ES, Weissman BA, eds. *Clinical Contact Lens Practice.* Philadelphia: JB Lippincott, 1991:1–14.

17. Hill RM, Brezinski SD. The center thickness factor. *Contact Lens Spectrum.* 1987;2:52–54.

18. Kalin NS, Maeda N, Klyce SD, et al. Automated topographic screening for keratoconus in refractive surgery candidates. *CLAO J.* 1996;22:164–167.

19. Ruiz-Montenegro J, Mafra CH, Wilson SE, et al. Corneal topographic alterations in normal contact lens wearers. *Ophthalmology.* 1993;100:128–134.

20. Weinstock FJ. *Contact Lens Fitting: A Clinical Text Atlas.* New York: JB Lippincott, 1989;11:10–11.

24

Lid and Conjunctival Complications Associated with Contact Lens Use

Cleusa Coral-Ghanem,
Newton Kara-José,
and LeVelle Jenkins

1. Why does ptosis occur in contact lens users, and how is it managed?

Ptosis generally occurs in association with inflammatory conditions related to blepharitis or meibomianitis, which leads to subclinical lid edema. Ptosis is most common in rigid contact lens users, principally in those whose contact lenses have a large diameter or a thick edge. One study by van der Bosch and Lemij[1] demonstrated that rigid contact lens users, when compared with a control group, had an overall 0.5-mm decrease in superior lid height. Ptosis has also been described in patients whose contact lenses were "lost" and remained for a period of time in the superior cul-de-sac.[2] In this position, the "lost" contact lens produced chronic irritation and subsequent ptosis. For this reason, whenever a patient has a history of contact lens use and the subsequent development of ptosis, the conjunctival fornices and tarsi should be carefully examined and stained with fluorescein. This may sometimes reveal the lost lens.

In the hydrophilic contact lens wearer, ptosis is most commonly due to giant papillary conjunctivitis in an advanced phase. Unilateral cases are diagnosed earlier because of the obvious difference between the two upper lids.

When a patient with ptosis wants contact lenses, it is better to correct the lid abnormality prior to the fitting, and, whenever possible, to opt for a hydrophilic lens.

Management

1. Revise the contact lens edge using a positive carrier.
2. Reduce contact lens thickness and/or decrease the overall diameter, making the fit interpalpebral.
3. Refit with a hydrophilic lens if the patient is using a rigid contact lens.
4. Refrain from contact lens use while the underlying problem is taken care of; for example, giant papillary conjunctivitis, meibomian gland dysfunction, blepharitis, or other local inflammatory disease.
5. Formulate a differential diagnosis that includes functional alterations of the levator muscles.

2. When do blepharitis and meibomianitis interfere with contact lens use, and how is this managed?

Seborrheic blepharitis is a local form of seborrheic dermatitis. It is a chronic inflammatory disease that affects different age groups.[3-6] It is generally classified in three categories: pure seborrheic blepharitis, mixed seborrheic blepharitis associated with staphylococcal infection, and seborrheic blepharitis with secondary meibomitis.[7,8]

Meibomian gland dysfunction can cause contact lens intolerance[9] by mechanical obstruction of the meibomian glands that results in alteration of the oil secretion and by the release of bacteria or toxic products into the precorneal tear film.

Meibomian gland dysfunction can be associated with development of deposits on soft contact lenses. The lipid content of these deposits is similar to the composition of meibomian gland secretions. For this reason, when the user presents with oil deposits on the contact lens, the examiner should look for the presence of meibomian gland dysfunction and initiate the appropriate treatment.

Symptoms and Signs

- Blurred vision
- Burning
- Foreign body sensation with rapid breakup of the tear film
- Decreased contact lens tolerance
- Changes in the transparency of the tear film
- Retained material in the meibomian glands
- Deposit on the contact lens
- Scales on the lid margin

Causes

There is excessive production of lipids in cases of blepharitis and meibomianitis that decreases the transparency of the tear film and coats the contact lens, producing a decrease in visual acuity and decreasing lens tolerance. The contact lens exacerbates the inflammation of the lid margins. In these cases, different factors may be involved:

- Mechanical irritation by the edge of the contact lens with blinking
- Chemical irritation from the contact lens material or maintenance solutions
- Deposits on the contact lens

Management

1. Stop contact lens use.
2. Perform lid massage and meibomian gland expression when there is an excess of lipids. If the exudate is milky white instead of clear, the bacteria have infected the gland itself, and an oral antibiotic is warranted.
3. Use warm compresses to increase the fluidity of the secretions.
4. Cleanse the upper and lower lid margins with diluted baby shampoo or commercial solutions. This treatment removes eyelash and skin debris laden with bacteria.
5. Treat with topical antibiotic in mixed forms of seborrheic blepharitis associated with staphylococcal disease or meibomianitis. Antibiotics are less effective in patients with pure seborrheic blepharitis.[7,10]
6. Prescribe systemic antibiotics such as doxycycline or tetracycline. In patients with meibomianitis who do not also have acre rosacea, the antibiotic dose can be diminished or discontinued after 3 months of treatment. The use of lipophilic antibiotics diminishes the production of bacterial lipases. Moreover, tetracycline reduces the production of cholesterol esters necessary for the development of blepharitis and inhibits the activity of collagenase, preventing corneal vascularization.[11]
7. A mild topical corticosteroid can be used for a short period of time in cases of severe inflammation and discomfort.
8. After regression of lid inflammation, one can refit the lens with the causative factors eliminated.

3. How does contact lens–induced superior limbic keratoconjunctivitis manifest itself; why does it occur; and how is it treated (Color Plate 27)?

Symptoms and Signs

- Photophobia
- Burning
- Excessive tearing
- Mild lid swelling
- Pseudoptosis
- Blepharospasm

- Foreign body sensation
- Decreased contact lens tolerance
- Sectoral inflammation of the superior bulbar conjunctiva with areas staining with rose bengal
- Punctate keratitis of the superior limbus and cornea
- Subepithelial opacification in the superior third of the cornea
- Superior corneal vascularization
- Mild papillary hypertrophy on the superior tarsal conjunctiva

Causes

- Sensitivity reaction to preservatives, especially thimerosal[12]
- Toxic reaction
- Hypoxia of the superior limbus
- Poor contact lens–cornea relationship, causing mechanical irritation of the superior limbal region

Management

1. Discontinue contact lens use temporarily.
2. Discontinue use of solutions containing thimerosal.
3. Start a preservative-free lubricant drop.
4. Consider the use of a mild topical corticosteroid, monitoring intraocular pressure carefully.
5. Refit with a thinner lens or with a different lens material.
6. Fit a rigid gas permeable contact lens to avoid pannus formation if the problem is recurrent.
7. Start a care system that does not contain a preservative.[13]

4. What is indicated in cases of infectious conjunctivitis?

- Temporary suspension of contact lens wear
- Disinfection or exchange of the contact lens
- Culture of the ocular secretions
- Antibiotic drops

Infectious conjunctivitis in contact lens users has similar characteristics as in non–contact lens wearers. The contamination may or may not be related to the contact lens. When it is directly contact lens related, the source of contamination is usually the same as is found in corneal ulcers in contact lens users.[14]

5. How and why does irritative conjunctivitis manifest itself in contact lens users, and what is the management?

Symptoms and Signs

- Tearing
- Conjunctival hyperemia

- Burning
- Foreign body sensation
- Punctate keratopathy and/or corneal erosion
- Fluorescein staining (generally in the paracentral cornea concentric to the limbus)

Causes

An improper lens–cornea relationship due to a large contact lens, a tight lens, a lens with surface deposits, poor centration, and lid eversion or inversion.

- *Alterations in the material.* Alterations in the material with breakage or deterioration of the contact lens can cause mechanical irritation.
- *Impurities.* Impurities within the contact lens may cause an immediate and intense conjunctival reaction as well as keratitis.
- *Deposits.* Deposits on the surface of the contact lens may make it rough or excessively tight and may accordingly diminish visual acuity as well as oxygen transmissibility to the cornea.
- *Contamination.* The surface of the lens can be contaminated by fungi or bacteria and can provoke an irritative conjunctivitis that disappears with removal of the contact lens.

An ocular infection can occur if there is a corneal abrasion. The hydrophilic contact lens for aphakia is the most susceptible to invasion with fungi.

Management

1. Refit with a new contact lens.
2. Remove the deposits with the help of an enzymatic cleaner.
3. Employ specific treatment in cases of compromise of the corneal surface.

6. How and why does mucoprotein conjunctivitis occur in the contact lens user, and what is its management?

Symptoms and Signs

- Ocular irritation
- Discharge
- Blurring of vision because of deposits
- Decreased contact lens tolerance

Causes

- Mucoprotein deposits on the contact lens surface
- Sensitivity to preservatives in contact lens maintenance solutions

Management

1. Have the patient temporarily discontinue contact lens wear.
2. Start steroid and antibiotic drops.
3. Remove deposits or exchange contact lenses.
4. Change the method of contact lens maintenance.
5. Refit with rigid gas permeable (RGP) lenses or lower water content soft lenses.

If the patient tends to be a deposit former, check for abnormalities in the tear film and the meibomian glands.

Mucoprotein conjunctivitis is most common in hydrophilic lens wearers, principally those using high-water-content lenses.

7. How does giant papillary conjunctivitis (GPC) manifest, and what are the causes?

Symptoms and Signs

Initial symptoms include decreased lens tolerance or loss of tolerance to contact lens wear, increased itching after lens removal, increased mucus discharge in the morning, and photophobia. Vision can be interrupted because of the deposits on the lens itself or the displacement of the lens due to superior lid papillary hypertrophy.

Contact Lens Deposits

There are a variety of morphologic characteristics of these deposits. They may be classified by their microscopic appearance as granular, trabecular, cellular, or mixed.[15] The higher the water content, the larger the amount of deposits and the more difficult it is to keep the contact lens clean.[16] It appears that there is no predisposition for the appearance of a specific type of protein deposit on the lens surface.[17,18] Although a deposit-coated contact lens does not necessarily lead to the occurrence of GPC,[19] patients with GPC characteristically have deposits on the lens surface.

Giant Papillae on the Superior Tarsus (Color Plates 35 and 36).

From 0.3 to 2 mm in diameter, tarsal papillae may frequently exceed 1 mm in diameter and are almost always found on the superior tarsus, their size generally reflecting the stage of the disease.[20] The initial presentation of giant papillae appears to be related to the type of contact lens used. The use of a rigid contact lens is associated initially with papillae at the lid margin, which then increase in the direction of the superior tarsus. The use of hydrophilic contact lenses is often associated with the opposite pattern, in which the papillae are generally seen at the superior tarsus and advance in the direction of the palpebral margin.[21,22] Fluorescein staining of the papillae occurs when the endothelial cells are mechanically damaged or when the apex is flattened in the form of a crater.[22,23] The patient with giant papillary conjunctivitis may have minimal or no symptoms, but the papillae may enlarge anew when exposed to the suspected allergic stimulus, specifically protein deposits on the surface of the contact lens.[24,25] Total regression of giant papillae may take months to years.[26] In the advanced stages, giant papillary conjunctivitis may cause ptosis of the lid.[27]

Causes of GPC

Giant papillary conjunctivitis is likely a delayed hypersensitivity response of a cutaneous basophilic type. The hypothesis is that the principal causes inciting antigen and disease are deposits on the contact lens or the lens material. In the majority of cases, a decrease in the reaction occurs with a new contact lens, even if it is the same material. The contact lens coated with deposits causes conjunctival trauma with liberation of neutrophilic chemotactic factors. The trauma is related also to the development of GPC encountered in patients submitted to surgery when the nylon suture remains exposed, causing mechanical irritation to the superior tarsal conjunctiva. One encounters similar manifestations in patients with prostheses, extrusion of scleral implants, keratinized dermoid cysts, and cyanoacrylate adhesives. Other forms of trauma include the edge of the contact lens that comes into contact with the superior tarsus. Chronic trauma predisposes the conjunctiva to a major absorption of antigen. The trauma is followed by hypersensitivity reaction of types I and IV. The histologic findings are similar to those in vernal conjunctivitis.[28]

8. What is the treatment of giant papillary conjunctivitis?

In early GPC with mild signs and symptoms, decreased wearing time is recommended; alternatively, disposable contact lenses with daily removal can be employed.

In patients with moderate signs and symptoms, it is advisable to discontinue use for 1 to 4 weeks, especially if there is fluorescein staining at the apices of the papillae. With the removal of the contact lens, the symptoms disappear almost immediately or within 4 to 5 days.[29] Removal of the traumatic agent produces an improvement in the clinical picture.[30] The papillae retain their form for weeks or months and very slowly become less elevated, eventually transforming into flattened disks approximately 1 mm in diameter.

Exchange of the contact lens for a new one of a different material and a different design is recommended. If possible, it is advisable to switch to disposable, frequent planned-replacement, or RGP lenses. One-day or 1- to 2-week disposable contact lenses are desirable in this situation because they can be disposed of frequently. The daily use of disposable contact lenses requires the daily use of a surfactant cleaner and daily disinfection, as with conventional hydrophilic lenses. Hydrogen peroxide is a disinfection solution without preservative that will eliminate the possibility of additional intolerance to preservative, and its use, together with enzymatic cleaner, is also beneficial.

Management

1. Increase the use of enzymatic agents to keep lens clean.
2. Discourage continuous wear because it favors greater deposit formation.

Topical Corticosteroids

Corticosteroids can be used in the initial phase of treatment. The limited use of topical steroids is suggested in cases of severe GPC to minimize the hyperproduction of mucus, extreme hyperemia, cellular infiltrates, and inflammatory mediators present in the lacrimal area in stage IV GPC, for which conventional therapy can be used. Corticosteroids do not treat the cause of GPC but rather reduce or eliminate the symptoms by controlling the inflammatory reaction. The patient should be alerted to the risk of prolonged use of corticosteroids, principally the development of secondary glaucoma or steroid-induced cataract.

Histamines and other vasoactive substances in the surrounding tissue require 2 weeks to be metabolized or destroyed by enzymes. In this interim, to alleviate symptoms, the patient can use vasoconstrictor substances, combined medicines such as olopatadine 0.1% drops, or corticosteroids.

Mast Cell Stabilizers

The use of these substances is an attempt to interfere with the cellular response to the antigenic stimulus.

Disodium Cromoglycate (2% to 4%)

Cromoglycate sodium stabilizes the membrane of mast cells, thereby avoiding the release of histamine and other biochemical mediators. When applied topically in stage I or II GPC, sodium cromoglycate prevents the signs and symptoms associated with type I allergic reactions, including GPC.[31]

The side effects of sodium cromoglycate are minimal. They include burning or stinging with application of the drops.[32] Two to four drops a day are recommended while the patient is using contact lenses.

Lodoxamide 0.1%

Lodoxamide 0.1% (Alomide™) acts to inhibit the degranulation of mast cells and the migration of eosinophils. It alleviates itching, photophobia, and decreases secretions. The recommended dose is four times per day for 3 months. It generally takes 7 to 14 days for significant effect, and it may be used with vasoconstrictors and antihistamines.

Mast Cell Stabilizer Plus Antihistamine

Olopatadine Chlorhydrate 0.1% (Patanol™)

Olopatadine acts to block H1 receptors, inhibiting the release of histamine and alleviating itching. It inhibits inflammatory mediators [triptase and prostaglandin D_2 (PGD_2)]. It stabilizes mast cell membranes, diminishing the recurrences. It also decreases hyperemia through its decongestant activity. Two drops daily are recommended at intervals of 6 to 8 hours.

    The treatment of GPC in rigid contact lens users is similar to that in hydrophilic lens users. The difference is that one can use a polish on rigid lenses to eliminate deposits without exchanging the lens. Thin and smooth-edged designs are less likely to incite mechanical lid irritation and the deposit of debris. There is an inverse relation between the oxygen permeability (Dk) of the material in an RGP lens and the time of onset of giant papillary conjunctivitis.[33] It may be necessary to change the design and the material of the RGP or move to a polymethylmethacrylate lens.

9. What are the principal causes of conjunctival hyperemia?

- Changes in tear film
- Changes in contact lens material
- Air conditioning
- Eye rubbing
- Insufficient blinking
- Contact lens deposits
- Corneal hypoxia
- Insufficient lubrication of contact lens
- Poor contact lens–cornea relationship
- Environmental pollution
- Allergic reactions to preservatives in solutions
- Toxic reactions to lens care solutions
- Traumatic insertion or removal of the contact lenses

10. How and why does acute early-morning red eye occur (Color Plate 30)?

Symptoms and Signs

- Unilateral ocular pain in the morning upon arising
- Intense photophobia and tearing
- Limbal and bulbar conjunctival injection
- Subepithelial or anterior stromal infiltrates a few millimeters from the limbus
- Absence of superficial punctate keratitis

Causes

- Drying of the tear film during sleep
- Toxic inflammatory effects by debris under the contact lens
- Irritative response from acute hypoxia or contact lens deposits
- Hypersensitivity to or toxicity from the preservatives used in contact lens care solutions
- Mechanical irritation due to the design of the contact lens
- Adherence of a tight hydrophilic contact lens. Different from a rigid contact lens, which with each blink exchanges 20% of the tear film under the lens, the hydrophilic contact lens exchanges only 0.5% to 1%.[34] This lacrimal stagnation, as such, may cause corneal edema aside from the retention of debris. The tight hydrophilic lens may also cause compression of the limbal and conjunctival vasculature near the edge of the lens.

An acute morning red eye is an inflammatory defense response encountered in patients who sleep with contact lenses. The inflammatory reaction in this syndrome normally presents with inflammatory infiltrates and is not accompanied by keratitis. However, infectious keratitis should be considered in the differential diagnosis. If there are epithelial defects with adjacent infiltrates, it is necessary to treat with antibiotics and to observe the patient closely, especially in the first 24 hours.

Management

1. Remove the contact lens; infiltrates will disappear in several weeks.
2. Use topical corticosteroid to reduce the inflammatory response; use with great caution, however, because hypoxia facilitates microbial infection.
3. Avoid the use of a contact lens, especially if inflammatory signs do not disappear.
4. Fit a new contact lens, preferentially one of a different design and material.
5. Discourage continuous use. With return of the syndrome, continuous wear is contraindicated.

References

1. Van Der Bosch W, Lemij H. Blepharoptosis induced by prolonged hard contact lens wear. *Ophthalmology.* 1993;99:1759.
2. Yassin J, White R, Shannon G. Blepharoptosis as a complication of contact lens migration. *Am J Ophthalmol.* 1971;72:536.
3. Smolin G, Okumoto M. Staphylococcal blepharitis. *Arch Ophthalmol.* 1977; 95:812.
4. Thygeson P. Complications of *Staphylococcus* blepharitis. *Am J Ophthalmol.* 1969;68:446.
5. Leibowitz HM, Capino D. Treatment of chronic blepharitis. *Arch Ophthalmol.* 1988;106:720.
6. Polack, FM, Goodman DF. Experience with a new detergent lid scrub in the management of chronic blepharitis. *Arch Ophthalmol.* 1988;106:719.

7. Dougherty JM, McCulley JP. Comparative bacteriology of chronic blepharitis. *Br J Ophthalmol.* 1984;68:524.

8. McCulley JP, Sciallis GF. Meibomian keratoconjunctivitis. *Am J Ophthalmol.* 1977;84:778.

9. Korb D, Henriquez A. Meibomian gland dysfunction and contact lens intolerance. *J Am Optom Assoc.* 1980;51:243.

10. Bowman RW, Dougherty JM, McCulley JP. Chronic blepharitis and dry eyes. *Int Ophthalmol Clin.* 1987;27:27.

11. Friedlaender MH, Ohashi Y, Kelley J. Diagnosis of allergic conjunctivitis. *Arch Ophthalmol.* 1984;102:1198–1199.

12. Sendale DD, Kenyon KR, Mobilia F, et al. Superior limbic keratoconjunctivitis in contact lens wearers. *Ophthalmology.* 1983;90:616.

13. Silbert JA. Contact lens-related pathology: part II. *Rev Optom.* 1984;121:51.

14. Stein H, Slatt BJ. *Fitting Guide for Rigid and Soft Contact Lenses.* St. Louis: CV Mosby, 1990.

15. Fowler SA, Greiner JV, Allansmith MR. Soft contact lenses from patients with giant papillary conjunctivitis. *Am J Ophthalmol.* 1979;88:1056.

16. Fowler SA, Korb DR, Allansmith MR. Deposits on soft contact lenses of various water contents. *CLAO J.* 1985;11:124.

17. Caroline PJ, et al. Microscopic and elemental analysis of deposits on extended wear soft contact lenses. *CLAO J.* 1985;1:311.

18. Gudmundsson OG, et al. Identification of proteins in contact lens surface deposits by immunofluorescence microscopy. *Arch Ophthalmol.* 1985; 103:196.

19. Ballow M, et al. Immunologic responses in cynomolgus monkeys to lenses from patients with contact lens-induced giant papillary conjunctivitis. *CLAO J.* 1989;15:64.

20. Allansmith MR, Korb DR, Greiner JV. Giant papillary conjunctivitis in contact lens wearers. *Am J Ophthalmol.* 1977;83:697.

21. Greiner JV, Covington HI, Allansmith MR. Surface morphology of giant papillary conjunctivitis in contact lens wearers. *Am J Ophthalmol.* 1985; 85:242.

22. Korb DR, Allansmith MR, Greiner JV, et al. Biomicroscopy of papillae associated with hard contact lens wearing. *Ophthalmology.* 1981;88:1132.

23. Greiner JV, Fowler SA, Allansmith MR. Giant papillary conjunctivitis. In: Dabezies O, ed. *Contact Lenses: The CLAO Guide to Basic Science and Clinical Practice.* Orlando, FL: Grune & Stratton, 1984:431.

24. Allansmith MR. Pathology and treatment of giant papillary conjunctivitis. I: the U.S. perspective. *Clin Ther.* 1987;9:443.

25. Donshik PC, Ballow M, Lustro A, Samartino L. Treatment of contact lens induced giant papillary conjunctivitis. *CLAO J.* 1984;10:346.

26. Allansmith MR. Giant papillary conjunctivitis. *J Am Optom Assoc.* 1990; 61(suppl): S42.

27. Luxenburg MN. Blepharoptosis associated with giant papillary conjunctivitis. *Arch Ophthalmol.* 1986;104:1706.

28. Nishiwaki-Dantas MC, Finzi S. Desordens imunologicas da conjuntiva—Conjuntivites alergicas. In: Lima ALH, Dantas MCN, Alves MR, eds. *Doencas Externas Oculares e Cornea,* vol 1. Rio de Janeiro: Editora Cultura Medica, 1999:210–221.

29. Hill DS, Molinari JF. A review of giant papillary conjunctivitis associated with soft contact lens wear. *Int Contact Lens Clin.* 1981;8:45.

30. Allansmith MR, Ross RN. Giant papillary conjunctivitis. *Int Ophthalmol Clin.* 1988;28:309.

31. Kruger CJ, Ehlers WH, Luistro AE, Donshik PC. Treatment of giant papillary conjunctivitis with cromolyn sodium. *CLAO J.* 1992;18:46.

32. Goen TM, Sieboldt K, Terry JE. Cromolyn sodium in ocular allergic diseases. *J Am Optom Assoc*. 1986;57:526.
33. Douglas JP, Lowder CY, Lazorik R, Meisler DM. Giant papillary conjunctivitis associated with rigid gas-permeable contact lenses. *CLAO J*. 1988; 14:143.
34. Polse KA. Tear flow under hydrogel contact lenses. *Invest Ophthalmol Vis Sci*. 1979;18:409–413.

25

AIDS and Contact Lenses

Cleusa Coral-Ghanem
and Cynthia H. Green

Human immunodeficiency virus (HIV) has been isolated in almost all body fluids, including tears,[1] and in the majority of ocular tissues,[2] for example, in the conjunctiva and the cornea of infected patients, albeit in very small quantities. To date, there has been no recognized case of transmission of HIV through these tissues.[3] There has been no HIV transmission from patient to eye care practitioner during ophthalmic surgery.[4] There have been no cases of HIV transmission from the donors in cases of corneal transplants involving an HIV-positive donor, unlike other organ transplants.[5,6]

The Centers for Disease Control (CDC) has excluded tears from its list of body fluids classified as potentially infectious, because the quantity of virus encountered in the tears of a patient with AIDS is extremely small. This consideration is quite important, because it frees the contact lens fitter from using gloves during the routine ophthalmic examination. Nonetheless, tears are considered a source of HIV contamination when they are mixed with blood, in which case gloves should certainly be used. Despite the low likelihood of contamination with HIV in the eye clinic, we provide some guidelines here for precautions in contact lens fitting.

1. How can one prevent contamination with HIV in the ophthalmic office?

In 1985, the CDC[7] published recommendations, which were corroborated in 1988 by the American Academy of Ophthalmology:

1. Wash hands with soap and dry them well.
2. Do not touch the eye with the tips of dropper bottles.
3. Disinfect all instruments that come in direct contact with the patient's eye, particularly the Goldmann tonometer tip.
4. Have two types of tonometer available for use in case one is being disinfected. Follow recommendations of the CDC and the American Academy of Ophthalmology (AAO) for disinfection. This can be achieved in several ways:

- Clean the tip of the tonometer vigorously with 70% isopropyl alcohol, rinse, and thoroughly dry.
- Immerse the tip of the tonometer for 5 minutes in commercial bleach solution (dilute 1:10, bleach to water). Following this, one should rinse thoroughly and dry.
- Soak in 3% hydrogen peroxide for 5 to 10 minutes.
5. Take special care with hand towels or whatever materials might come in direct contact with the patient's body.
6. Use gloves when the eye care professional:
    - Has a possibility of coming into contact with skin or mucous membrane on which there is blood or another potentially infectious fluid
    - Has a cut or dermatitis
    - May come into contact with a wound on the patient
    - Has to puncture a vein, such as in fluorescein angiography
    - Is manipulating cutting instruments, including a needle
    - Is planning to do any surgical procedure

Observations

It is not necessary to use gloves during a routine ophthalmic examination. Sound clinical judgment should be used. Should one accidentally injure oneself in the context of examining an AIDS patient, one should wash the wound vigorously with antiseptic for 5 minutes and contact the appropriate institution or public health agency.

2. How does one prevent a contamination with HIV in contact lens practice?

As has already been pointed out, the isolation of HIV in the tears of patients with AIDS[1] raised the concern about the possibility of HIV transmission during contact lens fitting. HIV has been found in high-water-content contact lenses[8] and in the rinsing solutions of AIDS patients. For this reason, in contact lens practice, the tears should be considered a potential source of HIV infection, albeit very unlikely.
To prevent contamination:

1. Wash and dry hands after each patient's appointment.
2. Disinfect all trial lenses.

It is not necessary to use gloves routinely. The recommendations made in 1995 by the CDC[7] were for disinfection of polymethyl methacrylate (PMMA), rigid gas permeable (RGP), and hydrophilic lenses using hydrogen peroxide or, if the contact lens material permits, thermal disinfection.

It has also been demonstrated that rubbing of the contact lens with surfactant cleaner followed by rinsing removes HIV particles from a contaminated contact lens.[9] The cleaning, rinsing, and disinfecting of the trial lenses using routine methods, including many chemical disinfectant solutions, destroy the virus and avoid transmission of HIV from one patient to the next.[9]

Fortunately, HIV is one of the most easily inactivated viruses. There are no documented cases of HIV transmission that can be linked to contact lens fitting. The risk of a patient transmitting HIV to the eye care professional through the contact lens or contact with the tears is virtually nonexistent.

3. What are the guidelines for the user infected with AIDS?

When the clinical diagnosis of AIDS has been made, normally it is because the individual has presented some medical evidence of systemic immunosuppression. The contact lens user with AIDS should be counseled to:[10]

- Use an FDA-approved disinfection system compatible with his contact lens.
- Not share the contact lens, the case, or solutions with any other user.
- Remove the contact lens with any abnormal ocular sign or symptom and seek out an eye care professional.

Additional considerations for contact lens wear in patients infected with HIV include:[11]

- Extended wear is contraindicated in patients infected with HIV.
- Daily-wear disposable lenses are a good alternative to allow minimal exposure to possible pathogens and reduce disinfection concerns.
- The contact lens case should be cleaned carefully.
- Careful and more numerous contact lens follow-up visits are indicated.
- Patients should be educated about the possibility of dry eye syndrome and ocular pathogens.
- The patient should never share his/her contact lenses with other individuals—even with careful disinfection.

The patient should be aware of the potential for developing diseases of the ocular surface related to AIDS, independent of the use of a contact lens. Such disorders may result in the need to stop contact lens use.

It is important to emphasize that the primary objective of contact lens and tonometer tip disinfection is to prevent secondary ocular infection during immunosuppression, not just to avoid contamination of the contact lens with HIV.

References

1. Fujikawa LS, Salahuddin SZ, Ablashi D, et al. HTLV-III in tears of AIDS patients. *Ophthalmology.* 1986;12:1479–1481.
2. Cantrill HL, Henry K, Jackson B, et al. Recovery of human immunodeficiency virus from ocular tissues in patients with acquired immune deficiency syndrome. *Ophthalmology.* 1988;10:158–162.
3. AIDS Task Force Policy Statement—Section on Public Health and Occupational Vision of the American Academy of Optometry. *Am J Optom Physiol Opt.* 1988;65:599–601.
4. American Academy of Ophthalmology. Updated recommendations for

ophthalmic practice in relation to the human immunodeficiency virus. Clinical Alert 2/4. San Francisco: AAO, August 1988.

5. Schwarz A, Hoffman F, Lage Stehe J, et al. Human immunodeficiency virus transmission by organ donation. Outcome in cornea and kidney recipients. *Transplantation.* 1987;44:21–24.

6. Heck E, Petty C, Palestine A, et al. ELISA HIV testing and viral culture in the screening of corneal tissue for transplantation from medical examiner cases. *Cornea.* 1989;8:77–80.

7. Centers for Disease Control. Recommendations for preventing possible transmission of human-T-lymphotropic virus type III. Lymphadenopathy-associated virus from tears. *MMWR.* 1985;34:533–534.

8. Tervo T, Lahdevirta J, Vaheri A, et al. Recovery of HTLV-III from contact lenses. *Lancet.* 1986;1:370–380.

9. Vogt MV, Ho DD, Bakar SR, et al. Safe disinfection of contact lenses after contamination with HTLV-III. *Ophthalmology.* 1986;93:771–774.

10. Slonim CB. AIDS and the contact lens practice. *CLAO J.* 1995;10:233–235.

11. Chronister C. Viral infections and the immunocompromised patient. In: Silbert J, ed. *Anterior Segment Complications of Contact Lens Wear,* 2nd ed. Boston: Butterworth-Heinemann, 2000:214.

Index